# Sudden Cardiac Death

*Guest Editors*

RAUL WEISS, MD
EMILE G. DAOUD, MD

# HEART FAILURE CLINICS

www.heartfailure.theclinics.com

*Consulting Editors*
RAGAVENDRA R. BALIGA, MD, MBA
JAMES B. YOUNG, MD

*Founding Editor*
JAGAT NARULA, MD, PhD
April 2011 • Volume 7 • Number 2

SAUNDERS an imprint of ELSEVIER, Inc.

**W.B. SAUNDERS COMPANY**
*A Division of Elsevier Inc.*

1600 John F. Kennedy Boulevard • Suite 1800 • Philadelphia, Pennsylvania 19103-2899

http://www.theclinics.com

**HEART FAILURE CLINICS Volume 7, Number 2**
**April 2011 ISSN 1551-7136, ISBN-13: 978-1-4557-0458-3**

Editor: Barbara Cohen-Kligerman
Developmental Editor: Jessica Demetriou

*Heart Failure Clinics* (ISSN 1551-7136) is published quarterly by Elsevier Inc., 360 Park Avenue South, New York, NY 10010-1710. Months of publication are January, April, July, and October. Business and editorial offices: 1600 John F. Kennedy Boulevard, Suite 1800, Philadelphia, PA 19103-2899. Periodicals postage paid at New York, NY, and additional mailing offices. Subscription prices are USD 207.00 per year for US individuals, USD 326.00 per year for US institutions, USD 70.00 per year for US students and residents, USD 248.00 per year for Canadian individuals, USD 374.00 per year for Canadian institutions, USD 264.00 per year for international individuals, USD 374.00 per year for international institutions, and USD 89.00 per year for Canadian and foreign students/residents. To receive student and resident rate, orders must be accompanied by name of affiliated institution, date of term, and the *signature* of program/residency coordinator on institution letterhead. Orders will be billed at individual rate until proof of status is received. Foreign air speed delivery is included in all *Clinics* subscription prices. All prices are subject to change without notice. **POSTMASTER:** Send address changes to *Heart Failure Clinics*, Elsevier Health Sciences Division, Subscription Customer Service, 3251 Riverport Lane, Maryland Heights, MO 63043. **Customer Service: 1-800-654-2452 (US and Canada). From outside of the US and Canada, call 314-447-8871. Fax: 314-447-8029. For print support, e-mail: JournalsCustomerService-usa@elsevier.com. For online support, e-mail: JournalsOnlineSupport-usa@elsevier.com.**

*Reprints.* For copies of 100 or more of articles in this publication, please contact the Commercial Reprints Department, Elsevier Inc., 360 Park Avenue South, New York, NY 10010-1710. Tel.: 212-633-3812; Fax: 212-462-1935; E-mail: reprints@elsevier.com.

*Heart Failure Clinics* is covered in *MEDLINE/PubMed (Index Medicus)*.

Printed and bound by CPI Group (UK) Ltd, Croydon, CR0 4YY
Transferred to Digital Print 2011
**Cover artwork courtesy of Umberto M. Jezek.**

# Contributors

## CONSULTING EDITORS

**RAGAVENDRA R. BALIGA, MD, MBA**
Professor of Internal Medicine;
Vice-Chief and Assistant Division Director,
Professor of Medicine, Division of
Cardiovascular Medicine, The Ohio State
University Medical Center, Columbus, Ohio

**JAMES B. YOUNG, MD**
Professor of Medicine and Executive Dean,
Cleveland Clinic Lerner College of Medicine;
George and Linda Kaufman Chair, Chairman,
Endocrinology and Metabolism Institute,
Cleveland Clinic, Cleveland, Ohio

## GUEST EDITORS

**RAUL WEISS, MD**
Associate Professor, Internal Medicine;
Director, Electrophysiology Fellowship,
Dorothy M. Davis Heart and Lung Research
Institute, Ohio State University Medical Center,
Ross Heart Hospital, Columbus, Ohio

**EMILE G. DAOUD, MD**
Professor, Internal Medicine; Chief, Cardiac
Electrophysiology Section, Dorothy M. Davis
Heart and Lung Research Institute, Ohio State
University Medical Center, Ross Heart
Hospital, Columbus, Ohio

## AUTHORS

**WILLIAM T. ABRAHAM, MD**
Department of Cardiovascular Medicine,
The Ohio State University Medical Center,
Columbus, Ohio

**KAMEL ADDO, MD**
Fellow in Electrophysiology, Division
of Cardiology, Rhode Island and Miriam
Hospitals, The Warren Alpert Medical
School of Brown University, Providence,
Rhode Island

**AMIN AL-AHMAD, MD, FACC**
Division of Cardiovascular Medicine,
Department of Internal Medicine, Cardiac
Arrhythmia Service, Stanford University
School of Medicine, Stanford, California

**TOM P. AUFDERHEIDE, MD, FACEP, FAHA**
Professor of Emergency Medicine and
Associate Chair of Research Affairs,
Department of Emergency Medicine,
Medical College of Wisconsin, Milwaukee,
Wisconsin

**MICHAEL L. BERNARD, MD, PhD**
Division of Cardiology, Medical University
of South Carolina, Charleston,
South Carolina

**ALFRED E. BUXTON, MD**
Director, Division of Cardiology, Rhode Island
and Miriam Hospitals; Ruth and Paul Levinger
Professor in Cardiology, The Warren Alpert
Medical School of Brown University,
Providence, Rhode Island

**DAVID J. CALLANS, MD, FAHA, FACC, FHRS**
Professor of Medicine, Electrophysiology
Section, Division of Cardiovascular Medicine,
Hospital of the University of Pennsylvania,
Philadelphia, Pennsylvania

**ADAM CHODOSH, MD**
Fellow in Electrophysiology, Division
of Cardiology, Rhode Island and Miriam
Hospitals, The Warren Alpert Medical
School of Brown University, Providence,
Rhode Island

**CHRISTOPHER DROOGAN, DO, FACC**
Attending Cardiologist, Department of
Cardiology, Main Line Health Heart Center
and Lankenau Hospital, Wynnewood; Clinical
Instructor of Medicine, Department of
Pharmacology, Jefferson Medical College,
Thomas Jefferson University Hospital,
Philadelphia; Department of Cardiology,
Lankenau Institute for Medical Research,
Wynnewood, Pennsylvania

**ANDREW E. EPSTEIN, MD, FAHA, FACC, FHRS**
Professor of Medicine, Electrophysiology
Section, Division of Cardiovascular Medicine,
Hospital of the University of Pennsylvania,
Philadelphia, Pennsylvania

**VERONICA FRANCO, MD**
Department of Cardiovascular Medicine,
The Ohio State University Medical Center,
Columbus, Ohio

**MICHAEL R. GOLD, MD, PhD**
Division of Cardiology, Medical University
of South Carolina, Charleston, South Carolina

**ANURAG GUPTA, MD**
Division of Cardiovascular Medicine,
Department of Internal Medicine, Cardiac
Arrhythmia Service, Stanford University School
of Medicine, Stanford, California

**AYESHA HASAN, MD, FACC**
Medical Director, Cardiac Transplant Program;
Director, Heart Failure Devices Clinic, Division
of Cardiovascular Medicine, Ohio State
University Medical Center, Columbus, Ohio

**MAHMOUD HOUMSSE, MD**
Assistant Professor of Internal Medicine,
Division of Cardiovascular Medicine,
Department of Cardiovascular Medicine, Davis
Heart and Lung Research Institute, The Ohio
State University Medical Center, Columbus,
Ohio

**VENKAT IYER, MD**
Fellow in Electrophysiology, Division of
Cardiology, Rhode Island and Miriam
Hospitals, The Warren Alpert Medical School
of Brown University, Providence,
Rhode Island

**KOSTANTINOS KOTSIFAS, MD**
Consultant Pulmonary Medicine, Department
of Pulmonary Medicine, Sotiria General
Hospital, Athens, Greece

**PETER R. KOWEY, MD**
Attending Cardiologist, Department
of Cardiology, Main Line Health Heart
Center and Lankenau Hospital, Wynnewood;
Professor of Medicine, Department of
Pharmacology, Jefferson Medical College,
Thomas Jefferson University Hospital,
Philadelphia; Department of Cardiology,
Lankenau Institute for Medical Research,
Wynnewood, Pennsylvania

**YOUNGHOON KWON, MD**
Staff Physician and Research Fellow,
Healthcare East System, Division of
Cardiology, Department of Medicine,
University of Minnesota, St Joseph Hospital,
St Paul, Minnesota

**PEEM LORVIDHAYA, MD**
Clinical Assistant Professor of Medicine,
Division of Cardiology, Rhode Island and
Miriam Hospitals, The Warren Alpert
Medical School of Brown University,
Providence, Rhode Island

**JEREMY LUM, MD**
Fellow in Electrophysiology, Division of
Cardiology, Rhode Island and Miriam
Hospitals, The Warren Alpert Medical
School of Brown University, Providence,
Rhode Island

**KEITH G. LURIE, MD**
Professor of Medicine and Emergency
Medicine, Hennepin County Medical Center,
Minneapolis Medical Research Foundation,
University of Minnesota, Minneapolis,
Minnesota

**RICHARD L. PAGE, MD**
George R. and Elaine Love Professor,
and Chair, Department of Medicine,
University of Wisconsin School
of Medicine & Public Health, Madison,
Wisconsin

**CHINMAY PATEL, MD**
Cardiology Fellow, Department of Cardiology,
Main Line Health Heart Center and Lankenau
Hospital, Wynnewood, Pennsylvania

**ROBERT W. RHO, MD**
Associate Professor of Medicine, Division
of Medicine, University of Washington;
Seattle; Division of Cardiology,
University of Washington Medical Center,
Seattle, Washington

**MELISSA R. ROBINSON, MD**
Assistant Professor of Medicine,
Electrophysiology Section, Division
of Cardiovascular Medicine, University
of Illinois, Chicago, Illinois

**SAMIR SABA, MD, FACC, FHRS**
Associate Professor of Medicine; Chief,
Cardiovascular Electrophysiology Section,
University of Pittsburgh Medical Center,
Pittsburgh, Pennsylvania

**S. ADAM STRICKBERGER, MD**
Washington Electrophysiology, and
Cardiovascular Research Institute,
Washington Hospital Center,
Washington, DC

**BENJAMIN SUN, MD**
Chair, Cardiac, Thoracic and Transplant
Surgery, Minneapolis Heart Institute, Allina
Health Systems, Minneapolis, Minnesota

**NIRAJ VARMA, MA, DM, FRCP**
Cardiac Pacing and Electrophysiology,
Department of Cardiovascular Medicine,
Cleveland Clinic, Cleveland, Ohio

**GANESH VENKATARAMAN, MD**
Washington Electrophysiology, and
Cardiovascular Research Institute, Washington
Hospital Center, Washington, DC

**PAUL J. WANG, MD, FACC**
Division of Cardiovascular Medicine,
Department of Internal Medicine, Cardiac
Arrhythmia Service, Stanford University School
of Medicine, Stanford, California

**BRUCE WILKOFF, MD, FHRS**
Cardiac Pacing and Electrophysiology,
Department of Cardiovascular Medicine,
Cleveland Clinic, Cleveland, Ohio

**GAN-XIN YAN, MD, PhD**
Attending Cardiologist, Department of
Cardiology, Main Line Health Heart Center and
Lankenau Hospital, Wynnewood; Professor of
Medicine, Department of Pharmacology,
Jefferson Medical College, Thomas Jefferson
University Hospital, Philadelphia; Department
of Cardiology, Lankenau Institute for Medical
Research, Wynnewood, Pennsylvania

**DEMETRIS YANNOPOULOS, MD**
Assistant Professor of Medicine, Department
of Medicine, Interventional Cardiology,
University of Minnesota, Minneapolis,
Minnesota

# Contents

Mortality in congestive heart failure (CHF) usually occurs from either progressive worsening of cardiac pump failure or sudden cardiac death (SCD). Medical interventions that counter neurohormonal changes slow the progression of CHF and also prevent SCD. The benefits of medical therapy on SCD prevention have been variable, depending on the type of medical therapy. This article discusses the incidence, prediction, and prevention of SCD in CHF due to ischemic and nonischemic cardiomyopathy.

The multiplicity of mechanisms contributing to arrhythmogenesis in patients with heart failure carries obvious implications for risk stratification. If patients having the propensity to develop arrhythmias by these different mechanisms are to be identified, tests must be devised that reveal the substrates or other factors that relate to each mechanism. In the absence of this, efforts to risk stratify patients are likely to be neither cost-effective nor accurate. This article reviews the current knowledge base of risk stratification for sudden death in patients with heart failure, while acknowledging several limitations in the studies examined.

Sudden cardiac death (SCD) is the prime cause of death in the United States. The trials that focus on identifying and protecting patients at risk of SCD have identified the left ventricular ejection fraction (EF) as the single clinical marker that is most useful for risk assessment and stratification in primary prevention. This article reviews the data from major randomized clinical trials of implantable cardioverter-defibrillator implantation in patients with low EF for the primary prevention of SCD and exposes some of the shortcomings of the EF as a stratifier of mortality risk.

Although most recent investigations into sudden cardiac death prevention in heart failure patients have been focused on primary prevention, secondary indications for defibrillators and medical therapy remain vitally important in this complex patient group. Antiarrhythmic therapy is currently used primarily as adjuvant therapy to implantable defibrillators. Secondary prophylaxis defibrillator trials have shown clear benefit in preventing recurrent sudden cardiac death, despite concern over inappropriate shocks and the potential detrimental effects of appropriate shocks. Device programming for secondary prophylaxis can help ameliorate these issues. This article discusses these issues as well as the continued underuse of defibrillators in specific populations.

The implantable cardioverter-defibrillator (ICD) is the standard of care in patients with ischemic and nonischemic cardiomyopathy who are at high risk for arrhythmic events and sudden cardiac death. Although an ICD saves life, ICD shocks are emotionally and physically debilitating. Most patients receive adjuvant antiarrhythmic drug therapy to circumvent episodes of recurrent ventricular and supraventricular arrhythmias. Antiarrhythmic drugs including β-blockers, sotalol, amiodarone, and azimilide are effective at reducing the shock burden. This article describes data supporting the need for and potential risks and benefits of adjuvant antiarrhythmic drug therapy and examines the benefits and pitfalls of the same in ICD-implanted patients.

Frequent shocks from an implantable defibrillator (ICD) can have adverse cardiac affects and lead to increased pain, anxiety, and a decreased quality of life. Pharmacologic attempts and ICD reprogramming strategies aimed at reducing ICD shocks have modest results, with frequent discontinuation of medicines because of side effects. Ventricular tachycardia (VT) ablation is recommended in the treatment of patients with frequent ICD shocks caused by VT. VT ablation may also be considered in patients with an initial ICD shock and as prophylactic treatment in patients with a history of sustained VT who are undergoing ICD implant.

Implanted devices in heart failure patients improve survival, but requires correct prescription, programming, and monitoring. Requirements change since heart failure is a dynamic condition. Repeated episodes of acute decompensation increase mortality. Events involve several processes converging to manifest with fluid congestion. Implantable devices identify changes such as those in rhythm, device function or hemodynamics. Incorporation of remote monitoring technology (TRUST Trial), enables tracking of these parameters and prompt notification of deviations, even if the patient remains asymptomatic. This may facilitate management of large patient volumes and enable pre-emptive treatment to improve outcomes in these high-risk patients.

Despite the positive impact of medical therapy, the burden of heart failure persists, with disease progression, frequent hospitalizations, and reduced survival. Mortality related to ventricular tachyarrhythmias and/or pump failure has led to the introduction of device therapy. Implantable cardioverter-defibrillators (ICDs) and cardiac resynchronization therapy (CRT) have now been established as the standard of care in selected patients with chronic heart failure. CRT and ICDs offer the opportunity to reduce morbidity and increase survival in patients with drug-refractory heart failure, and to retard, if not prevent, development of end-stage heart failure requiring cardiac transplantation.

Use of implantable cardioverter defibrillators (ICDs) and/or cardiac resynchronization therapy reduces mortality among several high-risk cohorts, primarily those with left ventricular systolic dysfunction and heart failure. Since the advent of these technologies, concerns regarding the high initial costs of device implantation have been considered a potential barrier to widespread adoption. Despite such concerns, the use of these devices for primary or secondary prevention of sudden cardiac death seems to be cost-effective when compared with national standards. Moreover, ICDs have been shown to be cost-effective in several health care systems and specialized populations such as those with high-risk long QT syndrome and hypertrophic cardiomyopathy.

This article focuses on important advances in the science of cardiopulmonary resuscitation in the last decade that have led to a significant improvement in understanding the complex physiology of cardiac arrest and critical interventions for the initial management of cardiac arrest and postresuscitation treatment. Special emphasis is given to the basic simple ways to improve circulation, vital organ perfusion pressures, and the grave prognosis of sudden cardiac death.

In the United States, 250,000 people die from a cardiac arrest every year. Despite a well established emergency medical response system, survival from out-of-hospital cardiac arrest remains poor in United States cities. Paramount to achieving successful resuscitation of a cardiac arrest victim is provision of early defibrillation. Among patients that arrest due to a ventricular fibrillation, the likelihood of survival decreases by 10% for every minute of delay in defibrillation. In 1995, the American Heart Association challenged the medical industry to develop a defibrillator that could be placed in public settings, used safely by lay responders, and provide earlier defibrillation to cardiac arrest victims. Over the last decade, there have been significant technological advancements in automated external defibrillators (AEDs), and clinical studies have demonstrated their benefits and limitations in various public locations. This article discusses the technologic features of the modern AED and the current data available on the use of AEDs in public settings.

The "chain of survival" (early access, early cardiopulmonary resuscitation, early defibrillation, and early advanced care) defines the proven interventions necessary for successful resuscitation and survival of patients with cardiac arrest. Low survival rates from cardiac arrest are not due to lack of understanding of effective interventions, but instead are due to weak links in the chain of survival and the inability of communities to make sure these links function in an efficient, timely, and coordinated fashion. This article reviews how quality is defined for each link, how communities can strengthen each link, and how communities can forge a strong relationship between each link. By optimizing local leadership and stakeholder collaboration, communities have the potential to vastly improve outcomes from this devastating disease.

The advent of subcutaneous implantable cardioverter-defibrillator (ICD) systems represents a paradigm shift for the detection and therapy of ventricular tachyarrhythmias. Despite advances in transvenous lead technology, problems remain that notably include requirement for technical expertise; periprocedural complications during implantation and explantation; and long-term lead failure. Although subcutaneous ICD systems may mitigate some of these risks, they provide new shortcomings, such as inability to provide pacing therapy for bradyarrhythmias, ventricular tachyarrhythmias, and cardiac resynchronization. Ongoing clinical evaluation and development are required before the role of subcutaneous ICDs as an adjunctive or primary therapy can be defined. This article examines studies investigating the subcutaneous ICD and discusses its possible advantages and disadvantages as compared with current transvenous ICD systems.

**Erratum**

An oversight was made in "Valvular and Hemodynamic Assessment with CMR," which was published in the July 2009 issue (volume 5, number 3) pages 389–400, in that a funder was not mentioned. Dr Saul Myerson would like to acknowledge support from the Oxford NIHR Biomedical Research Centre program.

# Heart Failure Clinics

**VISIT THE CLINICS ONLINE!**

Access your subscription at:
**www.theclinics.com**

# Editorial: Sudden Death in Heart Failure: An Ounce of Prediction is Worth a Pound of Prevention

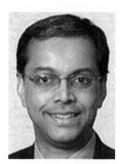 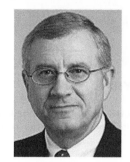

Ragavendra R. Baliga, MD, MBA      James B. Young, MD

*Consulting Editors*

Sudden cardiac death (SCD) is not only a clinical problem that is extraordinarily frightening for patients and their families but also a major and costly public health burden. Nearly 450,000 individuals die of SCD every year in the United States,[1] and SCD claims more lives every year in the United States than stroke, lung cancer, breast cancer, and AIDS combined. Unfortunately, there are few discernible risk factors in most patients with SCD. However, left ventricular (LV) systolic dysfunction, particularly because of coronary artery disease (CAD), identifies a group at particularly high risk of SCD.[2] The incidence of sudden death in patients with LV ejection fraction (LVEF) less than 0.30 is more than 15%. In the Metoprolol CR/XL Randomised Intervention Trial in Congestive Heart Failure (MERIT-HF) study, the proportion of sudden death was highest in relatively asymptomatic patients, that is, New York Heart Association (NYHA) class II patients, and sudden deaths generally decreased with increasing severity of heart failure according to the NYHA functional class (**Fig. 1**),[3] suggesting that the therapies targeted early in the course of the disease should get the "biggest bang for the buck".

Implantable cardioverter-defibrillators (ICDs), unlike antiarrhythmic drugs, are highly effective at reducing SCD risk in appropriately selected patients with both ischemic and nonischemic cardiomyopathy. In patients with CAD, nonsustained ventricular tachycardia (NSVT), and reduced ($\leq$40%) ventricular function, there is about a 2-fold increase in risk of SCD.[4–6] Several clinical trials have shown that using antiarrhythmic drugs to reduce mortality is not only ineffective but also, possibly, harmful.[7,8] Findings from 2 clinical trials, the MADIT (Multicenter Automatic Defibrillator Implantation Trial) 1[9] and MUSTT (Multicenter Unsustained Tachycardia Trial),[10] conducted in the 1990s suggested that approximately 4 patients with ischemic cardiomyopathy would need to undergo ICD implantation to save 1 life over a relatively short period of follow-up. These studies were conducted before the widespread use of beta-blockade in heart failure. MADIT 1 and MUSTT enrolled patients with prior myocardial infarction, LVEF less than 40%, NSVT, and ventricular tachycardia induced during electrophysiology study, who were then randomized to receive standard medical therapy, that is, antiarrhythmic therapy (primarily ICDs). Although several differences existed between these studies, the remarkable observation was a 23% reduction in absolute mortality in the patients treated with the ICD during 2 to 3 years of follow-up. Subsequent studies (MADIT 2[11,12] and the Sudden Cardiac Death Heart Failure Trial [SCD-HeFT][12]) eliminated the requirement for demonstrating ambient ventricular ectopy or sustained ventricular arrhythmia during invasive electrophysiologic testing. These trials also enrolled patients with lower EFs (LVEF$\leq$30% in MADIT 2 or $\leq$35% with clinical congestive heart failure in SCD-HeFT). MADIT 2 and SCD-HeFT

Heart Failure Clin 7 (2011) xiii–xviii
doi:10.1016/j.hfc.2011.02.001

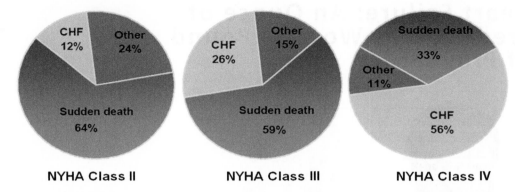

**Fig. 1.** Severity of heart failure and mode of death. CHF, congestive heart failure. (*From* Effect of metoprolol CR/XL in chronic heart failure: Metoprolol CR/XL Randomised Intervention Trial in Congestive Heart Failure (MERIT-HF). Lancet 1999;353(9169):2001–7; with permission.)

reported that the reduction in absolute mortality was more modest (5%–7%), although still significant. Results from both studies suggest that 11 to 17 patients required ICD implantation to save 1 life over a follow-up period of 1 to 2 years. When ICD implantation is limited only to patients who have decreased LV function but in addition have spontaneous NSVT on 24-hour continuous cardiac monitoring and inducible ventricular tachycardia on electrophysiologic study, a higher-risk population is identified, and only 4 ICDs will have to be inserted to save 1 life over 3 years of follow-up.[9] The latter approach, however, results in the omission of patients with decreased LV function but no inducible arrhythmias—a cohort that remains

at considerable risk of death (>40% at 5 years) if not treated with an ICD.[13]

On the other hand, ICD implantation is associated with a 12% risk of major complications,[14] making it important to develop better predictive algorithms to identify patients at risk for SCD. ICDs are also expensive, and although they offer substantive protection against arrhythmic death, SCD (both from malignant arrhythmias and other nonarrhythmogenic causes) can still occur in patients with ICDs.[15] One study suggests that ICD implantation is futile in an identifiable subgroup of patients in SCD-HeFT because their heart failure is simply too advanced,[16] which is not surprising given that sudden death is more

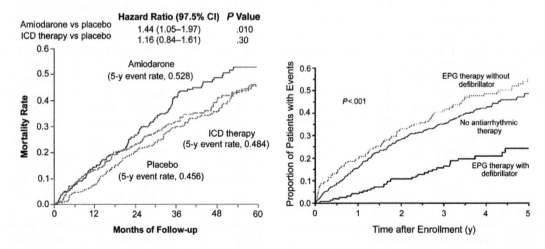

**Fig. 2.** Antiarrhythmic therapy can perform worse than placebo. Inferior performance of antiarrhythmic therapy compared with control group in the SCD-HeFT NYHA functional class III patients (*top*) and the MUSTT (*bottom*). CI, confidence interval; EPG, electrophysiology-guided. (*From* Tung R, Zimetbaum P, Josephson ME. A critical appraisal of implantable cardioverter-defibrillator therapy for the prevention of sudden cardiac death. J Am Coll Cardiol 2008;52(14):1111–21; with permission.)

**Table 1**
**Disparate rates of beta-blockade in major ICD trials**

| | ICD (%) | Control Group (%) |
|---|---|---|
| Significant mortality benefit demonstrated | | |
| AVID[a] (n = 1016) | 42 | 16 |
| MADIT 1[a] (n = 196) | 26 | 8 |
| MADIT 2 (n = 1232) | 70 | 70 |
| SCD-HeFT[a] (n = 2521) | 82 | 79 |
| Nonsignificant differences shown | | |
| CABG Patch (n = 900) | 19 | 16 |
| CAT (n = 104) | 4 | 4 |
| AMIOVERT (n = 103) | 53 | 50 |
| DEFINITE (n = 450) | 85 | 85 |
| DINAMIT (n = 674) | 87 | 86 |
| CIDS[b] (n = 659) | 37 | 21 |
| CASH (n = 288) | 0 | 96 |

*Abbreviations:* AMIOVERT, Amiodarone versus Implantable Defibrillator in Patients with Nonischemic Cardiomyopathy and Asymptomatic Nonsustained Ventricular Tachycardia study; AVID, Antiarrhythmics versus Implantable Defibrillators Trial; CABG Patch, Coronary Artery Bypass Graft Patch trial; CASH, Cardiac Arrest Study Hamburg; CAT, Cardiomyopathy Trial; CIDS, Canadian Implantable Defibrillator Study; DEFINITE, Defibrillator in Non-Ischemic Cardiomyopathy Treatment Evaluation trial; DINAMIT, Defibrillator in Acute Myocardial Infarction Trial.

[a] Statistical significance between groups.

[b] Treatment differences may be confounded by higher usage of sotalol and class I drugs in ICD group.

*From* Tung R, Zimetbaum P, Josephson ME. A critical appraisal of implantable cardioverter-defibrillator therapy for the prevention of sudden cardiac death. J Am Coll Cardiol 2008;52(14):1111–21; with permission.

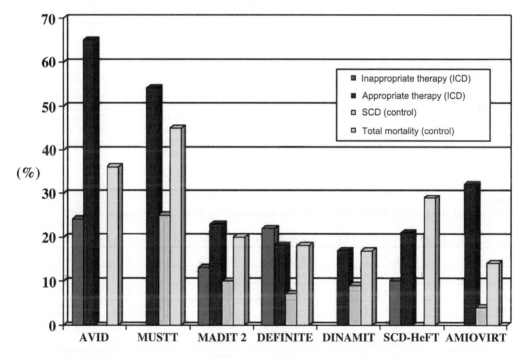

**Fig. 3.** Appropriate shocks outnumber control arrhythmic mortality in 6 of 7 trials. AMIOVIRT, Amiodarone versus Implantable Cardioverter Defibrillator Trial; AVID, Antiarrhythmics versus Implantable Defibrillators trial; DEFINITE, Defibrillators in Non-Ischemic Cardiomyopathy Treatment Evaluation trial; DINAMIT, Defibrillators in Acute Myocardial Infarction Trial. (*Adapted from* Germano JJ, Reynolds M, Essebag V, et al. Frequency and causes of implantable cardioverter-defibrillator therapies: is device therapy proarrhythmic? Am J Cardiol 2006;97(8): 1255–61; with permission; and Tung R, Zimetbaum P, Josephson ME. A critical appraisal of implantable cardioverter-defibrillator therapy for the prevention of sudden cardiac death. J Am Coll Cardiol 2008;52(14): 1111–21; with permission.)

likely to occur in NHYA class II patients than in those with more advanced heart failure (see **Fig. 1**). In the National Cardiovascular Data Registry's ICD Registry, among patients with ICD implants, 22.5% did not meet evidence-based criteria for implantation.[17] Moreover, patients and their relatives are avoiding implantation of devices despite physician recommendation and consensus guidelines.[18,19] A recent review[20] argued that (1) there has been an overestimation of the clinical benefit of ICDs in clinical trials through stacking the deck by using antiarrhythmic drugs as a control arm (**Fig. 2**) and β-blocker inequity (**Table 1**); (2) the adverse effects on morbidity, quality of life, and the potential for proarrhythmia have been underestimated because appropriate ICD shocks do not equal necessary life-saving shocks (**Fig. 3**) and pacemaker and lead malfunction; and (3) the unfavorable cost-effectiveness of ICD therapy is understated because it did not account for hospitalizations, recurrent shocks, and lead replacement.[21] During the 3.5-year period of the MADIT 2 study, the estimated cost per life-year saved by ICDs was relatively high[21]; the average survival gain for the defibrillator arm was 0.167 years (2 months), the additional costs were $39,200, and the incremental cost-effectiveness ratio was $235,000 per year-of-life saved. But when the cost was projected over the course of longer time horizons, the cost-effectiveness approached the accepted range of $50,000 to $100,000— in 3 alternative projections to 12 years, this ratio ranged from $78,600 to $114,000.

Better risk prediction may identify either presently indicated patients whose risk of ventricular

**Table 2**
**The Duke SCD risk score can be calculated by adding points for all risk factors**

| Risk Factor | Points |
|---|---|
| EF (%) | |
| 1–5 | 56 |
| 6–10 | 51 |
| 11–15 | 46 |
| 16–20 | 42 |
| 21–25 | 37 |
| 26–30 | 32 |
| 31–35 | 28 |
| 36–40 | 23 |
| 41–45 | 19 |
| 46–50 | 14 |
| 51–55 | 9 |
| 56–60 | 5 |
| >61 | 0 |
| No. of diseased arteries | |
| 1 | 0 |
| 2 | 6 |
| 3 | 13 |
| Cerebrovascular disease | 8 |
| Heart failure | 7 |
| Diabetes | 7 |
| Hypertension | 6 |
| Tobacco use | 4 |

*Data from* Atwater BD, Thompson VP, Vest RN 3rd, et al. Usefulness of the Duke Sudden Cardiac Death risk score for predicting sudden cardiac death in patients with angiographic (>75% narrowing) coronary artery disease. Am J Cardiol 2009;104:1624–30.

**Table 3**
**Correlation of the Duke SCD risk score with the estimated 1-, 3-, 5-, 7-, or 10-year SCD risk**

| Duke SCD Risk Score | 1-y Risk (%) | 3-y Risk (%) | 5-y Risk (%) | 7-y Risk (%) | 10-y Risk (%) |
|---|---|---|---|---|---|
| 0–10 | 0.2–0.3 | 0.3–0.6 | 0.5–0.9 | 0.8–1.3 | 1.2–1.9 |
| 11–20 | 0.3–0.4 | 0.7–0.9 | 1.1–1.4 | 1.6–2.1 | 2.5–3.2 |
| 21–30 | 0.6–0.7 | 1.2–1.5 | 1.8–2.3 | 2.3–3.4 | 4.0–5.1 |
| 31–40 | 0.9–1.2 | 1.9–2.4 | 3.0–3.8 | 4.3–5.5 | 6.5–8.3 |
| 41–50 | 1.5–1.9 | 3.1–4.0 | 4.9–6.2 | 6.9–8.8 | 10.5–13.2 |
| 51–60 | 2.4–3.1 | 5.1–6.5 | 7.9–10.0 | 11.1–14.0 | 16.6–20.8 |
| 61–70 | 4.0–5.0 | 8.2–10.4 | 12.6–15.8 | 17.6–22.0 | 25.8–31.8 |
| 71–80 | 6.4–8.2 | 13.1–16.5 | 19.8–24.6 | 27.3–33.5 | 38.7–46.6 |
| 81–90 | 10.3–13.0 | 20.6–25.6 | 30.4–37.1 | 40.7–48.8 | 55.3–64.3 |
| 91–100 | 16.4–20.5 | 31.5–38.4 | 44.8–53.3 | 57.6–66.7 | 73.3–81.6 |

*Data from* Atwater BD, Thompson VP, Vest RN 3rd, et al. Usefulness of the Duke Sudden Cardiac Death risk score for predicting sudden cardiac death in patients with angiographic (>75% narrowing) coronary artery disease. Am J Cardiol 2009;104:1624–30.

**Table 4**
**Distribution of patient outcomes by Duke SCD risk score quartile**

| Duke SCD Risk Score | Patients (n) | Alive (%) | SCD (%) | Other Deaths (%) | NNT to Prevent 1 SCD |
|---|---|---|---|---|---|
| 0–14 | 9570 | 7404 (77.4) | 138 (1.4) | 2028 (21.2) | 118 |
| 15–23 | 9230 | 6189 (67.1) | 265 (2.9) | 2776 (30.1) | 57 |
| 24–36 | 9534 | 5191 (54.4) | 403 (4.2) | 3940 (41.3) | 38 |
| 37–101 | 8924 | 2828 (31.7) | 762 (8.5) | 5334 (59.8) | 18 |

Median follow-up 6.2 y.
*Abbreviation:* NNT, number needed to treat.
*Data from* Atwater BD, Thompson VP, Vest RN 3rd, et al. Usefulness of the Duke Sudden Cardiac Death risk score for predicting sudden cardiac death in patients with angiographic (>75% narrowing) coronary artery disease. Am J Cardiol 2009;104:1624–30.

tachyarrhythmia is too low to benefit or those patients whose risk of death from competing comorbidities is too high to benefit. One such score is the Duke SCD risk score,[22] which is probably superior to the single dichotomous EF cutoff for the prediction of SCD. The Duke model includes the following 7 variables: depressed LVEF, number of diseased coronary arteries, diabetes mellitus, hypertension, heart failure, cerebrovascular disease, and tobacco use (**Table 2**). This model was internally validated with bootstrapping and externally validated in patients with ischemic cardiomyopathy from the SCD-HeFT database. In this model, the probability of SCD can be estimated by calculating the point total according to the presence or absence of the risk factors (**Table 3**) and then correlating that point total with the estimated 1-, 3-, 5-, 7-, or 10-year incidence of SCD (**Table 4**). The baseline Duke SCD risk score quartile listed in **Table 4** stratified observed patient outcomes. There was an increase in proportion of patients with SCD and increase in mortality by other causes across the SCD risk score quartiles. The creators of this risk model asserted that assuming ICD implantation reduces the risk of tachyarrhythmic death by 60% in at-risk patients,[23] the predicted number of patients that need to be treated to prevent 1 SCD over time using a prophylactic ICD implantation strategy decreased incrementally across the SCD risk quartiles. Eighteen patients would have required prophylactic ICD therapy to prevent 1 SCD in the greatest SCD risk quartile. Prospective studies are required to validate the ability of the Duke SCD risk score to improve the cost-effectiveness of prophylactic ICD implantation.

To discuss these and other challenges in the management of sudden death, Drs Raul Weiss and Emile Daoud have put together a group of world-class experts in the field. Patients and their relatives, payers, and physicians all want to optimize primary prevention ICD therapy. In our opinion, to do so, better predictors of SCD are required to avoid implantation in patients for whom ICD therapy is futile or even harmful, although their risk of ventricular tachyarrhythmia may be considerable—we need to strive toward better models for prediction—"An Ounce of Prediction Should be Worth More than a Pound of Prevention!"

Ragavendra R. Baliga, MD, MBA
Division of Cardiovascular Medicine
The Ohio State University Medical Center
Columbus, OH, USA

James B. Young, MD
Lerner College of Medicine
Endocrinology & Metabolism Institute
Cleveland Clinic
Cleveland, OH, USA

E-mail addresses:
Ragavendra.baliga@osumc.edu (R.R. Baliga)
youngj@ccf.org (J.B. Young)

**REFERENCES**

1. Zheng ZJ, Croft JB, Giles WH, et al. Sudden cardiac death in the United States, 1989 to 1998. Circulation 2001;104(18):2158–63.
2. Zipes DP, Camm AJ, Borggrefe M, et al. ACC/AHA/ESC 2006 guidelines for management of patients with ventricular arrhythmias and the prevention of sudden cardiac death: a report of the American College of Cardiology/American Heart Association Task Force and the European Society of Cardiology Committee for Practice Guidelines (Writing Committee to Develop Guidelines for Management of Patients With Ventricular Arrhythmias and the Prevention of Sudden Cardiac Death). J Am Coll Cardiol 2006;48(5):e247–346.

3. Effect of metoprolol CR/XL in chronic heart failure: Metoprolol CR/XL Randomised Intervention Trial in Congestive Heart Failure (MERIT-HF). Lancet 1999; 353(9169):2001–7.

4. The Multicenter Postinfarction Research Group. Risk stratification and survival after myocardial infarction. N Engl J Med 1983;309(6):331–6.

5. Josephson M, Wellens HJ. Implantable defibrillators and sudden cardiac death. Circulation 2004; 109(22):2685–91.

6. Tavazzi L, Volpi A. Remarks about postinfarction prognosis in light of the experience with the Gruppo Italiano per lo Studio della Sopravvivenza nell' Infarto Miocardico (GISSI) trials. Circulation 1997; 95(5):1341–5.

7. Echt DS, Liebson PR, Mitchell LB, et al. Mortality and morbidity in patients receiving encainide, flecainide, or placebo. The Cardiac Arrhythmia Suppression Trial. N Engl J Med 1991;324(12):781–8.

8. Julian DG, Camm AJ, Frangin G, et al. Randomised trial of effect of amiodarone on mortality in patients with left-ventricular dysfunction after recent myocardial infarction: EMIAT. European Myocardial Infarct Amiodarone Trial Investigators. Lancet 1997; 349(9053):667–74.

9. Moss AJ, Hall WJ, Cannom DS, et al. Improved survival with an implanted defibrillator in patients with coronary disease at high risk for ventricular arrhythmia. Multicenter Automatic Defibrillator Implantation Trial Investigators. N Engl J Med 1996;335(26):1933–40.

10. Buxton AE, Lee KL, Fisher JD, et al. A randomized study of the prevention of sudden death in patients with coronary artery disease. Multicenter Unsustained Tachycardia Trial Investigators. N Engl J Med 1999;341(25):1882–90.

11. Moss AJ, Zareba W, Hall WJ, et al. Prophylactic implantation of a defibrillator in patients with myocardial infarction and reduced ejection fraction. N Engl J Med 2002;346(12):877–83.

12. Bardy GH, Lee KL, Mark DB, et al. Amiodarone or an implantable cardioverter-defibrillator for congestive heart failure. N Engl J Med 2005;352(3):225–37.

13. Buxton AE, Lee KL, DiCarlo L, et al. Electrophysiologic testing to identify patients with coronary artery disease who are at risk for sudden death. Multicenter Unsustained Tachycardia Trial Investigators. N Engl J Med 2000;342(26):1937–45.

14. Kron J, Herre J, Renfroe EG, et al. Lead- and device-related complications in the antiarrhythmics versus implantable defibrillators trial. Am Heart J 2001; 141(1):92–8.

15. Mitchell LB, Pineda EA, Titus JL, et al. Sudden death in patients with implantable cardioverter defibrillators: the importance of post-shock electromechanical dissociation. J Am Coll Cardiol 2002;39(8): 1323–8.

16. Levy WC, Lee KL, Hellkamp AS, et al. Maximizing survival benefit with primary prevention implantable cardioverter-defibrillator therapy in a heart failure population. Circulation 2009;120(10):835–42.

17. Al-Khatib SM, Hellkamp A, Curtis J, et al. Non-evidence-based ICD implantations in the United States. JAMA 2011;305(1):43–9.

18. Butler K. What broke my father's heart. The New York Times June 18, 2010. Available at: http://www.nytimes.com/2010/06/20/magazine/20pacemaker-t.html. Accessed February 23, 2011.

19. Zimetbaum PJ. A 59-year-old man considering implantation of a cardiac defibrillator. JAMA 2007; 297(17):1909–16.

20. Tung R, Zimetbaum P, Josephson ME. A critical appraisal of implantable cardioverter-defibrillator therapy for the prevention of sudden cardiac death. J Am Coll Cardiol 2008;52(14):1111–21.

21. Zwanziger J, Hall WJ, Dick AW, et al. The cost effectiveness of implantable cardioverter-defibrillators: results from the Multicenter Automatic Defibrillator Implantation Trial (MADIT)-II. J Am Coll Cardiol 2006;47(11):2310–8.

22. Atwater BD, Thompson VP, Vest RN 3rd, et al. Usefulness of the Duke Sudden Cardiac Death risk score for predicting sudden cardiac death in patients with angiographic (>75% narrowing) coronary artery disease. Am J Cardiol 2009;104(12):1624–30.

23. Packer D, Bernstein R, Wood F, et al. Impact of amiodarone versus implantable cardioverter defibrillator therapy on the mode of death in congestive heart failure patients in the SCDHeFT trial. Heart Rhythm 2005;2(S38):AB20–2.

# Preface

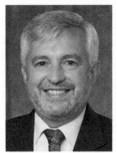 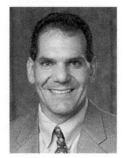

Raul Weiss, MD    Emile G. Daoud, MD
*Guest Editors*

This issue of *Heart Failure Clinics* focuses on sudden cardiac death (SCD) in patients with heart failure (HF). Given the magnitude of the number of individuals affected with HF and the high incidence of SCD, management of SCD in this patient population has become a major public health problem.

HF incidence and prevalence in the United States are quite high, 400,000 and 5,000,000, respectively. The reason for these high numbers, which also reflect a global trend, is twofold. First, there has been an increase in obesity, hypertension, and diabetes with subsequent development of HF. Second, better medical therapy has resulted in reduced mortality. However, even with reduced mortality, SCD remains a significant cause of death. Sudden cardiac death occurs without warning, can occur in young individuals (resulting in catastrophic impact on families and communities), and requires immediate therapy to offer any opportunity to minimize long-term morbidity. Perhaps the most frustrating thing about SCD is the difficulty in predicting who is at high risk. Paradoxically, patients with left ventricular dysfunction but with minimal HF symptoms are more likely to succumb to SCD than to progression of HF.

Implantable cardioverter defibrillators (ICDs) have been shown to be effective in preventing SCD and increase survival in primary and secondary prevention trials. Yet, even with the availability of ICD technology, identifying the individual patient who will benefit from ICD therapy remains challenging. Also, ICD therapy can be associated with significant morbidity related to complications from the implantation procedure, inappropriate ICD shocks, alteration of quality of life, and medical expenses. Moreover, ICD therapy is considered treatment for the entire life of the patient, thus having an even greater influence on younger patients.

For this volume of the *Heart Failure Clinics*, we have gathered expert opinions to help address management of SCD in HF. The first article, written by Dr Houmsse and colleagues, discusses the magnitude of the problem in the general population as well as in specific patient subgroups. Dr Lorvidhaya and coauthors provide an up-to-date review on tools available for risk stratification. Drs Saba and Robinson and colleagues evaluate and analyze trials for primary and secondary prevention, with focus on HF due to any etiology.

Given the importance and impact of ICD shock therapy, two articles are devoted to it. One discusses how to minimize shocks utilizing medical therapy (Dr Droogan and colleagues); the second discusses the utilization of radiofrequency ablation to reduce ICD shocks (Drs Venkataraman and Strickberger).

Drs Varma and Wilcoff discuss device-related features (eg, remote monitoring that may lead to early detection of arrhythmias, technical problems, or even subclinical HF) that may prompt early treatment and prevent progression of symptoms and hospitalization.

For those patients with advanced HF, the only hope of survival is cardiac transplantation; yet, due to organ shortage and the high mortality while waiting for an organ, bridge therapy with ICDs,

Heart Failure Clin 7 (2011) xix–xx
doi:10.1016/j.hfc.2011.01.002
1551-7136/11/$ – see front matter © 2011 Elsevier Inc. All rights reserved.

cardiac resynchronization therapy, and/or ventric-
ular assist devices is becoming more prevalent.
These treatment strategies are discussed by
Drs Hasan and Sun.

No issue is complete until there is some discussion regarding the economics of managing SCD.
Drs Bernard and Gold present an extensive and
thoughtful review of the literature.

Finally, the issue finishes with four excellent articles about SCD from *Cardiac Electrophysiology
Clinics*.

It is our goal to convey to the readers of this
issue of *Heart Failure Clinics* that SCD is a serious
and growing public health issue. Albeit not without
important limitations, ICDs, in conjunction with
medical therapy, have been shown to be the
best current therapy to manage SCD. Although
an ICD can be associated with complications,
this issue elucidates the advantages of ICD
therapy and helps readers understand that the
advancing ICD technology will become a valuable
tool for managing the broader spectrum of HF.

Raul Weiss, MD
Dorothy M. Davis Heart and Lung
Research Institute
Ohio State University Medical Center
Ross Heart Hospital
Suite 200
473 West 12th Avenue
Columbus, OH 43210-1252, USA

Emile G. Daoud, MD
Cardiac Electrophysiology Section
Dorothy M. Davis Heart and Lung
Research Institute
Ohio State University Medical Center
Ross Heart Hospital
Suite 200
473 West 12th Avenue
Columbus, OH 43210-1252, USA

E-mail addresses:
Raul.Weiss@osumc.edu (R. Weiss)
Emile.Daoud@osumc.edu (E.G. Daoud)

# Epidemiology of Sudden Cardiac Death in Patients with Heart Failure

Mahmoud Houmsse, MD[a],*, Veronica Franco, MD[b],
William T. Abraham, MD[b]

**KEYWORDS**

- Heart failure • Sudden cardiac death • Cardiomyopathy
- Predictor • Ejection fraction

Mortality in congestive heart failure (CHF) usually occurs from either progressive worsening of cardiac pump failure or sudden cardiac death (SCD). Medical interventions that counter neurohormonal changes slow the progression of CHF and also prevent SCD.[1] The benefits of medical therapy on SCD prevention have been variable, depending on the type of medical therapy:

1. β-Blocker use in patients after infarction and in patients with CHF decreases SCD by 44%[2] and 41%[3] and pump failure death by 26%[2] and 49%,[3] respectively.
2. Aldosterone antagonists initiated early after myocardial infarction (MI) and in advanced CHF decrease SCD and overall mortality in CHF.[4]
3. Angiotensin-converting enzyme (ACE) inhibitor and angiotensin receptor blocker significantly reduced total mortality and heart failure (HF) hospitalization,[5–7] and the effect improved much with the addition of β-blocker.[3]

SCD is also common among patients with a less severe degree of CHF, (New York Heart Association [NYHA] functional class II), whereas death from progressive pump failure increases as CHF becomes more severe.[8] Despite the advances in medical therapy for the treatment of HF, SCD continues to be the predominant mechanism of death, up to 60% of all cardiac mortality.[3] This result could be because of the shifting in the distribution of mortality by increasing SCD and decreasing death caused by progressive and worsening HF as a result of medical therapy.[9]

## DEFINITION OF SCD

The most accepted definition of SCD is the one used by the World Health Organization: SCD is a sudden unexpected death either within 1 hour of symptom onset (witnessed) or within 24 hours of having been observed alive without symptoms (unwitnessed).[10] The hallmark of the SCD definition is "unexpected," which allows the inclusion of a wider range of preceding clinical states with different levels of underlying risks.[11]

## INCIDENCE OF SCD

Because death certificates overestimate the incidence of SCD[10] and 40% of sudden deaths can be unwitnessed,[12] most of the epidemiologic data of SCD have reported a wide range of incidence of SCD from 184,000 to more than 400,000.[13–16] According to the 2006 American College of Cardiology guidelines for the management of patients with ventricular arrhythmias and prevention of SCD, 300,000 to 350,000 will die from SCD annually.[17,18] The percentage of SCD to all deaths has been influenced by the definition of SCD. About 13% and 18.5% of all deaths were

[a] Division of Cardiovascular Medicine, Department of Cardiovascular Medicine, Davis Heart and Lung Research Institute, The Ohio State University Medical Center, Suite 200, 473 West 12th Avenue, Columbus, OH 43210, USA

[b] Department of Cardiovascular Medicine, The Ohio State University Medical Center, Suite 200, 473 West 12th Avenue, Columbus, OH 43210, USA

* Corresponding author.

*E-mail address:* Mahmoud.houmsse@osumc.edu

Heart Failure Clin 7 (2011) 147–155
doi:10.1016/j.hfc.2010.12.008
1551-7136/11/$ – see front matter © 2011 Elsevier Inc. All rights reserved.

attributed to SCD when the definition of 1 hour and 24 hours were used, respectively. The higher percentage of SCD in the 24-hour category is likely to be related to deaths of noncardiac causes. The overall incidence of SCD in the United States is 0.1% to 0.2% per year among the population 35 years and older.[17] SCD could be the first manifestation of coronary heart disease and accounts for more than 50% of the mortality. From 1989 to 1998, SCD, compared with all cardiac deaths, increased by 12.4% (56.3%–63.9% of cardiac deaths). In 1998, mortality data for residents 35 years and older showed that SCD occurred in 456,076 of 719,456 annual cardiac deaths (63%).[14,19] SCD claimed more lives each year than stroke (167,366),[20] lung cancer (157,400),[21] AIDS (42,156),[22] and breast cancer (40,600) (**Fig. 1**).[21] The black population had higher death rates for SCD than the white, American Indian, Alaskan Native, or Asian/Pacific Islander populations. Studies comparing racial differences demonstrated excess risk of SCD among blacks compared with whites.[23,24] SCD rates among the Hispanic populations were lower[23] than in the non-Hispanic population. The rate of SCD increased with age and was higher in men than in women.

## PREDICTION OF SCD IN HF

Many clinical and pathologic conditions have been suggested as high-risk markers for SCD. Some of them include coronary artery disease, cardiomyopathy with or without symptoms, cardiac rhythm disturbances, and hypertensive heart disease.[25] Multiple clinical and laboratory parameters

(NYHA class, left ventricular ejection fraction [LVEF], systolic blood pressure, adherence to medication use [potassium-sparing diuretic use, statin use, allopurinol use, ACE inhibitor, angiotensin receptor blocker, β-blocker, and loop diuretic dose], hemoglobin, percentage of lymphocyte count, serum uric acid, serum sodium, serum cholesterol, B-type natriuretic peptide [BNP], ambulatory electrocardiographic monitoring, T-wave alternans analysis, heart rate variability measurement, and signal-averaged electrocardiography [SAECG]) have been evaluated as predictors of SCD in HF and cardiomyopathy.

### The Seattle HF Model

The Seattle HF Model (SHFM) was established after the retrospective analysis of the predictors of survival among 1125 patients with CHF in the Prospective Randomized Amlodipine Survival Evaluation Study-1 (PRAISE-1) (NYHA classes IIIB–IV, LVEF<30%, ACE inhibitor, diuretics, 403 deaths). A stepwise hazard model was used to develop a multivariate risk model, which identified clinical (age, gender, ischemic cause, NYHA class, LVEF, systolic blood pressure), pharmacologic (potassium-sparing diuretic use, statin use, allopurinol use, ACE inhibitor, angiotensin receptor blocker, β-blocker and loop diuretic dose), device (defibrillator, biventricular pacemaker, both, left ventricular assist device, or no device), and laboratory (hemoglobin, percentage of lymphocyte count, serum uric acid, serum sodium, and serum cholesterol) characteristics as significant predictors of survival. The SHFM score is calculated and graded from 0 to 4. To calculate the SHFM

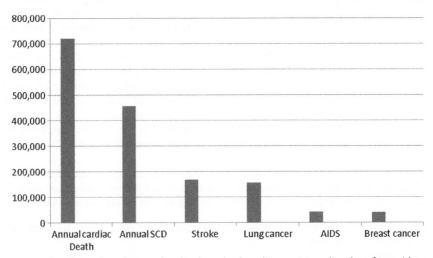

**Fig. 1.** SCD compared with total cardiovascular death and other disease. Mortality data for residents 35 years or older showed that annual SCD occurred in 456,076 of 719,456 (63%) cardiac deaths. SCD claimed more lives each year than stroke (167,366), lung cancer (157,400), AIDS (42,156), and breast cancer (40,600).

score, each variable in the multivariate model is incorporated in a special equation.[26,27] The SHFM score provides an accurate estimate of 1-, 2-, 3-, and 5-year survival. These data were prospectively evaluated in 10,538 ambulatory patients with NYHA classes II to IV HF and mainly systolic dysfunction enrolled in 6 randomized trials or registries. A total of 2014 deaths were reported, which included 1014 SCDs at lower SHFM scores (0–1) and 684 pump failure deaths at the highest score (4). SCD according to the SHFM was similar regardless of age, gender, cause of CHF, or LVEF. The SHFM has also shown that patients with a low NYHA class not taking β-blockers are at an increased risk for SCD.[25] Therefore, patients with NYHA class II, regardless of the cause of their cardiomyopathy, benefit from β-blocker therapy. This result was also reported in the Metoprolol CR/XL Randomized Intervention Trial in Congestive Heart Failure (MERIT-HF); the incidence of deaths that resulted from sudden death in patients with NYHA classes II, III, and IV was 64%, 57%, and 33%, respectively (**Fig. 2**).[3]

## LVEF

Left ventricular systolic dysfunction (LVSD) is an important predictor of SCD in symptomatic HF and asymptomatic CHF. It is estimated that 50% of patients with CHF have LVSD, which presents as a low LVEF without symptoms.[28] Despite optimal medical therapy in asymptomatic CHF, mortality is very high, with a rate of 20% (30% caused by SCD) in 4 to 5 years' follow-up.[29] This result led to the study of implantable cardioverter defibrillators (ICDs) as an adjunctive therapy in patients with CHF and LVSD. In the Multicenter Automatic Defibrillator Implantation Trial (MADIT),

the first SCD primary prevention trial, a group of patients with NYHA class I, II, or III with prior MI, an LVEF of 35% or less, ischemic cardiomyopathy, nonsustained ventricular tachycardia (NSVT), and inducible sustained monomorphic ventricular tachycardia (VT) that was not suppressed with intravenous procainamide identified as a high-risk group. Prophylactic ICDs reduced total mortality by 54% and SCD by 70%.[30] In the MADIT-II, 1232 patients with a month after a MI (and LVEF<30%) were randomized to conventional medical therapy plus ICD implantation or medical therapy alone. One-third of each group was asymptomatic. There was a 31% reduction in death in the ICD group compared with the group with medical therapy alone. The benefits included asymptomatic (NYHA class I) and symptomatic (NYHA classes II–IV) CHF.[31] Therefore, ICD implantation improves overall survival in patients with HF and LVSD 4 weeks post-MI; data for immediate ICD implantation after MI are not conclusive. The Defibrillators in Non-Ischemic Cardiomyopathy Treatment Evaluation (DEFINITE) study investigated the benefit of ICDs in nonischemic dilated cardiomyopathy in addition to ACE inhibitors and β-blocker therapy. The study concluded that ICD implantation significantly decreased the risk of SCD from arrhythmia and was associated with a nonsignificant reduction in the risk of death from any cause. Substudy analyses showed that ICD implantation decreased the risk of death among men with NYHA class III HF.[32]

### Tachycardia-Induced Cardiomyopathy

Tachycardia-induced cardiomyopathy (TIC) is considered a reversible condition if identified early, and once tachycardia resolved either by rate or rhythm control,[33,34] LVEF usually normalizes in weeks to months.[35–40] Recurrent tachycardia results in a drop in the LVEF and HF, as well as the long-term risk for SCD. Nerheim and colleagues[41] reported a series of 24 patients with TIC and NYHA class III HF. The LVEF of all patients improved or normalized after optimal rate control or correction of the rhythm within 6 months. Only 5 patients developed recurrent tachycardia (all atrial fibrillation), a drop in the LVEF, and HF within 6 months. Rate control eliminated HF and improved LVEF within 6 months. Of the 5 patients, 3 died suddenly.

### Diastolic HF

Diastolic HF has an increased risk of SCD. There is a 4-times increase in mortality in patients with HF

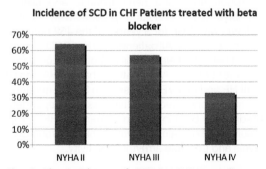

**Incidence of SCD in CHF Patients treated with beta blocker**

**Fig. 2.** The incidence of SCD in CHF according to NYHA. The incidence of deaths that resulted from sudden cardiac death in NYHA classes II, III, and IV patients was 64%, 57%, and 33% as reported by MERIT-HF.

and normal LVEF when compared with control subjects without CHF symptoms. However, the mortality risk in this group was only about half that in the group with CHF and a low LVEF. This result was reported for patients with CHF and preserved left ventricular systolic function in the veterans heart failure trial study.[42] Al-Khatib and colleagues[43] examined the incidence and predictors of SCD in patients with diastolic HF. They evaluated 2314 patients with a history of CHF and an LVEF of greater than 50% and then compared the baseline characteristics of patients who died suddenly with those who died of other causes. The predictors of patients with SCD (45 patients; 1.9%) in diastolic HF include male sex, history of an MI within 3 months, peripheral vascular disease, hyperlipidemia, higher body mass index, more advanced coronary arterial disease, mitral regurgitation, presence of an $S_3$ gallop, history of coronary artery bypass graft, and CHF severity according to the NYHA classification.

### Hypertrophic Cardiomyopathy

Hypertrophic cardiomyopathy (HCM) is considered the most common cause of SCD in young competitive athletes.[44] The annual cardiac mortality rate of patients with HCM is about 1%, with SCD comprising at least half and HF and stroke comprising the remainder.[45–47] The strongest predictors of SCD in HCM have been identified:

- History of SCD or sustained VT
  Prior SCD and spontaneous sustained VT are 2 major predictors for SCD. In a series of 33 patients who were successfully resuscitated, the survival rates free of recurrent cardiac arrest or death after 1, 5, and 10 years were 83%, 65%, and 53%, respectively.[48] These observations were supported with a higher incidence of appropriate defibrillator shocks in patients who received defibrillators for secondary prevention (6.3% and 11% per year in 2 different studies).[49,50]
- Family history of SCD
  Family history becomes much more important in the affected family members if there are multiple SCD events in a family and occurring at a young age.[51,52]
- Recurrent unexplained syncope
  Exertional syncope in young patients with HCM is a risk factor for SCD.[53]
- Multiple episodes of NSVT
  Patients with HCM and NSVT have an incidence of SCD of 8.6% per year compared with 1% per year in patients without NSVT.[54] The risk is higher in symptomatic and young patients. The odds ratio of

sudden death in patients younger than 30 years with NSVT was 4.35 (95% confidence interval [CI], 1.54–12.28; $P = .006$) compared with 2.16 (95% CI, 0.84–5.69; $P = .1$) in those older than 30 years.
- Abnormal blood pressure with exercise
  Either an increase of systolic blood pressure less than 20 mm Hg from rest to peak exercise or a decrease in systolic blood pressure of more than 20 mm Hg during exercise is associated with an increased risk for SCD.[55]
- Massive left ventricular hypertrophy (LVH) greater than 3 cm.
  LVH more than 30 mm in patients younger than 30 years has an increased risk of SCD.[56] There is no risk of SCD for a wall thickness of less than 15 mm compared with 1.8% per year for a wall thickness of greater than 30 mm.
- Genetic mutation in α-tropomyosin and β-myosin heavy chain has been associated with SCD.[57,58]

### Restrictive Cardiomyopathy

Restrictive cardiomyopathy (RCM) prognosis is poor. Rivens and colleagues[59] reported the risk of SCD in a series of 18 patients with RCM over 31 years. Most patients who developed SCD were women, had signs or symptoms of ischemia characterized by chest pain, syncope, or both at presentation, and did not have CHF.

### BNP

Multiple neurohormones have been evaluated to assess their values in predicting SCD, especially in mild to moderate symptoms of CHF. BNP levels have a powerful prognostic role in the care of patients with CHF.[60,61] Marked elevations in BNP levels during hospitalization for HF may predict rehospitalization and death.[1] Levels of BNP and other neurohormones and hemodynamic and clinical variables were evaluated prospectively in 452 patients with CHF for 3 years. Of the 452 patients, 44 died suddenly. All patients who had SCD, except 1, had persistent elevated levels of BNP compared with the survivors. All 44 patients had NYHA class II or III HF and an LVEF of less than 35%. Therefore, the study concluded that BNP was an independent predictor of SCD in mild to moderate CHF.[62] This result might explain the relationship between BNP levels and possible arrhythmic activity.

### Electrocardiographic Parameters

Routine use of ambulatory electrocardiographic monitoring, T-wave alternans analysis, heart rate variability measurement, and SAECG have not been shown to provide an incremental value in assessing the overall prognosis.[1,63] Huikuri and colleagues[63] assessed the power of noninvasive arrhythmia risk markers, including NSVT, LVEF, heart rate variability, baroreflex sensitivity, SAECG, QT dispersion, and QRS duration, to predict SCD after an acute MI (AMI) with 97% beta-blockade therapy at discharge. SCD was weakly predicted only by reduced LVEF, NSVT, and abnormal SAECG. The common arrhythmia risk variables, particularly the autonomic and standard electrocardiography markers, have limited predictive power in identifying patients at risk of SCD after AMI in the beta-blocking era.

## PREDICTING AND PREVENTING SCD IMMEDIATELY AFTER MI

Advances in the treatment of ST-segment elevation MI with primary percutaneous coronary intervention and pharmacologic therapy have resulted in a decrease in sudden death and total mortality.[64–66] The Valsartan in Acute Myocardial Infarction Trial (VALIANT) assessed the incidence and timing of SCD among survivors of AMI with reduced left ventricular systolic function. It concluded that the highest incidence of SCD occurs during the first 30 days after AMI despite optimal therapy. Therefore, earlier strategies need to be implemented to prevent SCD.[64] The LVEF has been established as a useful marker of increased mortality after MI, but it does not identify patients at an increased risk of arrhythmic death relative to total mortality. Patient with high rates of sudden death but low rates of nonsudden death, ICD therapy can provide effective and cost-effective therapy.[67] Multiple clinical trials have demonstrated that the ICD prevents SCD and significantly reduces mortality among patients with LVSD caused by ischemic heart disease but no recent MI.[29–31]

Wilber and colleagues[68] have evaluated the timing of SCD or ICD shocks after MI in the MADIT-II; they examined the effect of ICDs on survival in patients after MI and with an LVEF of less than 30%. A total of 1159 patients with a mean time from their recent MI of 81 ± 78 months were randomized to an ICD group (n = 699) or conventional optimal medical therapy group (n = 460). Mortality rates (deaths per 100 person-years of follow-up) in both arms of treatment were evaluated by time from MI and divided into quartiles (<18, 18–59, 60–119, and ≥120 months). In the conventional optimal medical therapy group, these rates increased as time from MI increased (7.8%, 8.4%, 11.6%, and 14.0%; $P$ = .03). A lower mortality rate in each

quartile as well as minimal increase over time was noticed in the ICD group (7.2%, 4.9%, 8.2%, and 9.0%; $P$ = .19) (see **Fig. 2**). The study concluded that the risk of death associated with ICD therapy was 0.97 for recent MI (<18 months) and 0.55 for remote MI (≥18 months). It also concluded that the mortality risk in MADIT-II population increased as a function of time from MI. The survival benefit associated with ICDs seemed to be greater for remote MI and remained substantial for up to 15 years or more after MI (**Fig. 3**).

By contrast, the trials assessing the role of the ICD in patients at high risk for SCD immediately after MI have failed to show survival benefits.[69–75] The Defibrillator in Acute Myocardial Infarction Trial (DINAMIT) assessed the strategy of ICD use within 4 to 40 days after an AMI with an LVEF of less than 35% and low heart rate variability; the trial did not identify any subsequent benefits from the use of ICD in these high-risk patients.[69]

The Immediate Risk-Stratification Improves Survival (IRIS) trial evaluated the strategy of early post-MI ICD implantation within 1 month of an AMI with an LVEF of less than 40% on optimal medical therapy.[70] Because of the increase in nonarrhythmic death, as in DINAMIT, the benefit of arrhythmic mortality did not affect the total mortality.[69,71] Therefore, there are 2 periods of risk for SCD with different underlying pathophysiologic conditions: an early period with ineffective preventive ICD therapy and a later period with effective preventive ICD therapy. In the early stage, an ongoing ventricular remodeling initiated with AMI followed by collagen deposition is the predominant pathologic process; therefore, treatment is aimed at affecting and possibly reversing ventricular remodeling, which is time dependent and might last over a period of years. This result has been supported by the findings of the Eplerenone Post-AMI Heart Failure Efficacy and Survival Study (EPHUSUS), with a 21% decline in SCD in patients with AMI, LVSD, and CHF who were treated with a selective aldosterone antagonist, eplerenone.[4] In the later period, fixed substrate and scar tissue resulted from remodeling.[76] Use of ICD prevents SCD because an arrhythmic substrate has been created. This process could be delayed by cardiac revascularization (CR) in addition to the optimal medical therapy; therefore, the benefit from ICD in CR is delayed up to more than 6 months. This result was confirmed during CR group analysis of ICD benefit in MADIT-II.[77] This AMI-SCD paradox has been firmly established. It is hoped that in the future, newer risk predictors will identify primary arrhythmic death post-MI because current arrhythmic markers do not predict

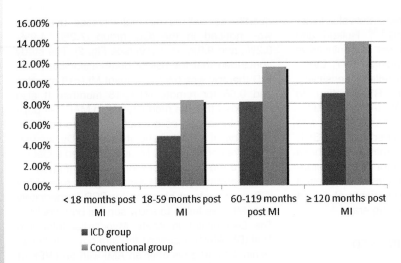

**Fig. 3.** Incidence of SCD in post-MI in-patients treated with conventional medical therapy alone or with ICD according to the time interval post-MI. Post-MI interval was classified to 4 quartiles (<18, 18–59, 60–119, and ≥120 months). In the conventional optimal medical therapy group, these rates increased as time from MI increased (7.80%, 8.40%, 11.60%, and 14.00%; $P = .03$). A lower mortality rate in each quartile as well as a minimal increase over time in the ICD group was noticed (7.2%, 4.9%, 8.2%, and 9.0%; $P = .19$). The risk of death associated with ICD therapy was 0.97 (7.2% vs 7.8%) for recent MI (<18 months) and 0.55 (4.9% vs 8.4%) for remote MI (≥18 months). The survival benefit associated with ICD seems to be greater for remote MI and remains substantial.

SCD.[64–67] Until that time, there is no benefit from early ICD implantation. There is possible deleterious effect of ICD implantation and testing in the early stage post-AMI.[76]

## DOES ICD SHOCK SHIFT THE MODE OF DEATH FROM SCD TO INCREASED HF EVENTS?

The Comparison of Medical Therapy, Pacing, and Defibrillation in Heart Failure (COMPANION) Trial demonstrated that cardiac resynchronization therapy decreases the combined risk of death or first hospitalization in patients with advanced HF and prolonged QRS duration.[78] There was an ICD shock in 142 of 595 (24%) patients. Eighty-eight (61%) shocks were due to appropriate shock for sensed VT and ventricular fibrillation (VF), and 54 (38%) were inappropriate shocks. An appropriate ICD shock does not imply sustained VT or VF or a surrogate for mortality. Patients with an ICD tend to have worse prognosis and more frequent HF after shocks,[78] which were attributed to myocardial damage that may contribute to heart failure decompensation.

## REFERENCES

1. Jessup M, Abraham WT, Casey D, et al. 2009 Focused update: ACCF/AHA Guidelines for the Diagnosis and Management of Heart Failure in Adults: a report of the American College of Cardiology Foundation/American Heart Association Task Force on Practice Guidelines: developed in collaboration with the International Society for Heart and Lung Transplantation. J Am Coll Cardiol 2009;53: 1343–82.
2. Lechat P, Brunhuber KW, Hofmann R, et al. The Cardiac Insufficiency Bisoprolol Study II (CIBIS-II): a randomized trial. Lancet 1999;353:9–13.
3. Hjalmarson A, Goldstein S, Fagerberg B, et al. Effect of metoprolol CR/XL in chronic heart failure: Metoprolol CR/XL Randomized Intervention Trial in Congestive Heart Failure (MERIT-HF). Lancet 1999; 353:2001–7.
4. Pitt B, Williams G, Remme W, et al. Eplerenone in patients with heart failure due to systolic dysfunction complicating acute myocardial infarction. Eplerenone Post-AMI Heart Failure Efficacy and Survival Study (EPHESUS trial). Cardiovasc Drugs Ther 2001;15:79–87.
5. Garg RG, Yusuf S. Overview of randomized trials of angiotensin converting enzyme inhibitors on mortality and morbidity in patients with heart failure. JAMA 1995;273:1450–6.
6. Yusuf S. Effect of enalapril on survival in patients with reduced left ventricular ejection fractions and congestive heart failure. N Engl J Med 1991;325: 293–302.
7. Pfeffer MA, Braunwald E, Moyé LA, et al. Effect of captopril on mortality and morbidity in patients with left ventricular dysfunction after myocardial infarction: results of the survival and ventricular enlargement trial. N Engl J Med 1992;327: 669–77.
8. Rankin AC, Cobbe SM. Arrhytmias and sudden death in heart failure: can we prevent them? In: McMurray JJ, Cleland JG, editors. Heart failure in clinical practice. London: Martin Dunitz Ltd; 1996. p. 189–205.

9. Goldstein S. The changing epidemiology of sudden death in heart failure. Curr Heart Fail Rep 2004;1: 93–7.

10. Chugh SS, Jui J, Gunson K, et al. Current burden of sudden cardiac death: multiple source surveillance versus retrospective death certificate-based review in a large U.S. community. J Am Coll Cardiol 2004; 44:1268–75.

11. Myerburg RJ, Castellanos A. Emerging paradigms of the epidemiology and demographics of sudden cardiac arrest. Heart Rhythm 2006;3(2):235–9.

12. de Vreede Swagemakers JJ, Gorgels AP, Dubois-Arbouw WI, et al. Out-of-hospital cardiac arrest in the 1990's: a population-based study in the Maastricht area on incidence, characteristics and survival. J Am Coll Cardiol 1997;30:1500–5.

13. Myerburg RJ. Scientific gaps in the prediction and prevention of sudden cardiac death. J Cardiovasc Electrophysiol 2002;13:709–23.

14. Zheng ZJ, Croft JB, Giles WH, et al. Sudden cardiac death in the United States, 1989 to 1998. Circulation 2001;104:2158–63.

15. Cobb LA, Fahrenbruch CE, Olsufka M, et al. Changing incidence of out-of-hospital ventricular fibrillation, 1980–2000. JAMA 2002;288:3008–13.

16. Escobedo LG, Zack MM. Comparison of sudden and nonsudden coronary deaths in the United States. Circulation 1996;93:2033–6.

17. Myerburg RJ, Kessler KM, Castellanos A. Sudden cardiac death: epidemiology, transient risk, and intervention assessment. Ann Intern Med 1993;119: 1187–97.

18. Zipes DP, Cam J, Borggrefe M, et al. ACC/AHA/ ESC 2006 guidelines for management of patients with ventricular arrhythmias and the prevention of sudden cardiac death—executive summary: a report of the American College of Cardiology/ American Heart Association Task Force and the European Society of Cardiology Committee for Practice Guidelines (Writing Committee to Develop Guidelines for Management of Patients with Ventricular Arrhythmias and the Prevention of Sudden Cardiac Death). Developed in collaboration with the European Heart Rhythm Association and the Heart Rhythm Society. J Am Coll Cardiol 2006;48: 1064–108.

19. Thom T, Haase N, Rosamond W, et al. Heart disease and stroke statistics—2006 update. Circulation 2006;113:e85–151.

20. American Heart Association. 2002 Heart and stroke statistical update. Dallas (TX): American Heart Association; 2001.

21. American Cancer Society. Surveillance research, cancer facts and figures 2001. Atlanta (GA): American Cancer Society, Inc; 2001.

22. Statistical Abstract of the United States: 2001. U.S. Census Bureau; 2001.

23. Gillum RF. Sudden cardiac death in Hispanic Americans and African Americans. Am J Public Health 1997;87:1461–6.

24. Becker LB, Han BH, Meyer PM, et al. Racial differences in the incidence of cardiac arrest and subsequent survival. The CPR Chicago Project. N Engl J Med 1993;329:600–6.

25. Mozaffarian D, Anker SD, Anand I, et al. Prediction of mode of death in heart failure: the Seattle Heart Failure Model. Circulation 2007;116:392–8.

26. Aaronson KD, Schwartz JS, Chen TM, et al. Development and prospective validation of a clinical index to predict survival in ambulatory patients referred for cardiac transplant evaluation. Circulation 1997;95: 2660–7.

27. Brophy JM, Dagenais GR, McSherry F, et al. A multivariate model for predicting mortality in patients with heart failure and systolic dysfunction. Am J Med 2004;116:300–4.

28. Goldberg LR, Jessup M. Stage B heart failure management of asymptomatic left ventricular systolic dysfunction. Circulation 2006;113:2851–60.

29. Buxton AE, Lee KL, Fisher JD, et al. Multicenter Unsustained Tachycardia Trial Investigators. A randomized study of the prevention of sudden death in patients with coronary artery disease. N Engl J Med 1999;341:1882–90.

30. Moss AJ, Hall WJ, Cannom DS, et al. Multicenter Automatic Defibrillator Implantation Trial Investigators. Improved survival with an implanted defibrillator in patients with coronary disease at high risk for ventricular arrhythmia. N Engl J Med 1996;335: 1933–40.

31. Moss AJ, Zareba W, Hall WJ, et al. Prophylactic implantation of a defibrillator in patients with myocardial infarction and reduced ejection fraction. N Engl J Med 2002;346:877–83.

32. Kadish A, Dyer A, Daubert JP, et al. Prophylactic defibrillator implantation in patients with nonischemic dilated cardiomyopathy. N Engl J Med 2004; 350:2151–8.

33. Packer DL, Bardy GH, Worley SJ, et al. Tachycardia-induced cardiomyopathy: a reversible form of left ventricular dysfunction. Am J Cardiol 1986; 57:563–70.

34. Rosenqvist M, Lee MA, Moulinier L, et al. Long-term follow-up of patients after transcatheter direct current ablation of the atrioventricular junction. J Am Coll Cardiol 1990;16:1467–74.

35. Gillette PC, Smith RT, Garson A Jr, et al. Chronic supraventricular tachycardia: a curable cause of congestive cardiomyopathy. JAMA 1985;253:391–2.

36. Wu EB, Chia HM, Gill JS. Reversible cardiomyopathy after radiofrequency ablation of lateral free-wall pathway-mediated incessant supraventricular tachycardia. Pacing Clin Electrophysiol 2000;23: 1308–10.

37. Ott P, Kelly PA, Mann DE, et al. Tachycardia-induced cardiomyopathy in a cardiac transplant recipient: treatment with radiofrequency catheter ablation. J Cardiovasc Electrophysiol 1995;6:391–5.

38. Harrigan JT, Kangos JJ, Sikka A, et al. Successful treatment of fetal congestive heart failure secondary to tachycardia. N Engl J Med 1981;304:1527–9.

39. Manolis AG, Katsivas AG, Lazaris EE, et al. Ventricular performance and quality of life in patients who underwent radiofrequency AV junction ablation and permanent pacemaker implantation due to medically refractory atrial tachyarrhythmias. J Interv Card Electrophysiol 1998;2:71–6.

40. Grogan M, Smith HC, Gersh BJ, et al. Left ventricular dysfunction due to atrial fibrillation in patients initially believed to have idiopathic dilated cardiomyopathy. Am J Cardiol 1992;69:1570–3.

41. Nerheim P, Birger-Botkin S, Piracha L, et al. Heart failure and sudden death in patients with tachycardia-induced cardiomyopathy and recurrent tachycardia. Circulation 2004;110:247–52.

42. Cohn JN, Johnson G. Heart failure with normal ejection fraction: the V-HEFT study. Circulation 1990; 81(2 Suppl):III48–53.

43. Al-Khatib SM, Shaw LK, O'Connor CM, et al. Sudden cardiac death in patients with diastolic heart failure [abstract]. Circulation 2006;114:II405.

44. Maron BJ, Shirani J, Poliac LC, et al. Sudden death in young competitive athletes. Clinical, demographic, and pathological profiles. JAMA 1996;276: 199–204.

45. Maron BJ, Olivotto I, Spirito P, et al. Epidemiology of hypertrophic cardiomyopathy-related death: revisited in a large non-referral-based patient population. Circulation 2000;102:858–64.

46. Kofflard MJ, Ten Cate FJ, van der Lee C, et al. Hypertrophic cardiomyopathy in a large community-based population: clinical outcome and identification of risk factors for sudden cardiac death and clinical deterioration. J Am Coll Cardiol 2003;41:987–93.

47. Maron BJ. Hypertrophic cardiomyopathy: a systematic review. JAMA 2002;287:1308–20.

48. Cecchi F, Maron BJ, Epstein SE. Long-term outcome of patients with hypertrophic cardiomyopathy successfully resuscitated after cardiac arrest. J Am Coll Cardiol 1989;13:1283–8.

49. Maron BJ, Shen WK, Link MS, et al. Efficacy of implantable cardioverter defibrillators for the prevention of sudden death in patients with hypertrophic cardiomyopathy. N Engl J Med 2000;342:365–73.

50. Primo J, Geelen P, Brugada J, et al. Hypertrophic cardiomyopathy: role of the implantable cardioverter-defibrillator. J Am Coll Cardiol 1998;31:1081–5.

51. Mckenna WJ, Deanfield J, Faruqui A, et al. Prognosis in hypertrophic cardiomyopathy. Role of age and clinical, electrocardiographic and hemodynamic features. Am J Cardiol 1981;47:532–8.

52. Maron BJ, Lipson LC, Roberts WC, et al. "Malignant" hypertrophic cardiomyopathy: Identification of a subgroup of families with unusually frequent premature deaths. Am J Cardiol 1978;41:1133–40.

53. Priori SG, Aliot E, Blomstrom-Lundqvist C, et al. Task Force on Sudden Cardiac Death of the European Society of Cardiology. Eur Heart J 2001;22:1374–450.

54. Maron BJ, Savage DD, Wolfson JK, et al. Prognostic significance of 24 hour ambulatory electrocardiographic monitoring in patients with hypertrophic cardiomyopathy: a prospective study. Am J Cardiol 1981;48:252–7.

55. Sadoul N, Prasad K, Elliott PM, et al. Prospective prognostic assessment of blood pressure response during exercise in patients with hypertrophic cardiomyopathy. Circulation 1997;96:2987–91.

56. Spirito P, Bellone P, Harris KM, et al. Magnitude of left ventricular hypertrophy and risk of sudden cardiac death in hypertrophic cardiomyopathy. N Engl J Med 2000;342:1778–85.

57. Marian AJ, Roberts R. Molecular genetic basis of hypertrophic cardiomyopathy: genetic markers for sudden cardiac death. J Cardiovasc Electrophysiol 1998;9:88–99.

58. Spirito P, Seidman CE, McKenna WJ, et al. The management of hypertrophic cardiomyopathy. N Engl J Med 1997;336:775–85.

59. Rivenes SM, Kearney DL, O'Brian Smith E, et al. Sudden death and cardiovascular collapse in children with restrictive cardiomyopathy. Circulation 2000;102:876–82.

60. Tsutamoto T, Wada A, Maeda K, et al. Attenuation of compensation of endogenous cardiac natriuretic peptide system in chronic heart failure: prognostic role of plasma brain natriuretic peptide concentration in patients with chronic symptomatic left ventricular dysfunction. Circulation 1997;96:509–16.

61. Stanek B, Frey B, Huelsmann M, et al. Prognostic evaluation of neurohumoral plasma levels before and during beta-blocker therapy in advanced left ventricular dysfunction. J Am Coll Cardiol 2001;38: 436–42.

62. Berger R, Huelsman M, Strecker K, et al. B-type natriuretic peptide predicts sudden death in patients with chronic heart failure. Circulation 2002;105: 2392–7.

63. Huikuri HV, Tapanainen JM, Lindgren K, et al. Prediction of sudden cardiac death after myocardial infarction in the beta-blocking era. J Am Coll Cardiol 2003;42:652–8.

64. Solomon SD, Zelenkofske S, McMurray JJ, for the Valsartan in Acute Myocardial Infarction, et al. Sudden death in patients with myocardial infarction and left ventricular dysfunction, heart failure, or both. N Engl J Med 2005;352:2581–8.

65. Ottervanger JP, Ramdat Misier AR, Dambrink JH, et al. Mortality in patients with left ventricular ejection

fraction <30% after primary percutaneous coronary intervention for ST-elevation myocardial infarction. Am J Cardiol 2007;100:793–7.

66. Hohnloser SH, Gersh BJ. Changing late prognosis of acute myocardial infarction: impact on management of ventricular arrhythmias in the era of reperfusion and the implantable cardioverter-defibrillator. Circulation 2003;107:941–6.

67. Goldberger JJ, Cain ME, Hohnloser SH, et al. American Heart Association/American College of Cardiology Foundation/Heart Rhythm Society scientific statement on noninvasive risk stratification techniques for identifying patients at risk for sudden cardiac death: a scientific statement from the American Heart Association Council on Clinical Cardiology Committee on Electrocardiography and Arrhythmias and Council on Epidemiology and Prevention. Circulation 2008;118:1497–518.

68. Wilber DJ, Zareba W, Hall WJ, et al. Time dependence of mortality risk and defibrillator benefit after myocardial infarction. Circulation 2004;109:1082–4.

69. Hohnloser SH, Kuck KH, Dorian P, et al. Prophylactic use of an implantable cardioverter defibrillator after acute myocardial infarction. DINAMIT Investigators. N Engl J Med 2004;351:2481–8.

70. Steinbeck G. A randomized study of defibrillator implantation early after myocardial infarction in high-risk patients on optimal medical therapy. Paper presented at American College of Cardiology 2009 Scientific Sessions. Orlando: March 31, 2009.

71. Bardy GH, Lee KL, Mark DB, et al. Home use of automated external defibrillators for sudden cardiac arrest. N Engl J Med 2008;358:1793–804.

72. Uther JB, Richards JB, Dennis AR, et al. The prognostic significance of programmed ventricular stimulation after myocardial infarction. Circulation 1987; 75:1161–5.

73. Denniss AR, Richards DA, Cody DV, et al. Prognostic significance of ventricular tachycardia and fibrillation induced at programmed stimulation and delayed potentials detected on the signal-averaged electrocardiograms of survivors of acute myocardial infarction. Circulation 1986;74: 731–45.

74. Bhandarhi IA, Hong R, Kotelski A, et al. Prognostic significance of programmed ventricular stimulation in survivors of acute myocardial infarction. Br Heart J 1989;61:410–6.

75. Raviele A, Bongiorni MG, Brignole M, et al. Early EPS/ICD strategy in survivors of acute myocardial infarction with severe left ventricular dysfunction on optimal beta-blocker treatment: the BEtablocker STrategy plus ICD trial. Europace 2005;7:327–37.

76. Goldberger JJ, Passman R. Implantable cardiovertor-defibrillator therapy after acute myocardial infarction. J Am Coll Cardiol 2009;54:2001–5.

77. Goldenberg I, Moss AJ, McNitt S, for the MADIT-II Investigators, et al. Time dependence of defibrillator benefit after coronary revascularization in the Multicenter Automatic Defibrillator Implantation Trial (MADIT)-II. J Am Coll Cardiol 2006;47:1811–7.

78. Saxon LA, Bristow MR, Boehmer J, et al. Predictors of sudden cardiac death and appropriate shock in the comparison of medical therapy, pacing, and defibrillation in heart failure (COMPANION) trial. Circulation 2006;114:2766–72.

# Sudden Cardiac Death Risk Stratification in Patients with Heart Failure

Peem Lorvidhaya, MD, Kamel Addo, MD,
Adam Chodosh, MD, Venkat Iyer, MD, Jeremy Lum, MD,
Alfred E. Buxton, MD*

## KEYWORDS
- Heart failure • Risk stratification • Sudden cardiac death
- Ventricular premature depolarization

Patients with heart failure present a complex set of problems with regard to sudden cardiac death. Clinical heart failure represents the end point of a variety of disease processes. In Western societies heart failure is most often the result of coronary heart disease, followed by nonischemic cardiomyopathy, the latter often related to hypertension. Thus, it is obvious that cardiac arrhythmias in patients with heart failure may result from the original disease process as well as the arrhythmogenic effects of heart failure. Patients with coronary disease may be at risk for cardiac arrest as a result of acute severe ischemia, or reentrant ventricular tachycardia, as well as other mechanisms. Recent studies of patients with nonischemic cardiomyopathy make it clear that scar may form the basis for ventricular tachycardia (VT) in that setting, too. Furthermore, left ventricular hypertrophy is arrhythmogenic and may be present in patients with both coronary disease and nonischemic cardiomyopathies. Superimposed on pathology resulting from the underlying disease processes are the proarrhythmic effects of heart failure; the abnormal intracellular calcium handling, and abnormalities of autonomic tone.

The preceding remarks pertain to tachyarrhythmic mechanisms contributing to cardiac arrest and sudden death in heart failure patients. However, one must remember that sudden death

in this setting may also result from bradyarrhythmias. The authors suspect that the latter occur primarily in patients with end-stage heart failure, and probably do not represent primary arrhythmic events. Rather, the bradyarrhythmic events most likely reflect end-stage mechanical dysfunction. As such, they are less likely to be reversible, and have not been the prime objects of research into risk factors. It seems likely that antiarrhythmic therapies, such as the implantable cardioverter-defibrillator (ICD), are less likely to prevent sudden death caused by such events.

The multiplicity of mechanisms contributing to arrhythmogenesis in patients with heart failure carries obvious implications for risk stratification. If clinicians are to identify patients having the propensity to develop arrhythmias by these different mechanisms, tests must be devised that reveal the substrates or other factors that relate to each mechanism. In the absence of this, our efforts to risk stratify patients are likely to be neither cost-effective nor accurate. In this article the authors review the current knowledge base of risk stratification for sudden death in patients with heart failure. Several limitations in this task are acknowledged. First, most of the studies cited were not restricted to patients with heart failure. Second, in many trials that did require patients to have symptomatic heart failure, the causes of

Division of Cardiology, Rhode Island and Miriam Hospitals, The Warren Alpert Medical School of Brown University, 2 Dudley Street, Suite 360, Providence, RI 02905, USA
* Corresponding author.
E-mail address: Alfred_Buxton@Brown.edu

Heart Failure Clin 7 (2011) 157–174
doi:10.1016/j.hfc.2010.12.001
1551-7136/11/$ – see front matter © 2011 Elsevier Inc. All rights reserved.

heart failure were mixed (ischemic and nonischemic disease). In general, these trials were not powered to determine whether the tests perform differently, depending on the underlying heart disease. Nonetheless, existing data in patients with left ventricular dysfunction due to prior myocardial infarction (MI) are summarized, as well as data for patients with nonischemic dilated cardiomyopathies.

The studies are divided into several categories, recognizing that these distinctions are somewhat artificial and often overlap. These categories include tests that assess measures of left ventricular function and structure (ejection fraction [EF], magnetic resonance imaging [MRI]), autonomic nervous system function (baroreflex sensitivity [BRS], heart rate variability (HRV), heart rate turbulence (HRT), metaiodobenzylguanidine [MIBG] scans), measures of the presumed triggers of VT and ventricular fibrillation (VF) (spontaneous ventricular ectopy and nonsustained VT), measures of the substrate to support reentrant VT (signal-averaged electrocardiography [ECG], electrophysiologic testing), and measures of repolarization reserve (T wave alternans [TWA], QT duration, dispersion, and variability). Also evaluated are aspects of specific tests, such as ECG, recognizing that it may be used to evaluate intraventricular conduction (bundle branch blocks) and left ventricular hypertrophy, as well as repolarization (QT parameters).

## MEASURES OF GLOBAL VENTRICULAR FUNCTION AND STRUCTURE
### Ejection Fraction

EF has traditionally been regarded as the best marker of total mortality.[1] However, over the past decade there has been increasing recognition that functional status is just as important prognostically. This concept is supported by observations of mortality in patients with heart failure and preserved EF that is similar to that of heart failure patients with reduced EF.[2,3] One limitation of our current base is a lack of data regarding mode of death in patients with heart failure and preserved EF. The authors are not aware of studies that have compared the relative prevalence of sudden versus nonsudden death in persons with heart failure and preserved EF.

With regard to coronary heart disease, in studies performed before the advent of reperfusion therapy, as well as those performed in patients treated with thrombolytic therapy or primary angioplasty, total mortality risk increases steadily for patients with EF of 40% or less.[1] At present, for all practical purposes, reduced EF is the only

risk factor used to determine whether to implant an ICD for primary prevention of sudden death.[4] This practice has several limitations. First, fewer than 50% of patients that experience sudden death have an EF less than 30% to 35%.[5,6] Second, the relative prevalence of sudden versus nonsudden death is actually higher in patients with less severe degrees of heart failure (who are likely to have higher EF).[7] In addition, EF does not influence the mode of death (sudden vs nonsudden) in post-MI patients.[8,9] Third, in MI survivors, although those with lower EF (eg, <40%) have higher individual risk of morality, the total number of patients that die after MI is significantly greater (roughly double) among those with EF greater than 40%.[10] Finally, a substudy of the Multicenter Automatic Defibrillator Implantation Trial (MADIT-II) examined factors that influenced survival benefit from ICD therapy in patients with EF of 30% or less.[11] This study demonstrated that using only low EF as a criterion to implant ICDs after MI, approximately one-half of patients derived no survival benefit. The explanation for this was based on 2 observations: not all patients with low EF are at high risk for arrhythmic death, and many patients with low EF are at high risk for nonarrhythmic death (competing risk for death from heart failure, and so forth), and are thus not likely to benefit from ICD therapy. It is concluded that EF is neither sensitive nor specific for identifying patients with heart failure at risk for sudden death.

### Cardiac Magnetic Resonance Imaging

Cardiac MRI has recently emerged as a noninvasive imaging modality capable of providing high-resolution images of the heart. Delayed contrast-enhanced (DE) MRI can be used for noninvasive myocardial tissue characterization. Delayed myocardial enhancement MRI is performed after administration of a paramagnetic contrast agent, usually gadolinium. The addition of delayed enhancement to MRI allows visualization of scar or fibrosis. These areas appear as high signal intensity that is typically subendocardial or transmural in a coronary artery distribution. However, delayed myocardial enhancement is not specific for MI and can occur in a variety of other disorders, such as inflammatory or infectious diseases of the myocardium, as well as nonischemic cardiomyopathies. In nonischemic myocardial disease, the delayed enhancement usually does not occur in a coronary artery distribution and is often mid-wall rather than subendocardial or transmural.[12] The mechanism of DE is related to increased volume of distribution of the gadolinium contrast agent, due to disruption of cell membranes associated with myocardial necrosis.[12] The importance of the scar detected by DE MRI images relates to the fact that myocardial fibrosis can form the substrate for reentrant ventricular tachyarrhythmias.[13]

Increasing data support the potential utility for MRI to identify the substrate to support reentrant VT or VF after MI. Bello and colleagues[14] demonstrated that scar mass and surface area were significantly larger in patients with coronary artery disease (CAD) who had inducible monomorphic VT than in those without inducible ventricular tachycardia. Furthermore, this study showed that these scar characteristics detected by MRI are significantly better than EF in predicting inducible VT. Another measure of potential utility is tissue heterogeneity in areas of infarction. Tissue heterogeneity is likely to form the substrate to support reentry.[15] In MI, areas with enhancement of a lower intensity can often be found in the zone around the infarct borders. Schmidt and colleagues[16] demonstrated that heterogeneity at the infarct periphery was strongly associated with inducibility for monomorphic VT in patients with left ventricular dysfunction. In addition, a small prospective study has demonstrated that the extent of the peri-infarct border zone correlates with cardiovascular mortality, even after adjustment for left ventricular volume and EF.[17]

Wu and colleagues[18] studied the value of DE MRI to predict a composite end point of hospitalization for heart failure, appropriate ICD therapy, or sudden death in patients with nonischemic cardiomyopathy. Sixty-five patients who received an ICD for primary prevention of sudden cardiac death were studied. The presence of DE was associated with a higher risk of the combined end point. However, the absence of scar did not predict a follow-up free of ventricular arrhythmia. In the group with DE, 4 (15%) patients experienced appropriate ICD therapy, compared with 3 (9%) in the group without DE. These results contrast with those of a British study, demonstrating (despite relatively small size and small numbers of events) that mid-wall DE in patients with nonischemic dilated cardiomyopathy was predictive of the combined end point of total mortality and cardiovascular hospitalization, as well as predicting the occurrence of ventricular arrhythmias.[19] The finding that significant arrhythmic risk may exist in nonischemic cardiomyopathy patients without DE is not surprising, because fibrosis leading to macro-reentry is not the only mechanism for ventricular arrhythmias. Other mechanisms in the absence of fibrosis include bundle branch or interfascicular reentry and exaggerated

spatial dispersion of repolarization, as well as abnormal impulse initiation.[5]

Other investigators have focused not only on the presence of DE or scar but also the importance of its location. Nazarian and colleagues[20] were able to demonstrate that the distribution of scar in patients with nonischemic cardiomyopathies, identified by MRI, is predictive of inducible VT. These investigators found that predominance of scar distribution involving 26% to 75% of wall thickness was significantly more likely to be associated with inducible VT than scar that occupied 25% or less or greater than 75% wall thickness. This relation remained after adjustment for left ventricular ejection fraction (LVEF).

The role of MRI in risk stratification is promising; however, more research is needed to evaluate the ability to predict clinically important ventricular arrhythmia in ischemic and nonischemic cardiomyopathy. As is the case with most potential risk markers, the authors are aware of no study that has yet tested whether the use of abnormalities detected by MRI when used to guide ICD therapy will reduce mortality. In addition, the prognostic significance, especially for prediction of sudden death, has not been tested in large numbers of patients (especially in patients with coronary disease) to date.

## MEASURES OF AUTONOMIC FUNCTION

The sympathetic and parasympathetic innervation of the heart plays a major role in the regulation of myocardial function, heart rate, and coronary artery blood flow.[21] Abnormalities of adrenergic innervation and catecholamine stores in patients with heart failure have been recognized since the 1960s. In chronic heart failure, abnormalities in cardiac autonomic control, characterized by sympathetic overactivity and parasympathetic withdrawal, contribute to the progression of the disease and are associated with a worse prognosis.[22–24] Numerous studies have demonstrated increased central sympathetic activity, decreased myocardial catecholamine levels, desensitization of β-adrenoreceptors, and elevation of plasma norepinephrine levels in patients with congestive heart failure.[25–27] These abnormalities of autonomic control may also relate to the genesis of arrhythmias in patients with heart failure. Increased sympathetic activity can modulate basic arrhythmia mechanisms of reentry, automaticity, and triggered activity to help provoke spontaneous ventricular arrhythmias. Prior studies have found an association between markers of excess of sympathetic tone over parasympathetic tone, and increased mortality especially after MI (vide infra). Studies in canine models have shown that animals with markers of excess sympathetic tone have increased susceptibility to ventricular arrhythmias during myocardial ischemia.[28]

## Heart Rate Variability

One commonly used marker of autonomic balance is HRV, which is a measure of beat to beat variation in heart rate over time. HRV can be measured by either time-domain variables or frequency-domain variables. Time domain measures the variation in the RR interval whereas frequency domain measures the variation in frequency of the ECG signal. Most often, HRV is expressed as the standard deviation of RR intervals over a time period. This beat to beat variation is primarily related to respiration, whereby inspiration causes an increase in vagal tone whereas expiration results in a decrease in vagal activity. Therefore it is thought that a decrease in HRV is a reflection of decreased parasympathetic activity.

Limitations to the use of HRV include that it cannot be interpreted in patients in atrial fibrillation, those with frequent atrial or ventricular ectopy, and patients who are persistently paced.

Abnormal HRV has correlated with increased overall mortality in patients with prior MI, as well as chronic heart failure. In the Autonomic Tone and Reflexes After Myocardial Infarction (ATRAMI) study, the use of HRV and BRS were compared prospectively to assess their utility as predictors of cardiac mortality.[29] In this study, 1284 patients with a recent myocardial infarction were enrolled. Over the mean follow-up of 21 months, HRV was an independent predictor of cardiac mortality. In addition, in those patients with an EF of 35% or less, an abnormal HRV was predictive of increased arrhythmic events. Of note, patients with an EF greater than 35% and abnormally low HRV did not experience increased risk for sudden death.

The predictive value of HRV in patients with chronic heart failure was evaluated in a multicenter Italian study.[30] In this study of approximately 400 patients with a dilated cardiomyopathy and heart failure, after a follow-up of 3 years abnormal HRV was an independent predictor of sudden death. By contrast, a study of similar size conducted in the United Kingdom failed to find any significant relationship between HRV and sudden death, although abnormally low HRV was a significant predictor of total mortality.[31] The apparent contradiction between the results of these two studies may lie in part in differences between the two study populations. The average EF in the Italian study was 24%, whereas the mean EF in the UK study was 41%. Entry criteria for UK study included EF les than 45% and New York Heart Association (NYHA) Class I to III, whereas precise entry criteria in the Italian study are not stated.

Of note, no study that has analyzed the relation between HRV and both sudden death and total mortality has found the relative risk for sudden death to exceed the relative risk for total cardiovascular mortality, except for one older study in post-MI patients. The importance of this observation relates to the fact that if a parameter has a causal relation to arrhythmogenesis, one would expect patients with abnormal values for that variable to exhibit risk for arrhythmic sudden death to exceed their risk for total cardiovascular mortality. If abnormal results for a given marker only identify patients with more advanced disease, and therefore at increased risk for both sudden and nonsudden death, the relative risk should be similar for sudden and nonsudden death in patients with abnormal results for that variable. The importance of this relation is as follows. If we are to use ICDs in a cost-effective manner, we should identify patients specifically at significantly increased risk for sudden death. Otherwise ICDs will be implanted in many patients at high risk for nonsudden death, in whom the ICD is unlikely to prolong life.[11] Thus, at this time there is little reason to support the use of HRV for sudden death risk stratification in heart failure patients.

## Baroreflex Sensitivity

The baroreceptor reflex mechanism refers to the body's ability to regulate changes in systemic blood pressure (BP) in response to postural change. Elevation in systemic BP causes activation of the reflex to decrease the heart rate, thereby restoring BP to baseline levels. Hypotension depresses the reflex mechanism, causing an increase in the heart rate and increase in systemic BP. The baroreceptor reflex mechanism regulates the parasympathetic and sympathetic inputs to the heart and blood vessels.

BRS refers to the beat to beat adaptation (measured by the RR interval duration in milliseconds) to alterations in BP. BRS is usually assessed by the phenylephrine method. Phenylephrine (an $\alpha$-agonist) is infused at a dose of 25 to 100 $\mu$g to increase the systolic BP by 15 to 30 mm Hg. Beat to beat changes in the ECG-derived RR intervals and systemic BP are measured simultaneously. The slope of the linear regression line fitting the relationship between BP and RR intervals defines BRS.[32] BRS determined by a noninvasive finger cuff has been shown to provide data comparable to direct intra-arterial

BP measurements.[33] This advantage widens the potential applicability of BRS as a tool for risk stratification of patients with heart failure or MI.

Extensive work has linked the relationship between abnormally low BRS to increased likelihood for both total cardiac mortality and sudden cardiac death.[34–36] The multicenter, prospective ATRAMI study mentioned earlier evaluated the utility of BRS in predicting cardiac mortality after recent MI.[37] Depressed BRS (defined as <3 ms/mm Hg) was associated with significantly higher risk for total cardiac mortality (2.8, 95% confidence interval [CI]: 1.2–6.2) compared with patients with preserved BRS (≥3 ms/mm Hg) during a mean follow-up of 21 months. Of note, patients with low LVEF (<35%) and depressed BRS had a relative risk of 8.7 compared with patients with LVEF of 35% or more and preserved BRS. In addition, mortality of patients with abnormal BRS whose EF was greater than 35% did not have increased mortality risk in comparison with patients with preserved BRS. In contrast, patients with low LVEF (<35%) and abnormally low BRS had significantly higher mortality than those with preserved BRS, despite the reduced EF (18% vs 4.6%, $P<.05$).[29]

In the Canadian REFINE study, Exner and colleagues[38] studied 322 patients after an index MI, with a median follow-up of 47 months. Serial measurements of autonomic tone, electrical substrate, and LVEF were performed. In this study, measures of BRS performed within 1 month of the acute MI had no predictive utility. Also noteworthy is that these observers used a different standard for normal BRS than the Italian group, because they found improved sensitivity over the Italian cutoff value of 3 mm/ms. Patients with impaired BRS (defined as <6.1 ms/mm Hg when measured 10–14 weeks after index MI) had a significantly higher independent risk of the primary outcome (cardiac death or resuscitated cardiac arrest) when compared with patients with preserved BRS (hazard ratio 2.71, 95% CI 1.10–6.67 $P = .03$). The combination of impaired BRS plus abnormal exercise TWA (n = 52) predicted patients at significantly increased risk for the primary outcome (hazard ratio 3.27, 95% CI 1.42–7.00, $P = .005$). Furthermore, when this was combined with LVEF of less than 50%, the same held true (hazard ratio 5.22, 95% CI 2.25–12.13, $P<.0001$).

Depressed BRS has also been shown to be an independent predictor of mortality in heart failure patients.[39,40] La Rovere and colleagues[41] studied BRS in relation to β-adrenergic therapy in heart failure patients in an observational study. The study evaluated 103 patients receiving β-blockers and 144 not taking β-blockers to determine if the prognostic significance of BRS would be less in patients taking β-blockers. The end point was a combination of cardiac death, appropriate defibrillator discharge, or urgent transplant. During a median follow-up of 29 months, a total of 72 patients had a cardiac event (17 taking β-blockers and 55 not taking β-blockers). A depressed BRS was significantly associated with the cardiac event, independent of β-blocker treatment (adjusted hazard ratio 3.0, 95% CI 1.5–5.9, $P<.001$), thus suggesting that depressed BRS is a strong predictor of cardiovascular mortality in heart failure patients despite β-blocker therapy.

In conclusion, these initial studies suggest BRS may prove to be a useful instrument for the prediction of cardiovascular mortality in patients with heart failure as well as after MI in the β-blocker era. However, the technique has several limitations. It cannot be used in patients with atrial fibrillation, those that are pacer dependent, or patients with very frequent ectopy. In addition, it requires that a physician be present to administer phenylephrine and observe the patient. Furthermore, these studies have not shown any clear causal relation between abnormal BRS and sudden death. That is, the increased mortality in patients with reduced BRS was accounted for equally by sudden and nonsudden death. Nonetheless, there is abundant evidence that abnormal neural remodeling after MI and with heart failure plays an important role in the genesis of lethal arrhythmias. As a result, this technique warrants serious attention and further investigation.

### Heart Rate Turbulence

Schmidt and colleagues[42] first described HRT as the fluctuation (early acceleration and then deceleration) in sinus cycle length following a ventricular premature complex (VPC). Although the exact mechanism is unknown, it is thought to represent baroreflex response activity, similar to BRS.

As a result of the VPC, stroke volume decreases and the heart rate increases, due to transient vagal withdrawal in response to the decreased stroke volume causing decreased cardiac output. Following the VPC and compensatory pause, there is a sympathetically-mediated increase in cardiac output and BP, and subsequent decrease in the heart rate due to increased vagal tone. HRT is measured by 2 parameters: turbulence onset (TO) and turbulence slope (TS). TO is defined as the difference between the mean of the first 2 sinus RR intervals after a VPC and the last 2 sinus RR intervals before the VPC divided by the mean of the last 2 sinus RR intervals before the VPC. TS is defined as the maximum positive slope of a regression line assessed over any sequence of 5 subsequent sinus-rhythm RR intervals within the first 20 sinus-rhythm intervals after a VPC.[42]

For most clinical and risk stratification studies, TO less than 0% and TS greater than 2.5 ms/RR interval are considered to be normal, and have been validated. HRT values are usually classified into 1 of 3 categories: HRT category 0 means TO *and* TS are normal; HRT category 1 means one of TO *or* TS is abnormal; and HRT category 2 means both TO *and* TS are abnormal. If no or too few suitable VPC tachograms are found in the Holter recording and HRT cannot be calculated, these patients are classified as HRT category 0.[42,43]

Impaired HRT, specifically HRT category 2, has been shown to be the strongest predictor of subsequent death in univariate analyses of patients enrolled in post-infarction studies. Patients with HRT category 2 (TO>0% and TS≤2.5 ms/RR interval) had a 4.4- to 11.3-fold increased risk of death in univariate analyses and 3.5- to 5.9-fold increased risk of death in multivariate analyses compared with category 0.[44,45] Although the prognostic significance of HRT was similar to that of left ventricular dysfunction, it was independent of LVEF. Similar to BRS, the prognostic significance of HRT has been shown to be unaffected by use of β-blockers in the aforementioned studies.

In the REFINE study, Exner and colleagues[38] included 322 patients after a recent MI with a median follow-up of 47 months. Serial measurements of autonomic tone, electrical substrate, and LVEF were done. Measurements of HRT performed within 1 month of the MI had no prognostic significance. Patients with HRT category 1 compared with HRT category 0 had a significantly higher independent risk of the primary outcome (cardiac death or resuscitated cardiac arrest) when measured 10 to 14 weeks after index MI (hazard ratio 2.91, 95% CI 1.13–7.48, $P = .026$). Patients with impaired HRT plus abnormal TWA (n = 93) measured at 10 to 14 weeks after MI significantly predicted patients at risk for the primary outcome (hazard ratio 4.18, 95% CI 2.06–8.32, $P = .0001$).

Impaired HRT is seen in a large percentage of patients with heart failure, but the prognostic significance has been stronger for patients with congestive heart failure caused by prior MI and CAD rather than nonischemic cardiomyopathies.[46–49] However, as with most other prognostic variables, the relative risk for sudden death has not exceeded the relative risk for nonsudden death. Thus, abnormal degrees of HRT seem to identify patients at increased mortality risk, but not solely because of arrhythmic death.

Although the prognostic significance of impaired HRT has been established in post-MI patients and patients with heart failure, more data are needed in order to establish the utility in predicting those patients who will die suddenly. Limitations of HRT, as with other measures of autonomic tone, include inability to be measured in patients with atrial fibrillation and those that are pacer dependent. In addition, HRT cannot be measured in patients with very infrequent ectopy (<5 VPCs/24 h). There also remains some uncertainty as to the optimal time for measurement of HRT after an MI.

### Metaiodobenzylguanidine

MIBG is an analogue of the false neurotransmitter guanethidine that is taken up by adrenergic neurons in a similar fashion to norepinephrine.[1,6–8,15] When tagged with [123]I it can be used to image adrenergic receptors in many organs, including the heart, with conventional planar or single-photon emission computed tomography (SPECT) techniques. Such imaging allows the evaluation of receptor density and sympathetic innervation. Initial uptake of MIBG by diseased myocardium does not appear to be dramatically different from uptake by normal myocardium. However, the retention of the MIBG within abnormal myocardium is significantly different. After allowing for a "washout" period, the distribution of MIBG within the myocardium is significantly more "patchy" or heterogeneous in patients with both ischemic and nonischemic cardiomyopathy.[1,6–8]

Several studies have examined the results of MIBG imaging in patients with congestive heart failure. Patients with dilated cardiomyopathy in general have reduced MIBG uptake, and an increased washout rate compared with healthy subjects. MIBG abnormalities correlate with LVEF, plasma norepinephrine levels, and NYHA functional class, all variables associated with prognostic importance in patients with heart failure.[9–16] The relation of [123]I-MIBG uptake to myocardial histopathology was studied in 24 patients with nonischemic cardiomyopathy. MIBG uptake imaging was associated with myocyte hypertrophy, myocardial fibrotic change, myocyte degeneration and necrosis, mononuclear cell infiltration, and myocyte disarray.[12]

The use of MIBG imaging to predict outcome in patients with heart failure due to coronary and nonischemic cardiomyopathy has also been examined. An abnormally low ratio of MIBG uptake in the heart to that in the mediastinum (H/M ratio), as well as more rapid washout rate of MIBG are independent predictors of death in several studies.[9–11] Furthermore, the H/M ratio and washout rate were better predictors of sudden death than LVEF, norepinephrine serum levels, HRV, signal average ECG, QT dispersion, and TWA. Most of these studies are limited by small numbers.[15–19] However, a recent prospective study of 937 patients with NYHA Class II/III heart failure due to ischemic or nonischemic cardiomyopathy demonstrated the capacity of MIBG for predicting prognosis for significant cardiac events in this patient population. This study found a highly significant relationship between time to heart failure–related deaths and the H/M ratio. Furthermore, a clear association between severity of myocardial sympathetic neuronal dysfunction and risk for sudden cardiac death was exposed.[27] Another limitation of many studies investigating MIBG is the exclusion of patients taking medications known to interfere with MIBG uptake (eg, β-blockers).[13,15–19]

Although several publications have investigated the potential utility of MIBG scans for risk stratification, currently, [123]I-MIBG is not approved by the Food and Drug Administration for cardiac imaging in the United States. It is not clear that abnormal MIBG scan results identify patients whose risk of sudden death significantly exceeds their total mortality risk. Noteworthy potential advantages of MIBG scans over many other risk stratification techniques include that they can be performed in patients with atrial fibrillation, bundle branch block, and ventricular pacing, and do not require a stress test.

## VENTRICULAR PREMATURE DEPOLARIZATIONS AND NONSUSTAINED VENTRICULAR TACHYCARDIA

Most ventricular premature depolarizations (VPDs) and nonsustained ventricular tachycardia (NSVT) do not cause symptoms. Thus, their discovery requires the clinician to address the following questions: Is the patient symptomatic? What are the prognostic implications of ventricular ectopy in this patient? What interventions, if any, are warranted?

### Recognition of the Origin of Ectopy

The first step in evaluating a patient with ectopy is to be certain one correctly identifies the origin of ectopy (supraventricular vs ventricular). The ECG characteristics of a VPD include a QRS duration of at least 120 milliseconds, bizarre morphology, and T-wave in the opposite direction from the main QRS vector. However, a VPD originating from the contralateral ventricle in a patient with a preexisting bundle branch block may result in a QRS complex narrower than that of the sinus, and a pseudonormalized T-wave in a patient with a prior MI. This consideration is an important one to keep in mind when initializing the origin of ectopy and nonsustained tachycardias.

VPDs may be followed by pauses, and the pause may or may not be fully compensatory. If the VPD conducts retrogradely to the atrium and resets the sinus node, the pause will not be fully compensatory. If the VPD does not penetrate to the atrium, and the atrioventricular node is refractory at the time of the next sinus impulse, a fully compensatory pause results (ie, the RR interval surrounding the VPD is twice the normal sinus RR interval).

NSVT is most commonly defined as a run of 3 or more consecutive ventricular complexes at a rate greater than 100 beats per minute that terminates spontaneously within 30 seconds.

NSVT may be an important marker of increased risk for subsequent tachyarrhythmias capable of causing syncope, cardiac arrest, or sudden cardiac death in some settings. Of note, it is not entirely clear whether episodes of NSVT bear a cause and effect relationship with sustained tachyarrhythmias and sudden cardiac death, or if they are simply a surrogate marker of advanced cardiac dysfunction and electrical instability.

### Prevalence

The prevalence of VPDs and NSVT is directly related to the methods that are used to detect them and to the patient population that is studied. On a resting 12-lead ECG, patients with no known heart disease have been noted to have VPDs less than 5% of the time.[50,51] When the ECG is sampled for longer periods, for example using a 24-hour continuous ambulatory monitoring, VPDs are found in 50% of apparently healthy individuals, suggesting that VPD frequency is in part a function of sampling time.[52,53]

The prevalence of VPDs and NSVT in patients with nonischemic dilated cardiomyopathy is much higher than in healthy individuals, on average. In this case, almost all patients have ventricular ectopy, and up to 80% have NSVT.[54–60] Several factors have been implicated as contributing to the occurrence of ventricular arrhythmias in patients with ventricular dysfunction and heart failure, including the presence of localized fibrosis, abnormal wall stress, heightened sympathetic tone, and electrolyte abnormalities.

### Mechanisms

Triggered activity seems to be responsible for VPDs and NSVT development in 2 principal clinical settings. Early afterdepolarizations arising in Purkinje cells or ventricular myocardium are responsible for the initiation of most episodes of polymorphic VT (torsade de pointes) associated with congenital or acquired long QT syndrome.[61] If repetitive firing allows these afterdepolarizations to reach threshold potential, VPDs and NSVT can be generated and perpetuate in a reentrant pattern.[62] This mechanism may also hold in hypertrophied ventricles in which the action potential duration is prolonged. The second setting in which triggered activity appears to be responsible for NSVT is in the syndrome of right ventricular outflow tract arrhythmias.[63] Increased intracellular calcium via cyclic adenosine monophosphate has been shown to mediate this type of triggered activity.[64]

Other settings in which experimental data suggest focal, non-reentrant mechanisms underlying NSVT are dilated nonischemic and ischemic cardiomyopathies. NSVT in a rabbit model of dilated cardiomyopathy appears to originate in the subendocardium[65] as in the canine model of ischemic cardiomyopathy.[66]

### Prognostic Significance

In general, patients with dilated cardiomyopathy are at considerable risk of sudden death. Older studies reported 1-year mortality rates as high as 40% to 50%.[57,67–69] However, total mortality with modern pharmacologic therapy is much lower, approximating 7% yearly.[70,71] The prognostic significance of VPDs and NSVT is variable, with little evidence that the occurrence of these arrhythmias are related specifically to an increased risk for sudden death, although they do correlate with increased overall cardiac mortality.[55,56,59,60,67–69,72–75] This lack of direct association with sudden death may be due to the ubiquitous nature of VPDs and NSVT in this population and the high overall mortality rates. However, the GESICA investigators found that the relative risk of sudden cardiac death was significantly increased (compared with nonsudden death) in patients with NSVT.[59] In contrast, the Veterans Administration trial (CHF-STAT) investigators did not find a specific increased risk for sudden cardiac death associated with NSVT.[60] A recent analysis suggests that the prognostic significance of NSVT in patients with dilated cardiomyopathy is dependent on EF.[27] In this analysis, NSVT did not contribute prognostic information to patients with EF of 35% or less. However, in patients with EF greater than 35%, there was a threefold increased risk of arrhythmic events.[76]

## SUBSTRATE FOR REENTRANT VT
### Signal-Averaged ECG

The signal-averaged ECG (SAECG) is a high-resolution signal-processing technique developed to detect microvolt-level electrical potentials primarily in the terminal QRS complex, known as late potentials.[77–79] These potentials typically arise from areas in which myocardial fibrosis causes local conduction slowing, resulting in delayed activation, which may be the source of reentrant ventricular arrhythmias.[80] An abnormally prolonged duration of the filtered QRS complex on SAECG or the presence of late potentials has been established as a predictor of arrhythmic events and total mortality after MI.[81–86]

There are limited data regarding the predictive value of the SAECG specifically in patients with heart failure. Mancini and colleagues[87] examined the SAECG as a means of predicting the immediate need for transplantation or death in 114 patients with nonischemic cardiomyopathy, NYHA Classes I to IV. Survival curves over a 12-month period revealed the SAECG to be a powerful predictor of both events. After 12 months, the survival of patients with normal SAECG findings was 95%, compared with 39% for those with SAECG abnormalities. However, a similar, albeit much smaller (22 patients) study by Middlekauff and colleagues[88] did not confirm these findings. Likewise in a study by Silverman and colleagues,[89] of 112 patients with dilated cardiomyopathy the SAECG also failed to predict total mortality.

Several studies have examined the predictive utility of the SAECG in patients with abnormal left ventricular function after MI. Gomes and colleagues[90] analyzed SAECG recordings from 1925 patients enrolled in the Multicenter Unsustained Tachycardia Trial (MUSTT) with NSVT, CAD, and LVEF of 40% or less. A filtered QRS duration greater than 114 milliseconds (the best parameter for prediction from the SAECG) independently predicted arrhythmic death or cardiac arrest (primary end point), as well as cardiac death and total mortality. With an abnormal SAECG, the 5-year mortality rate for the primary end point was 28% versus 17% ($P = .0001$). Sixty-three percent of patients enrolled in that trial had congestive heart failure. One advantage of the SAECG is that in most studies, the negative predictive value has exceeded 90%. Thus, patients with normal SAECG results are probably at relatively low risk. Unfortunately, although somewhat counterintuitive, no study has found the relative risk for sudden death to significantly exceed the relative risk for overall cardiovascular mortality in patients with abnormal values of the SAECG. Thus, it is unlikely to identify patients who will derive significant survival benefit from ICD therapy.

Limitations of the SAECG include that normal values are not established in patients with bundle branch block or ventricular pacing. Advantages over some other risk stratification techniques include the fact that it can be interpreted in patients with atrial fibrillation and frequent ventricular ectopy. Furthermore, it is noninvasive, inexpensive to perform, and easily repeated, with reproducible results.

To summarize, in most post-MI studies a normal SAECG is a marker of patients having low risk for total and sudden cardiac death. In patients with heart failure caused by nonischemic cardiomyopathy, its value is uncertain.

## Programmed Electrical Stimulation (Electrophysiologic Study)

The ability to induce sustained monomorphic VT is a powerful risk stratification tool. It is the only direct indication of the presence of a reentrant VT circuit (and possibly VT due to triggered activity). All other tests discussed herein are surrogate measures of various kinds. However, it has several limitations. Evaluation of the role of programmed electrical stimulation of the ventricles (PES) in patients with heart failure is limited by similar factors noted earlier for most other risk stratification tests: a lack of data. The authors are not aware of any studies specifically evaluating PES in patients with heart failure. However, there is an abundance of data on the prognostic significance of PES in patients with nonischemic dilated cardiomyopathy, as well as in patients with left ventricular dysfunction after MI.

Relatively few studies have evaluated the performance of PES in asymptomatic patients (those without history of spontaneous sustained VT/VF or syncope) with idiopathic dilated cardiomyopathy; those reported are limited by relatively small size (<200 patients) and relatively short follow-up, on average.[91–93] However, the results are fairly consistent. Sustained monomorphic VT is induced in 10% or fewer of patients, and the presence of inducible VT does not predict sudden death.[91–93] Of interest, there is some indication that inducible rapid polymorphic VT/VF may actually be more likely to predict spontaneous occurrence of VT/VF in series that include patients with history of spontaneous VT/VF.[94]

The utility of PES for risk stratification of patients with coronary heart disease has been studied in 2 populations of patients. First is a series of studies of patients with recent (<1 month, and in many cases within 2 weeks) acute MI. Second are studies in patients with left ventricular dysfunction. Most of these studies also required patients to have NSVT. Studies evaluating PES in the second patient population typically involve patients who are several years removed (3–4 years on average) from their most recent MI. The distinction between these characteristics is important for several reasons. Event rates are markedly different between these 2 populations, because the period of highest risk is the first 3 months after acute MI. Another difference is that the patients enrolled in the studies of patients with remote MI typically have much higher prevalence of symptomatic heart failure.

The most significant studies (by virtue of numbers of patients enrolled and uniform protocol) evaluating PES early after MI are a series of studies from Australia and Germany.[95–99] These studies found sustained monomorphic VT inducible in 6% to 22% of patients. The relative risk for sudden cardiac death for patients with inducible VT ranged from 4 to 15. Of note, in each case the relative risk for sudden cardiac death exceeded the risk for nonsudden cardiac death. Because most of these studies were performed prior to widespread adaptation of primary reperfusion for acute MI, as well as use of long term β-adrenergic blockade after MI, these results may not be directly applicable to today's practice. Most recently, the Australian group has published a new prospective observational study. This study of 689 patients studied early after an ST-elevation acute MI was divided into patients by EF less than 40% versus those with EF greater than 40% between 2004 and 2007.[100] EF was measured 2 days after percutaneous intervention for the acute MI. Patients with an EF greater than 40% were discharged, with no further assessment, and followed prospectively. Those with EF 40% or less underwent PES. The stimulation protocol was quite simple: one right ventricular site was studied with a drive train of 400 milliseconds, and up to 4 extrastimuli. The stimulation protocol was repeated if initially negative. Induction of monomorphic VT lasting longer than 10 seconds, with a cycle length 200 milliseconds or longer being considered a positive result. All other PES results were classified as negative. Patients with a positive result were treated with an ICD and those with a negative result were followed prospectively. The patients were divided into 3 groups based on EF and outcomes of PES: Group 1 patients were those with EF above 40%, Group 2 patients were those with EF 40% or below, and negative PES, whereas Group 3 consisted of patients with EF 40% or less and positive PES. After a median follow-up of 12 months, total mortality was similar in all

3 groups: 3%, 3%, and 5.6% for Groups 1 to 3, respectively. The impact of this study is limited by it not being a randomized controlled trial. However, the observations provide useful and provocative information in a population with recent ST elevation MI (STEMI) that uniformly received contemporary management with acute percutaneous intervention. The event rates for total mortality and ventricular arrhythmias were low, over the short-term follow-up reported, and the PES results alone seem reasonably accurate.

It should be noted that another recent trial of PES-guided ICD therapy in patients with recent MI, the BEST+ICD Trial, failed to show a survival benefit from PES-guided therapy.[101] This trial was very small, involving only 143 patients with a mean follow-up of 18 months. Of note, the sudden death rate in patients treated with the PES-guided strategy was 5% versus 9% in patients assigned to conventional therapy (P not significant).

The second group of studies in patients with coronary disease involves patients not required to have a recent MI. Earlier studies showed a trend toward lower rates of inducible sustained VT in patients with EF greater than 40%, as well as lower rates of SCD.[102] As a result, most recent studies (since 1990) have only included patients with EF of 40% or less. The largest study to date evaluating the prognostic significance of the PES in patients with coronary heart disease and abnormal left ventricular function was the MUSTT trial.[103] This randomized trial of patients with EF 40% or less and NSVT found that patients with inducible VT treated without ICD therapy had an 18% risk of sudden death over 2 years, versus 12% for patients without inducible VT (P<.001). The significance of this trial for contemporary management is influenced by the fact that β-blocker therapy was underutilized: only 51% and 35% of patients with and without inducible VT, respectively, were treated with β-blockers, likely increasing the observed event rates. This trial also demonstrated that using PES to guide pharmacologic antiarrhythmic therapy does not reduce mortality.[104] A substudy of this trial suggested that the results of PES are more accurate in patients with EF of 30% to 40%, compared with those with EF less than 30%.[8]

The Multicenter Automatic Defibrillator Implantation Trial used PES for risk stratification after remote MI in patients with EF 35% or less and NSVT.[105] The study demonstrated that patients with inducible VT have high total mortality (32% at 2 years in the group without ICDs) and arrhythmic deaths (half of deaths were sudden). Unfortunately, only 8% of the non-ICD treated patients received β-blockers. In addition, there was no control group of patients without inducible VT included in the trial.

Another recent trial of PES was the Alternans Before Cardioverter Defibrillator Trial (ABCD) that compared PES with TWA to guide ICD therapy for patients with remote MI and EF of 40% or less.[106] Patients with coronary disease, EF les than 40%, and NSVT were included. This trial was also limited by failure to systematically include a group without ICD therapy. The primary end point was a composite of sudden death and the surrogate end point of ICD discharge. Nonetheless, the trial showed that the negative predictive value of PES alone was 95% and 90% at 1- and 2-year follow-up, respectively. The event rate in patients with abnormal PES was 18% at 2 years, identical to that observed in the MUSTT trial (86% of patients in this study received β-blockers).

Thus, PES has good capacity to distinguish patients at high versus low risk for sudden death. PES is the only test (apart from left ventricular hypertrophy) that has the capacity to identify patients whose risk for sudden death exceeds overall mortality risk, suggesting it would be cost-effective in assigning ICD use. The major limitation of PES is its requirement to perform a venous catheterization. However, it is not encumbered by limitations of several other tests. It can be performed in patients in atrial fibrillation, bundle branch block, and with frequent ventricular ectopy. It does not require that patients be able to exercise.

Several important questions remain unanswered regarding PES; these include uncertainty of the optimal stimulation protocol, as well as the prognostic significance of induced rapid polymorphic VT/VF versus monomorphic sustained VT. Most workers believe that induced rapid (CL <220 milliseconds) monomorphic VT and polymorphic VT/VF are associated with significantly lower risk of spontaneous arrhythmic events than induction of sustained monomorphic VT. Such questions require future study.

## THE STANDARD ELECTROCARDIOGRAM

Several conventional ECG features have been identified as independent predictors of overall mortality. The major ones are conduction delay (manifest by QRS duration), QT interval prolongation, QT dispersion, QT variability, and left ventricular hypertrophy (LVH). While several studies have examined the role of these ECG features in predicting the risk of sudden cardiac death, most studies have not focused on heart failure patients. Some insight can be gained into the relevance of these predictive features in heart failure patients by examining the prevalence of heart failure in the study populations. The task of assessing the predictive value of ECG features is further complicated by the observation that, of the few studies that addressed the role of the conventional ECG in risk stratification of heart failure patients, the focus was on all-cause mortality and not on sudden cardiac death.

## Conduction Delay

Heart failure is frequently associated with QRS prolongation beyond 120 milliseconds, an abnormality observed in 14% to 47% of patients in the study by Kashani and Barold.[107] Zimetbaum and colleagues[108] performed an analysis of the relation between ECG abnormalities and the occurrence of arrhythmic and total mortality in a subgroup of patients enrolled in the MUSTT trial. This cohort of patients had documented CAD, NSVT, and LVEF 40% or less, and did not receive any antiarrhythmic therapy. The investigators demonstrated that the presence of left bundle branch block and nonspecific intraventricular conduction delay (IVCD) was independently associated with an approximately 1.5-fold-increased risk of both cardiac arrest and total mortality. Right bundle branch block either alone or in association with left-axis deviation failed to predict either arrhythmic death or all-cause mortality. In this study, nearly 80% of the patients with left bundle branch block or IVCD had congestive heart failure. Of note, only 63% of all patients enrolled in the MUSTT trial had symptomatic heart failure. These results are consistent with those from a multivariable analysis from the CASS registry.[109]

## Left Ventricular Hypertrophy

In the analysis by Zimetbaum and colleagues,[108] ECG evidence of LVH was independently associated with a 35% increase in the risk of arrhythmic death, but was not a predictor of overall mortality. In this cohort, the patients with LVH had more severe left ventricular dysfunction and more congestive heart failure but fewer MIs than those without LVH. The findings of this analysis are consistent with other studies demonstrating an association between ECG evidence of LVH in patients without structural heart disease and risk of sudden death.[110] Proarrhythmia related to LVH may occur through the development of non-reentrant arrhythmias secondary to early afterdepolarizations.[111]

## QT Interval Prolongation

Prolongation of the QT interval is associated with increased mortality in population-based studies and in a variety of cardiac disorders, including heart failure.[112] Two studies have examined the prognostic implications of QT prolongation in patients with heart failure and left ventricular dysfunction. One study enrolled 554 ambulatory patients with congestive heart failure.[112] Both corrected QT interval (QTc) and QT dispersion (QTd) were found to be predictors of mortality only in univariate, but not in multivariate, analysis. In the second and larger study, Padmanabhan and colleagues[113] enrolled 2265 patients with left ventricular dysfunction.[113] Their findings strongly support the prognostic value of QTc prolongation for total mortality in patients with left ventricular dysfunction.

## QT Dispersion

QTd is an approximate measure of the spatial inhomogeneity of ventricular repolarization from the surface ECG. QTd is quantified by the maximum QT interval minus the minimum QT interval on a standard ECG in which all 12 leads are recorded simultaneously. Compared with QT interval, the impact of increased QT dispersion on prognosis in heart failure patients is less certain. Although QTd has been associated with increased mortality in small series of patients with heart failure, larger prospective studies have not confirmed these findings.[114–117] One of the larger studies is the Diamond-CHF study, in which 1518 patients were enrolled.[114] QTd was measurable in 703 patients, and QTd was not predictive of mortality. In the study by Padmanabhan and colleagues,[113] patients with a QTd greater than the mean value of 35 milliseconds had a 5-year mortality rate of 58%, compared with 45% for the remaining patients. The mortality rate impact of increased QTd was more striking in patients with LVEF 30% or less and in patients with a QTc 450 milliseconds or less. However, QTd was not related to mortality after correcting for these variables.

## QT Variability

Whereas QT dispersion is a measurement of the spatial variability of ventricular repolarization, QT variability is a measurement of temporal variability, and is quantified by measurement of the beat to beat QT interval variability during continuous measurement over a 5- to 15-minute period. In a study of patients with dilated cardiomyopathy, Berger and colleagues[118] showed that increased QT variability is present in this cohort, and that the degree of QT variability increases with worsening functional class but is independent of EF. Several studies have examined the predictive value of increased QT variability for arrhythmic death. In a substudy of the MADIT-II trial, Haigney and colleagues[119] showed that in postinfarction patients with severe left ventricular dysfunction, the presence of increased QT variability is associated with a nearly twofold increase in the 2-year risk of VT/VF. Seventy-one percent of the patents with the highest quartile of QT variability had NYHA Class II to IV heart failure symptoms. In summary, the body of evidence indicates that QT variability may be a strong predictor of risk of sudden cardiac death in heart failure patients. QT variability would appear to warrant further investigation to verify its clinical utility for risk stratification.

## T WAVE ALTERNANS

Microvolt TWA describes beat to beat changes in the amplitude or morphology of the T wave. It is thought that TWA results from repolarization changes in myocardial cells secondary to abnormal intracellular calcium handling. Measurement of TWA requires a modest elevation in the heart rate to 105–115 bpm that is usually achieved by exercise or atrial pacing. One of the major limitations of this test is that it cannot be performed during atrial fibrillation or frequent ventricular ectopy. The results of the test are usually broken down into positive, negative and indeterminate. Indeterminate results have been found to carry similar prognostic information as positive results with regard to total mortality. As a result, many studies combine positive and indeterminate results during analysis in order to achieve statistically significant outcomes.

Earlier (primarily single center) studies of TWA suggested that an abnormal result was highly predictive of increased mortality and arrhythmic events. A meta-analysis that combined data from 19 prospective studies is useful, although limited in relevance for the current chapter because heart failure was not an inclusion criterion for all the studies.[120] Overall the positive predictive value of TWA for arrhythmic events was 19% at an average follow up of 21 months, with a negative predictive value of 97%. There was significant variability in the predictive value of TWA, depending on the population of patients being studied. In contrast, the findings of a high negative predictive value seemed to be more consistent across the studies.

Recent studies of TWA testing in patients with heart failure or markedly abnormal left ventricular systolic function have been disappointing. A substudy of the Sudden Cardiac Death in Heart Failure (SCD-HeFT) trial (in which enrolled patients were evenly distributed between coronary disease and non-ischemic cardiomyopathy) examined the ability of TWA to predict arrhythmic events in this population of patients with EF ≤35% and NYHA

Class 2 or 3 symptoms.[121] The analysis included nearly 500 patients. The primary end point was a composite of the first occurrence of sudden cardiac death, sustained ventricular tachycardia/fibrillation, or appropriate implantable cardioverter defibrillator discharge. The authors found that at a mean follow-up of 30 months TWA testing was not predictive of the primary endpoint.

In contrast to the SCD-HeFT substudy, the ALPHA (TWA in patients with heart failure) study examined nearly 450 patients with a nonischemic cardiomyopathy, LVEF ≤40%, and NYHA functional classes II-III.[122] An abnormal TWA result predicted a 4-fold higher risk of the primary endpoint, which was cardiac death or life-threatening arrhythmia. The negative predictive value of a normal TWA result was high at 97%.

The Microvolt TWA Testing for Risk Stratification of Post MI Patients (MASTER) study evaluated TWA in patients with a prior myocardial infarction and depressed ejection fraction (≤30%). The primary endpoint was a composite of arrhythmic death or appropriate defibrillator shock.[123] Similar to the findings in SCD-HeFT, in this study the results of TWA testing did not predict the primary endpoint over an average follow-up of 2.1 years.

The ABCD study examined 566 patients with prior MI, LVEF ≤40% and spontaneous nonsustained ventricular tachycardia.[100] The goal of this study was to compare the predictive ability of TWA testing to electrophysiologic testing for arrhythmic events. Most patients in this study received ICDs, regardless of the results of the TWA or electrophysiology tests. After a median follow up of 1.9 years TWA testing and electrophysiological study (EPS) were comparable in their ability to predict sudden death or appropriate defibrillator discharge. However, it is noteworthy that while TWA discriminated between patients with and without arrhythmic events at one year follow-up, by 2 years TWA had largely lost its discriminatory value. The findings also suggested that EPS and TWA testing provided complimentary information in that if both results were positive, the event rate was significantly higher than in those patients with only one positive result.

Thus, at present the role of TWA testing in heart failure patients is unclear. In contrast to very favorable early results in patients with LVEF above 40% in post-infarction patients,[124] most recent large multicenter studies of patients with heart failure or markedly reduced EF suggest limited utility. Part of the difficulty interpreting and comparing the results of the multiple studies the heterogeneity of the patient populations that have been examined. In addition a significant number of the studies have used total mortality as their endpoint rather than arrhythmic or sudden death. The main utility of TWA testing may be its high negative predictive value. But whether this value is strong enough to warrant withholding an ICD in someone who would otherwise meet criteria is not known. In addition it is unclear how often reassessment with TWA testing needs to be performed.

## SUMMARY AND FUTURE DIRECTIONS

Despite the multitude of studies evaluating the prognostic significance of a variety of potential risk predictors, current guidelines for assigning ICD therapy for primary prevention of sudden death remain dependent on measures that bear no direct relation to arrhythmogenesis: left ventricular EF and NYHA functional class. Why do we find ourselves in this situation? There are several reasons for this. First, trials such as the second MADIT-II and SCD-HeFT used EF as the major entry criterion, and showed mortality reduction in the study population with ICD therapy. Second, there is a paucity of trials evaluating outcome when specific risk stratification tests guide antiarrhythmic therapy. Of note, EF has never been subjected to such a trial, and as such its utility as a risk stratification test is not yet proven. The authors suspect that until trials testing the ability of individual risk stratification tests to determine ICD therapy are performed, no other guidelines will emerge. This challenge is the most important in the arena of sudden death prevention.

Finally, the reader will note that none of the tests described here address mechanisms thought to contribute to arrhythmogenesis specifically in heart failure. The characteristic electrophysiologic alteration in heart failure is disordered intracellular calcium handling, leading to triggered arrhythmias.[125,126] While it is true that PES has the capability to induce triggered tachycardias, little is known of the characteristics of such behavior. It stands to reason that a search for clinical markers of the propensity for disordered intracellular calcium handling in individual patients may provide a more physiologic approach to risk stratification in heart failure.

## REFERENCES

1. Rouleau JL, Talajic M, Sussex B, et al. Myocardial infarction patients in the 1990s—their risk factors, stratification and survival in Canada: The Canadian Assessment of Myocardial Infarction (CAMI) study. J Am Coll Cardiol 1996;27:1119–27.

2. Lee DS, Gona P, Vasan RS, et al. Relation of disease pathogenesis and risk factors to heart failure with preserved or reduced ejection fraction: insights from the Framingham Heart Study of the National Heart, Lung, and Blood Institute. Circulation 2009;119:3070–7.

3. Tribouilloy C, Rusinaru D, Mahjoub H, et al. Prognosis of heart failure with preserved ejection fraction: a 5 year prospective population-based study. Eur Heart J 2008;29:339–47.

4. Epstein AE, DiMarco JP, Ellenbogen KA, et al. ACC/AHA/HRS 2008 guidelines for device-based therapy of cardiac rhythm abnormalities: executive summary: a report of the American College of Cardiology/American Heart Association Task Force on practice guidelines (writing committee to revise the CC/AHA/NASPE 2002 guideline update for implantation of cardiac pacemakers and antiarrhythmia devices). J Am Coll Cardiol 2008;51:2085–105.

5. Gorgels APM, Gijsbers C, de Vreede-Swagemakers J, et al. Out-of-hospital cardiac arrest-the relevance of heart failure. The Maastricht Circulatory Arrest Registry. Eur Heart J 2003;24:1204–9.

6. Stecker EC, Vickers C, Waltz J, et al. Population-based analysis of sudden cardiac death with and without left ventricular systolic dysfunction. Two-year findings from the Oregon Sudden Unexpected Death Study. J Am Coll Cardiol 2006;47:1161–6.

7. MERIT-HF Study Group. Effect of metoprolol CR/XL in chronic heart failure: metoprolol CR/XL randomised intervention trial in congestive heart failure (MERIT-HF). Lancet 1999;353:2001–7.

8. Buxton AE, Hafley GE, Lee KL, et al; MUSTT Investigators. Relation of ejection fraction and inducible ventricular tachycardia to mode of death in patients with coronary artery disease. Circulation 2002;106:2466–72.

9. Yap YG, Duong T, Bland M, et al. Temporal trends on the risk of arrhythmic vs. non-arrhythmic deaths in high-risk patients after myocardial infarction: a combined analysis from multicentre trials. Eur Heart J 2005;26:1385–93.

10. Ross AM, Coyne KS, Moreyra E, et al. Extended mortality benefit of early postinfarction reperfusion. Circulation 1998;97:1549–56.

11. Goldenberg I, Vyas AK, Hall WJ, et al, Madit II Investigators. Risk stratification for primary implantation of a cardioverter-defibrillator in patients with ischemic left ventricular dysfunction. J Am Coll Cardiol 2008;51:288–96.

12. Vogel-Claussen J, Rochitte C, Wu K, et al. Delayed enhancement MR imaging: Utility in myocardial assessment. Radiographics 2006;26:795–810.

13. Wu TJ, Ong JJ, Hwang C, et al. Characteristics of wave fronts during ventricular fibrillation in human hearts with dilated cardiomyopathy: role of increased fibrosis in the generation of reentry. J Am Coll Cardiol 1998;32:187–96.

14. Bello D, Fieno DS, Kim RJ, et al. Infarct morphology identifies patients with substrate for sustained

ventricular tachycardia. J Am Coll Cardiol 2005;45: 1104–8.

15. Hsia HH, Lin D, Sauer WH, et al. Anatomic characterization of endocardial substrate for hemodynamically stable reentrant ventricular tachycardia: identification of endocardial conducting channels. Heart Rhythm 2006;3:503–12.

16. Schmidt A, Azevedo CF, Cheng A, et al. Infarct tissue heterogeneity by magnetic resonance imaging identifies enhanced cardiac arrhythmia susceptibility in patients with left ventricular dysfunction. Circulation 2007;115:2006–14.

17. Yan AT, Shayne AJ, Brown KA, et al. Characterization of the peri-infarct zone by contrast-enhanced cardiac magnetic resonance imaging is a powerful predictor of post-myocardial infarction mortality. Circulation 2006;114:32–9.

18. Wu K, Weiss R, Thiemann D, et al. Late gadolinium enhancement by cardiovascular magnetic resonance heralds an adverse prognosis in nonischemic cardiomyopathy. J Am Coll Cardiol 2008;51: 2414–21.

19. Assomull RG, Prasad SK, Lyne J, et al. Cardiac magnetic resonance, fibrosis, and prognosis in dilated cardiomyopathy. J Am Coll Cardiol 2006; 48:1977–85.

20. Nazarian S, Bluemke DA, Lardo AC, et al. Magnetic resonance assessment of the substrate for inducible ventricular tachycardia in nonischemic cardiomyopathy. Circulation 2005;112:2821–5.

21. Baumgart D, Haude M, Gorge G, et al. Augmented alpha-adrenergic constriction of atherosclerotic human coronary arteries. Circulation 1999;99:2090–7.

22. Cohn J, Levine T, Olivari M, et al. Plasma norepinephrine as a guide to prognosis in patients with chronic congestive heart failure. N Engl J Med 1984;311:819–23.

23. Floras J. Clinical aspects of sympathetic activation and parasympathetic withdrawal in heart failure. J Am Coll Cardiol 1993;22:72–84.

24. Packer M. The neurohumoral hypothesis: a theory to explain the mechanism of disease progression in heart failure. J Am Coll Cardiol 1992;20:248–54.

25. Bristow M, Anderson F, Port J, et al. Differences in beta-adrenergic neuroeffector mechanisms in ischemic versus idiopathic dilated cardiomyopathy. Circulation 1991;84:1024–39.

26. Bristow MR, Minobe W, Rasmussen R, et al. Beta-adrenergic neuroeffector abnormalities in the failing human heart are produced by local rather than systemic mechanisms. J Clin Invest 1992;89:803–15.

27. Ungerer M, Bohm M, Elce J, et al. Altered expression of beta-adrenergic receptor kinase and beta 1-adrenergic receptors in the failing human heart. Circulation 1993;87:454–63.

28. Schwartz P, Billman G, Stone H. Autonomic mechanisms in ventricular fibrillation induced by myocardial ischemia during exercise in dogs with healed myocardial infarction. An experimental preparation for sudden cardiac death. Circulation 1984;69:790–800.

29. La Rovere M, Pinna G, Hohnloser S, et al. The Autonomic Tone and Relfexes After Myocardial Infarction (ATRAMI) Investigators. Baroreflex sensitivity and heart rate variability in the identification of patients at risk for life-threatening arrhythmias: Implications for clinical trials. Circulation 2001;103:2072–7.

30. La Rovere MT, Pinna GD, Maestri R, et al. Short-term heart rate variability strongly predicts sudden cardiac death in chronic heart failure patients. Circulation 2003;107:565–70.

31. Nolan J, Batin PD, Andrews R, et al. Prospective study of heart rate variability and mortality in chronic heart failure: results of the United Kingdom Heart Failure Evaluation and Assessment of Risk trial (UK-HEART). Circulation 1998;98:1510–6.

32. Eckberg DL, Sleight P. Human baroreflexes in health and disease. Oxford (UK): Clarendon Press; 1992.

33. Pinna G, LaRovere M, Maestri R, et al. Comparison between invasive and non-invasive measurements of baroreflex sensitivity. Implications for studies on risk stratification after a myocardial infarction. Eur Heart J 2000;21:1522–9.

34. Farrell TG, Odemuyiwa O, Bashir Y, et al. Prognostic value of baroreflex sensitivity testing after acute myocardial infarction. Br Heart J 1992;67:129–37.

35. La Rovere MT, Specchia G, Mortara A, et al. Baroreflex sensitivity, clinical correlates, and cardiovascular mortality among patients with a first myocardial infarction. A prospective study. Circulation 1988;78:816–24.

36. Schwartz PJ, La Rovere MT, Vanoli E. Autonomic nervous system and sudden cardiac death. Experimental basis and clinical observations for post-myocardial infarction risk stratification. Circulation 1992;85:I77–91.

37. La Rovere M, Bigger JT Jr, Marcus F, et al. Baroreflex sensitivity and heart-rate variability in prediction of total cardiac mortality after myocardial infarction. ATRAMI (Autonomic Tone and Reflexes After Myocardial Infarction) Investigators. Lancet 1998;351:478–84.

38. Exner DV, Kavanagh KM, Slawnych MP, et al, REFINE Investigators. Noninvasive risk assessment early after a myocardial infarction: the REFINE study. J Am Coll Cardiol 2007;50:2275–84.

39. Mortara A, La Rovere MT, Pinna GD, et al. Arterial baroreflex modulation of heart rate in chronic heart failure: clinical and hemodynamic correlates and prognostic implications. Circulation 1997;96: 3450–8.

40. Osterziel K, Hanlein D, Willenbrock R, et al. Baroreflex sensitivity and cardiovascular mortality in

patients with mild to moderate heart failure. Br Heart J 1995;73:517–22.

41. La Rovere M, Pinna G, Maestri R, et al. Prognostic implications of baroreflex sensitivity in heart failure patients in the beta-blocking era. J Am Coll Cardiol 2009;53:193–9.

42. Schmidt G, Malik M, Barthel P, et al. Heart-rate turbulence after ventricular premature beats as a predictor of mortality after acute myocardial infarction. Lancet 1999;353:1390–6.

43. Barthel P, Schneider R, Bauer A, et al. Risk stratification after acute myocardial infarction by heart rate turbulence. Circulation 2003;108:1221–6.

44. Bauer A, Barthel P, Muller A, et al. Risk prediction by heart rate turbulence and deceleration capacity in postinfarction patients with preserved left ventricular function retrospective analysis of 4 independent trials. J Electrocardiol 2009;42:597–601.

45. Ghuran A, Reid F, La Rovere MT, et al; on behalf of the ATRAMI investigators. Heart rate turbulence-based predictors of fatal and nonfatal cardiac arrest (The Autonomic Tone and Reflexes After Myocardial Infarction Substudy). Am J Cardiol 2002;89:184–90.

46. Zhong J-H, Chen X-P, Zeng C-F, et al. Effect of benazepril on heart rate turbulence in patients with dilated cardiomyopathy. Clin Exp Pharmacol 2007;34:612–6.

47. Moore RK, Groves DG, Barlow PE, et al. Heart rate turbulence and death due to cardiac decompensation in patients with chronic heart failure. Eur J Heart Fail 2006;8:585–90.

48. Cygankiewicz I, Zareba W, Vazquez R, et al. Heart rate turbulence predicts all-cause mortality and sudden death in congestive heart failure patients. Heart Rhythm 2008;5:1095–102.

49. Stein PK, Deedwania P. Usefulness of abnormal heart rate turbulence to predict cardiovascular mortality in high-risk patients with acute myocardial infarction and left ventricular dysfunction (from the EPHESUS study). Amer J Cardiol 2009;103:1495–9.

50. Chiang B, Perlman L, Ostrander L Jr, et al. Relationship of premature systoles to coronary heart disease and sudden death in the Techumseh epidemiologic study. Ann Intern Med 1969;70:1159–66.

51. Hiss R, Lamb L. Electrocardiographic findings in 122,043 individuals. Circulation 1962;25:947–61.

52. Brodsky M, Wu D, Denes P, et al. Arrhythmias documented by 24 hour continuous electrocardiographic monitoring in 50 male medical students without apparent heart disease. Am J Cardiol 1977;39:390–5.

53. Sobotka PA, Mayer JH, Bauernfeind RA, et al. Arrhythmias documented by 24-hour continuous ambulatory electrocardiographic monitoring in young women without apparent heart disease. Am Heart J 1981;101:753–9.

54. Suyama A, Anan T, Araki H, et al. Prevalence of ventricular tachycardia in patients with different underlying heart diseases: a study by Holter ECG monitoring. Am Heart J 1986;112:44–51.

55. Neri R, Mestroni L, Salvi A, et al. Arrhythmias in dilated cardiomyopathy. Postgrad Med J 1986;62: 593–7.

56. Meinertz T, Hofmann T, Kasper W, et al. Significance of ventricular arrhythmias in idiopathic dilated cardiomyopathy. Am J Cardiol 1984;53:902–7.

57. Huang SK, Messer JV, Denes P. Significance of ventricular tachycardia in idiopathic dilated cardiomyopathy: observations in 35 patients. Am J Cardiol 1983;51:507–12.

58. Olshausen KV, Stienen U, Schwarz F, et al. Long-term prognostic significance of ventricular arrhythmias in idiopathic dilated cardiomyopathy. Am J Cardiol 1988;61:146–51.

59. Doval HC, Nul DR, Grancelli HO, et al. Nonsustained ventricular tachycardia in severe heart failure. Independent marker of increased mortality due to sudden death. GESICA-GEMA Investigators. Circulation 1996;94:3198–203.

60. Singh SN, Fisher SG, Carson PE, et al. Prevalence and significance of nonsustained ventricular tachycardia in patients with premature ventricular contractions and heart failure treated with vasodilator therapy. Department of Veterans Affairs CHF STAT Investigators. J Am Coll Cardiol 1998;32:942–7.

61. Roden DM, Lazzara R, Rosen M, et al. Multiple mechanisms in the long-QT syndrome. Current knowledge, gaps, and future directions. The SADS foundation task force on LQTS. Circulation 1996;94:1996–2012.

62. el-Sherif N, Turitto G. The long QT syndrome and torsade de pointes. Pacing Clin Electrophysiol 1999;22:91–110.

63. Buxton AE, Waxman HL, Marchlinski FE, et al. Right ventricular tachycardia: clinical and electrophysiologic characteristics. Circulation 1983;68:917–27.

64. Lerman BB, Stein K, Engelstein ED, et al. Mechanism of repetitive monomorphic ventricular tachycardia. Circulation 1995;92:421–9.

65. Pogwizd SM. Nonreentrant mechanisms underlying spontaneous ventricular arrhythmias in a model of nonischemic heart failure in rabbits. Circulation 1995;92:1034–48.

66. Pogwizd SM. Focal mechanisms underlying ventricular tachycardia during prolonged ischemic cardiomyopathy. Circulation 1994;90:1441–58.

67. Holmes J, Kubo SH, Cody RJ, et al. Arrhythmias in ischemic and nonischemic dilated cardiomyopathy: prediction of mortality by ambulatory electrocardiography. Am J Cardiol 1985;55:146–51.

68. Gradman A, Deedwania P, Cody R, et al. Predictors of total mortality and sudden death in mild to moderate heart failure. Captopril-Digoxin Study

Group. J Am Coll Cardiol 1989;14:564–70 [discussion: 571–2].

69. Wilson JR, Schwartz JS, Sutton MS, et al. Prognosis in severe heart failure: relation to hemodynamic measurements and ventricular ectopic activity. J Am Coll Cardiol 1983;2:403–10.

70. Kadish A, Dyer A, Daubert JP, et al. Prophylactic defibrillator implantation in patients with nonischemic dilated cardiomyopathy. N Engl J Med 2004; 350:2151–8.

71. Bardy GH, Lee KL, Mark DB, et al. Amiodarone or an implantable cardioverter-defibrillator for congestive heart failure. N Engl J Med 2005;352:225–37.

72. Pantano JA, Oriel RJ. Prevalence and nature of cardiac arrhythmias in apparently normal well-trained runners. Am Heart J 1982;104:762–8.

73. Teerlink JR, Jalaluddin M, Anderson S, et al. Ambulatory ventricular arrhythmias in patients with heart failure do not specifically predict an increased risk of sudden death. PROMISE (Prospective Randomized Milrinone Survival Evaluation) Investigators. Circulation 2000;101:40–6.

74. Thanavaro S, Kleiger RE, Miller JP, et al. Coupling interval and types of ventricular ectopic activity associated with ventricular runs. Am Heart J 1983;106:484–91.

75. Unverferth DV, Magorien RD, Moeschberger ML, et al. Factors influencing the one-year mortality of dilated cardiomyopathy. Am J Cardiol 1984;54: 147–52.

76. Zecchin M, Di Lenarda A, Gregori D, et al. Are non-sustained ventricular tachycardias predictive of major arrhythmias in patients with dilated cardiomyopathy on optimal medical treatment? Pacing Clin Electrophysiol 2008;31:290–9.

77. Berbari EJ. High resolution electrocardiography. In: Zipes DP, Jalife J, editors. Cardiac electrophysiology: from cell to bedside. Philadelphia: Saunders; 2009. p. 793–802.

78. Berbari E, Scherlan R, Hope R, et al. Recordings from body surface of arrhythmogenic ventricular activity during the ST segment. Am J Cardiol 1978;41:697–702.

79. Cain ME, Anderson JL, Arnsdorf MF, et al. ACC expert consensus document: Signal-averaged electrocardiography. J Am Coll Cardiol 1996;27:238–49.

80. Simpson M. Use of signals in the terminal QRS complex to identify patients with recurrent ventricular tachycardia after myocardial infarction. Circulation 1981;64:235–42.

81. Breithardt G, Becker R, Seipel L, et al. Non-invasive detection of late potentials in man: a new marker for ventricular tachycardia. Eur Heart J 1981;2:1–11.

82. El-Sherif N, Denes P, Katz R, et al. Definition of the best prediction criteria of the time domain signal-averaged electrocardiogram for serious arrhythmic events in the postinfarction period. J Am Coll Cardiol 1995;25:908–14.

83. Gomes J, Mehra R, Barreca P, et al. Quantitative analysis of the high frequency components of the signal-averaged QRS complex in acute myocardial infarction. Circulation 1985;72:105–11.

84. Gomes J, Winters S, Martinson M, et al. The prognostic significance of quantitative signal-averaged variables relative to clinical variables, site of myocardial infarction, ejection fraction and ventricular premature beats: a prospective study. J Am Coll Cardiol 1988;13:377–84.

85. Gomes JA, Winters S, Stewart D, et al. A new noninvasive index to predict sustained ventricular tachycardia and sudden death in the first year after myocardial infarction: based on signal-average electrocardiogram, radionuclide ejection fraction and Holter monitoring. J Am Coll Cardiol 1987;10:349–57.

86. Kuchar DL, Thorburn CW, Sammel NL. Prediction of serious arrhythmic events after myocardial infarction: signal-averaged electrocardiogram, Holter monitoring and radionuclide ventriculography. J Am Coll Cardiol 1987;9:531–8.

87. Mancini D, Wong K, Simson M. Prognostic value of an abnormal signal-averaged electrocardiogram in patients with nonischemic congestive cardiomyopathy. Circulation 1993;87:1083–92.

88. Middlekauff H, Stevenson W, Woo M, et al. Comparison of frequency of late potentials in idiopathic dilated cardiomyopathy and ischemic cardiomyopathy with advanced congestive heart failure and their usefulness in predicting sudden death. Am J Cardiol 1990;66:1113–7.

89. Silverman M, Pressel M, Brackett J, et al. Prognostic value of the signal-averaged electrocardiogram and a prolonged QRS in ischemic and nonischemic cardiomyopathy. Am J Cardiol 1995;75:460–4.

90. Gomes J, Cain M, Buxton A, et al. Prediction of long-term outcomes by signal-averaged electrocardiography in patients with unsustained ventricular tachycardia, coronary artery disease, and left ventricular dysfunction. Circulation 2001;104:436–41.

91. Brembilla-Perrot B, Donetti J, de la Chaise AT, et al. Diagnostic value of ventricular stimulation in patients with idiopathic dilated cardiomyopathy. Am Heart J 1991;121:1124–31.

92. Grimm W, Hoffmann J, Menz V, et al. Programmed ventricular stimulation for arrhythmia risk prediction in patients with idiopathic dilated cardiomyopathy and nonsustained ventricular tachycardia. J Am Coll Cardiol 1998;32:739–45.

93. Becker R, Haass M, Ick D, et al. Role of nonsustained ventricular tachycardia and programmed ventricular stimulation for risk stratification in patients with idiopathic dilated cardiomyopathy. Basic Res Cardiol 2003;98:259–66.

94. Rolf S, Haverkamp W, Borggrefe M, et al. Induction of ventricular fibrillation rather than ventricular tachycardia predicts tachyarrhythmia recurrences in patients with idiopathic dilated cardiomyopathy and implantable cardioverter defibrillator for secondary prophylaxis. Europace 2009;11:289–96.

95. Andresen D, Steinbeck G, Bruggemann T, et al. Risk stratification following myocardial infarction in the thrombolytic era: a two-step strategy using noninvasive and invasive methods. J Am Coll Cardiol 1999;33:131–8.

96. Bhandari AK, Rose JS, Kotlewski A, et al. Frequency and significance of induced sustained ventricular tachycardia or fibrillation two weeks after acute myocardial infarction. Am J Cardiol 1985;56:737–42.

97. Bourke JP, Richards DA, Ross DL, et al. Routine programmed electrical stimulation in survivors of acute myocardial infarction for prediction of spontaneous ventricular tachyarrhythmias during follow-up: results, optimal stimulation protocol and cost-effective screening. J Am Coll Cardiol 1991; 18:780–8.

98. Richards DA, Byth K, Ross DL, et al. What is the best predictor of spontaneous ventricular tachycardia and sudden death after myocardial infarction? Circulation 1991;83:756–63.

99. Brembilla-Perrot B, de la Chaise AT, Briancon S, et al. Programmed ventricular stimulation in survivors of acute myocardial infarction: long-term follow-up. Int J Cardiol 1995;49:55–65.

100. Zaman S, Sivagangabalan G, Narayan A, et al. Outcomes of early risk stratification and targeted implantable cardioverter-defibrillator implantation after ST-elevation myocardial infarction treated with primary percutaneous coronary intervention. Circulation 2009;120:194–200.

101. Raviele A, Bongiorni MG, Brignole M, et al, BES-T+ICD Trial Investigators. Early EPS/ICD strategy in survivors of acute myocardial infarction with severe left ventricular dysfunction on optimal beta-blocker treatment. The Beta-Blocker Strategy plus ICD trial. Europace 2005;7:327–37.

102. Buxton AE, Marchlinski FE, Flores BT, et al. Nonsustained ventricular tachycardia in patients with coronary artery disease: role of electrophysiologic study. Circulation 1987;75:1178–85.

103. Buxton AE, Lee KL, DiCarlo L, et al. Electrophysiologic testing to identify patients with coronary artery disease who are at risk for sudden death. Multicenter Unsustained Tachycardia Trial Investigators. N Engl J Med 2000;342:1937–45.

104. Buxton AE, Lee KL, Fisher JD, et al. A randomized study of the prevention of sudden death in patients with coronary artery disease. Multicenter Unsustained Tachycardia Trial Investigators. N Engl J Med 1999;341:1882–90.

105. Moss AJ, Hall WJ, Cannom DS, et al. Improved survival with an implanted defibrillator in patients with coronary disease at high risk for ventricular arrhythmia. Multicenter Automatic Defibrillator Implantation Trial Investigators. N Engl J Med 1996;335:1933–40.

106. Costantini O, Hohnloser SH, Kirk MM, et al, ABCD Trial Investigators. The ABCD (alternans before cardioverter defibrillator) trial: strategies using T-wave alternans to improve efficiency of sudden cardiac death prevention. J Am Coll Cardiol 2009; 53:471–9.

107. Kashani A, Barold SS. Significance of QRS complex duration in patients with heart failure. J Am Coll Cardiol 2005;46:2183–92.

108. Zimetbaum PJ, Buxton AE, Batsford W, et al. Electrocardiographic predictors of arrhythmic death and total mortality in the multicenter unsustained tachycardia trial. Circulation 2004;110:766–9.

109. Freedman RA, Alderman EL, Sheffield LT, et al. Bundle branch block in patients with chronic coronary artery disease: angiographic correlates and prognostic significance. J Am Coll Cardiol 1987; 10:73–80.

110. Siscovick DS, Raghunathan TE, Rautaharju P, et al. Clinically silent electrocardiographic abnormalities and risk of primary cardiac arrest among hypertensive patients. Circulation 1996;94:1329–33.

111. Almendral J, Villacastin J, Arenal A, et al. Evidence favoring the hypothesis that ventricular arrhythmias have prognostic significance in left ventricular hypertrophy secondary to systemic hypertension. Am J Cardiol 1995;76:60D–3D.

112. Brooksby P, Batin PD, Nolan J, et al. The relationship between QT intervals and mortality in ambulant patients with chronic heart failure. The United Kingdom Heart Failure Evaluation and Assessment of Risk Trial (UK-heart). Eur Heart J 1999;20:1335.

113. Padmanabhan S, Silvet H, Amin J, et al. Prognostic value of QT interval and QT dispersion in patients with left ventricular systolic function: Results from a cohort of 2265 patients with an ejection fraction of ≤ 40%. Am Heart J 2003;145:132–8.

114. Brendorp B, Elming H, Jun L, et al. QT dispersion has no prognostic information for patients with advanced congestive heart failure and reduced left ventricular systolic function. Circulation 2001;103:831–5.

115. Fei L, Goldman J, Prasad K, et al. QT dispersion and RR variations on 12-lead ECGs in patients with congestive heart failure secondary to idiopathic dilated cardiomyopathy. Eur Heart J 1996; 17:258–63.

116. Galinier M, Vialette JC, Fourcade J, et al. QT interval dispersion as a predictor of arrhythmic events in congestive heart failure: importance of aetiology. Eur Heart J 1998;19:1054–62.

117. Pinsky D, Sciacca R, Steinberg J. QT dispersion as a marker of risk in patients awaiting heart transplantation. J Am Coll Cardiol 1997;29:1576–84.

118. Berger RD, Kasper EK, Baughman KL, et al. Beat-to-beat QT interval variability: novel evidence for repolarization lability in ischemic and nonischemic dilated cardiomyopathy. Circulation 1997;96:1557–65.

119. Haigney MC, Zareba W, Gentlesk PJ, et al. QT interval variability and spontaneous ventricular tachycardia or fibrillation in the multicenter automatic defibrillator implantation trial (MADIT) II patients. J Am Coll Cardiol 2004;44:1481–7.

120. Gehi AK, Stein RH, Metz LD, et al. Microvolt T-wave alternans for the risk stratification of ventricular tachyarrhythmic events: a meta-analysis. J Am Coll Cardiol 2005;46:75–82.

121. Gold MR, Ensley D, Chilson D, et al. T-wave alternans SCD HeFT study: primary endpoint analysis. Circulation 2007;114:428.

122. Salerno-Uriarte JA, De Ferrari GM, Klersy C, et al. Prognostic value of T-wave alternans in patients with heart failure due to nonischemic cardiomyopathy: results of the ALPHA study. J Am Coll Cardiol 2007;50:1896–904.

123. Chow T, Kereiakes DJ, Onufer J, et al; on behalf of the MASTER Trial Investigators. Does microvolt T-wave alternans testing predict ventricular tachyarrhythmias in patients with ischemic cardiomyopathy and prophylactic defibrillators?: The MASTER (microvolt T wave alternans testing for risk stratification of post-myocardial infarction patients) trial. J Am Coll Cardiol 2008;52:1607–15.

124. Ikeda T, Yoshino H, Sugi K, et al. Predictive value of microvolt T-wave alternans for sudden cardiac death in patients with preserved cardiac function after acute myocardial infarction: results of a collaborative cohort stud. J Am Coll Cardiol 2006;48:2268–74.

125. Pogwizd SM, Bers DM. Calcium cycling in heart failure: the arrhythmia connection. J Cardiovasc Electrophysiol 2002;13:88–91.

126. Pogwizd SM, Bers DM. Na/Ca exchange in heart failure. Contractile dysfunction and arrhythmogenesis. Ann N Y Acad Sci 2002;976:454–65.

# Sudden Cardiac Death Risk Stratification and Assessment: Primary Prevention Based on Ejection Fraction Criteria

Samir Saba, MD, FHRS

## KEYWORDS

- Sudden cardiac death • Primary prevention
- Left ventricular ejection fraction

Sudden cardiac death (SCD) is the prime cause of death in adults in industrialized countries.[1–3] It is estimated that in the United States, more than 300,000 Americans die every year from SCD, a staggering number, surpassing the total annual number of deaths from all cancers. It is established that malignant ventricular arrhythmias, namely ventricular fibrillation, constitute the most common mechanism of SCD (**Fig. 1**).[1–3]

The term sudden cardiac arrest (SCA) is used to describe aborted SCD. The survival of SCA survivors depends primarily on the time to defibrillation and to return to a hemodynamically perfusing rhythm.[4,5] Because of the hurdles hindering prompt defibrillation, survival of SCA survivors to hospital discharge continues to be very poor.[6]

Implantable cardioverter-defibrillators (ICDs) are devices that are implanted in high-risk patients to protect them against SCD (**Fig. 2**). Large randomized trials have demonstrated the benefits of the ICD in reducing total mortality in survivors of SCA.[7–9] These secondary prevention trials led the way to the more recent primary prevention trials, which evaluated the benefits of the ICD in patients at high risk of SCD who have not, however, previously had an SCA.[10–21]

Identifying those high-risk patients who may benefit from an ICD implantation has been the subject of multiple clinical trials over the past 10 to 15 years. Indices of electrical instability or alternans[22,23] and autonomic tone[24] to mention a few, have been proposed as markers of high-risk substrate with varying degrees of accuracy in predicting clinical events. To date, however, only the measure of left ventricular function as assessed by the ejection fraction (EF) has been established as a clinical tool to determine eligibility for ICD implantation.[25] This article reviews the clinical ICD trials for the primary prevention of SCD with special attention to the value and shortcomings of the EF as a clinical tool for the assessment and stratification of the risk of SCD.

## CLINICAL TRIALS IN PATIENTS WITH ISCHEMIC CARDIOMYOPATHY

Survivors of myocardial infarctions (MIs) who have established severe cardiomyopathy are at a significantly higher risk of death compared with the general population,[26] despite the salutary effects of pharmacologic therapy with medications such as β-adrenergic receptor blockers[27] or

Disclosures: Dr Saba has received research grants from Medtronic Inc, Boston Scientific, and St Jude Medical and is a consultant for Boston Scientific, St Jude Medical, and Spectranetics Inc.
Cardiovascular Electrophysiology Section, University of Pittsburgh Medical Center, 200 Lothrop Street, PUH B535, Pittsburgh, PA 15213, USA
E-mail address: sabas@upmc.edu

Heart Failure Clin 7 (2011) 175–183
doi:10.1016/j.hfc.2010.12.004

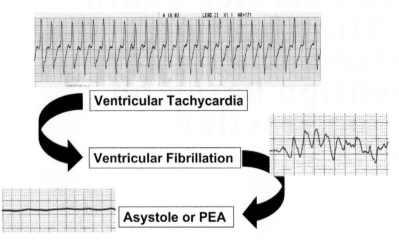

**Fig. 1.** The progression of arrhythmic mechanism leading to SCD. The defibrillator can intervene and possibly terminate these mechanisms through antitachycardia pacing, shock therapy, or backup pacing for bradycardia or asystole. PEA, pulseless electrical activity.

angiotensin-converting enzyme inhibitors.[28,29] Although there is a clustering of death early after MI,[30] higher mortality rates continue to plague MI survivors years after the acute coronary event. It is estimated that a large proportion of those patients succumb to SCD, whereas others die of heart failure (HF).

Evaluating the role of the defibrillator in patients with a history of MI was studied extensively, with varying results being attributed primarily to the timing of ICD implantation with respect to the index MI or revascularization procedures. The following sections discuss the highlights from the largest randomized ICD trials in patients with ischemic heart disease (**Table 1**).

### CABG-Patch

The Coronary Artery Bypass Graft Patch (CABG-Patch) trial[9] evaluated the role of ICDs in a population of patients with coronary artery disease undergoing elective coronary artery bypass grafting. Eligible patients had to have a decreased left ventricular cardiac function (EF<36%) and an abnormal signal-averaged electrocardiogram, which is used as a marker for higher risk of ventricular arrhythmias. All patients (n = 900) received epicardial defibrillator patches at the time of surgery and were randomized to receiving an ICD versus no ICD. After a mean follow-up of 32 months, there was no difference in the survival of patients with or without ICD (101 deaths in the ICD group compared with 95 deaths in the control arm). Although the risk of arrhythmic death was decreased in the ICD arm, nonarrhythmic deaths dominated the event rates in this study, which is one of the few negative primary prevention ICD studies in the population with ischemic cardiomyopathy.[10,11] The presence of surgical revascularization and perhaps the

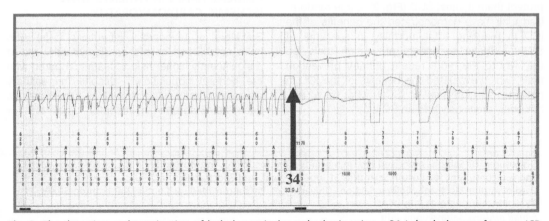

**Fig. 2.** The detection and termination of lethal ventricular arrhythmia using a 34-J shock therapy from an ICD. Red arrow indicates the time of shock delivery that terminates the lethal ventricular arrhythmia.

**Table 1**
**Summary of primary prevention clinical trials of defibrillators**

| Trials | N | ICM vs NICM | Study Arms | Inclusion | Relative Reduction in Total Mortality with ICD (*P* value) |
|---|---|---|---|---|---|
| CABG-PATCH[9] | 900 | ICM | ICD<br>Medical Rx | EF<36%<br>Elective CABG<br>SAECG abnormal | −7% (.64) |
| DINAMIT[10] | 674 | ICM | ICD<br>Medical Rx | 6–40 d after MI<br>EF≤35%<br>Decreased HRV | −8% (.66) |
| IRIS[11] | 898 | ICM | ICD<br>Medical Rx | 5–31 d after MI<br>EF≤40%<br>HR>90 or NSVT | −4% (.78) |
| MADIT[12] | 196 | ICM | ICD<br>Medical Rx<br>AAD | EF<35%<br>NSVT<br>EPS+ | 54% (.009) |
| MUSTT[13] | 704 | ICM | EP-guided Rx<br>AAD<br>ICD<br>Medical Rx | EF≤40%<br>NSVT<br>EPS+ | 76% (<.001) |
| MADIT II[14] | 1232 | ICM | ICD<br>Medical Rx | EF≤30% | 31% (.016) |
| SCD-HeFT[15] | 2521 | ICM/NICM | ICD<br>Amiodarone<br>Placebo | EF≤35%<br>NYHA class 2 & 3 | 23% (.007) |
| AMIOVIRT[16] | 103 | NICM | ICD<br>Amiodarone | EF≤35%<br>NYHA class 1–3<br>NSVT | 7% (.8) |
| CAT[17] | 104 | NICM | ICD<br>Medical Rx | EF≤30%<br>NYHA class 2 & 3<br>Diagnosis<9 mo | 7% (.554) |
| DEFINITE[18] | 458 | NICM | ICD<br>Medical Rx | EF<36%<br>NYHA class 1–3<br>PVC/NSVT | 35% (.08) |
| CARE-HF[19] | 813 | ICM/NICM | CRT-P<br>Medical Rx | EF≤35%<br>NYHA class 3 & 4<br>QRS≥120 ms | 36% (<.002) |
| COMPANION[20] | 1520 | ICM/NICM | CRT-D<br>CRT-P<br>Medical Rx | EF≤35%<br>NYHA class 3 & 4<br>QRS≥120 ms | 36% (.003) |
| MADIT-CRT[21] | 1820 | ICM/NICM | CRT-D<br>ICD only | EF≤30%<br>NYHA class 1 & 2<br>QRS≥130 ms | 7% (.99) |

N=total number of patients enrolled in study.

*Abbreviations:* AAD, antiarrhythmic drug; AMIOVIRT, Amiodarone versus Implantable Defibrillator Trial; CABG, coronary artery bypass graft; CABG-PATCH, Coronary Artery Bypass Graft Patch Trial; CARE-HF, Cardiac Resynchronization–Heart Failure Study; CAT, Cardiomyopathy Trial; COMPANION, Comparison of Medical Therapy, Pacing, and Defibrillation in Heart Failure Trial; CRT-D, cardiac resynchronization therapy defibrillator; CRT-P, cardiac resynchronization therapy pacemaker; DEFINITE, Defibrillators in Non-Ischemic Cardiomyopathy Treatment Evaluation; DINAMIT, Defibrillator in Acute Myocardial Infarction Trial; EP, electrophysiology; EPS, electrophysiological study; HR, heart rate; HRV, heart rate variability; ICM, ischemic cardiomyopathy; IRIS, Immediate Risk-Stratification Improves Survival Trial; MADIT, Multicenter Automatic Defibrillator Implantation Trial; MADIT-CRT, Multicenter Automatic Defibrillator Implantation Trial–Cardiac Resynchronization Therapy; MUSTT, Multicenter Unsustained Tachycardia Trial; NICM, nonischemic cardiomyopathy; NSVT, nonsustained ventricular tachycardia; NYHA, New York Heart Association; PVC, premature ventricular complex; Rx, therapy; SAECG, signal-averaged electrocardiography; SCD-HeFT, Sudden Cardiac Death in Heart Failure Trial.

poor performance of the signal-averaged electro-cardiogram as a tool for risk stratification are thought to be responsible for the negative results of this trial. Based on the results of this study, the left ventricular EF may need to be reevaluated within few months after coronary revascularization before an ICD is implanted.[25]

## DINAMIT

The Defibrillator in Acute Myocardial Infarction Trial (DINAMIT)[10] addressed the question of the timing of the implantation of the ICD after acute MI. Given the high risk of SCD early after MI (valiant) and the positive results of previously published primary prevention ICD trials (Multicenter Automatic Defibrillator Implantation Trial [MADIT], Multicenter Unsustained Tachycardia Trial [MUSTT]), DINAMIT tested the hypothesis that an ICD implanted shortly after MI (within 6–40 days) decreases the risk of death. Eligible patients had to have a recent MI, a decreased left ventricular function (EF≤35%), and reduced heart rate variability used as a marker of higher risk of lethal arrhythmias. Patients who underwent coronary revascularization were appropriately excluded from this study, given the results of CABG-Patch.[9] A total of 674 patients were enrolled and randomized to receiving a prophylactic ICD versus no ICD. After a mean follow-up of 30 months, there was no difference in the survival of patients with or without ICD (62 deaths in the ICD group compared with 58 deaths in the control arm). Although the ICD reduced the risk of arrhythmic death by about 58% (P = .009), there was an unexplained excess of nonarrhythmic deaths in the ICD arm, which eliminated the effect of the ICD in reducing total mortality. There are a lot of speculations regarding the negative results of DINAMIT on reducing total mortality. The implantation of ICD early after MI may increase the risk of nonarrhythmic death to the patient. Also, several patients in DINAMIT may have had recurrent ischemia or MI after the index event, thus leading to death that could not necessarily be prevented by the ICD.

## IRIS

The Immediate Risk-Stratification Improves Survival (IRIS) trial[11] examined a similar clinical question as DINAMIT, namely, if the use of a prophylactic ICD conferred a survival benefit in patients with recent MI. To answer this question, IRIS randomized a total of 898 patients to ICD or standard medical therapy. Eligible patients had to be within 5 to 31 days from the index MI, have an EF less than or equal to 40%, and have a heart rate greater than 90 beats per minute or nonsustained ventricular tachycardia (VT) on the first available electrocardiogram or Holter monitor recorded after the MI. After a mean follow-up of 37 months, IRIS failed to demonstrate a survival benefit with the ICD (P = .78). As seen in DINAMIT, although there was a significant decrease in SCD with the ICD (27 deaths in the ICD group vs 60 deaths in the control group, P = .049), the incidence of non-SCDs was higher in the ICD group (68 deaths in the ICD group vs 39 deaths in the control group, P = .001). Based on the results of this confirmatory study as well as DINAMIT,[10] implanting a prophylactic ICD within 40 days of an acute MI is contraindicated according to the published guidelines.[25]

## MADIT

The MADIT[12] was the first published ICD trial showing a benefit of the ICD on total mortality in a primary prevention population. The MADIT enrolled patients with a history of MI, a depressed left ventricular function (EF<35%), a history of asymptomatic nonsustained VT, and an inducible sustained VT during invasive electrophysiological (EP) testing, which could not be suppressed by the use of antiarrhythmic medications (mainly procainamide). A total of 196 patients were enrolled in this trial and randomized to receiving a prophylactic ICD versus antiarrhythmic medications (mainly amiodarone). After a mean follow-up of 27 months, there was a significant reduction in total mortality in the ICD compared with the control arm (15 deaths in the ICD group vs 39 deaths in the control group), mainly accounted for by a reduction in arrhythmic deaths.

## MUSTT

The MUSTT[13] examined the merits of 2 clinical approaches to the patient with ischemic cardiomyopathy (EF≤40%) who has inducible VT or ventricular fibrillation during invasive EP testing: (1) EP-guided antiarrhythmic therapy with medications belonging to both class I and class III categories according to the Vaughn Williams classification versus (2) standard medical therapy. In the first arm of the study, if all antiarrhythmic drugs failed to suppress the inducibility of ventricular arrhythmia during EP testing, then an ICD was implanted. A total of 704 eligible patients were enrolled in this study and randomized to its 2 arms. Of the 351 patients assigned to the EP-guided antiarrhythmic therapy, 161 received an ICD before discharge. Although there was no difference in total mortality between the 2 arms of the study at a median follow-up duration of 39 months, there was a significant reduction in total mortality among ICD recipients compared with patients discharged with no ICD (5-year mortality of 24% in ICD group compared with 55% in the non-ICD group, P<.001). Thus, although not designed to examine the value of ICD therapy in patients with ischemic cardiomyopathy, the MUSTT trial ended up confirming the previously published results of MADIT.[12] Based on the results of these 2 studies, implanting a prophylactic ICD in patients with prior MI, nonsustained VT, and an EF less than or equal to 40% in whom sustained ventricular arrhythmia can be induced during invasive EP testing is a class I indication for ICD implantation.[25]

## MADIT II

The MADIT II[14] was designed with the intent of simplifying eligibility criteria for implanting defibrillators in patients with ischemic cardiomyopathy and ventricular dysfunction and expanding the target population that may benefit from a prophylactic ICD. For these reasons, eligibility criteria in the MADIT II did not include the need for an invasive EP study or inducibility of ventricular arrhythmias. Inclusion into the MADIT II was simply based on a history of MI with low EF ($\leq$30%). Patients with very advanced symptoms of HF (New York Heart Association class IV) were excluded from this trial. A total of 1232 patients were enrolled and randomized to receiving an ICD versus standard medical therapy. At a mean follow-up of 20 months, there was a significant 31% relative reduction in total mortality in the patients who received ICD compared with the control patients (mortality of 14.2% in the ICD arm compared with 19.8% in the control arm, P = .016).

## SCD-HeFT

The SCD-HeFT[15] is the largest of all primary prevention trials examining the role of the ICD in reducing total mortality. SCD-HeFT enrolled patients with cardiomyopathy (EF$\leq$35%) of both ischemic and nonischemic etiologies and class II or III symptoms of HF, according to the New York Heart Association classification. Eligible patients were then randomized into 1 of the 3 groups: (1) standard medical therapy versus (2) antiarrhythmic therapy with amiodarone versus (3) ICD implantation. A total of 2521 patients were enrolled and followed up for a median of 45.5 months. amiodarone and conventional therapy were administered in a double-blinded manner. As compared with the placebo and amiodarone arms, the patients who received ICD had significant 23% reductions in the risk of death from any cause (total mortality of 22% in the ICD

group compared with 28% in the amiodarone group and 29% in the placebo group, P = .007). The results of the SCD-HeFT were consistent with the findings of the MADIT II[14] in the population with ischemic cardiomyopathy. The SCD-HeFT trial was the first to show a benefit of the ICD in reducing total mortality in a population with nonischemic cardiomyopathy (see later). Based on the results of these 2 studies,[13,14] patients with ischemic or nonischemic cardiomyopathy with EF less than or equal to 35% and class II or III symptoms of HF and patients with ischemic cardiomyopathy with EF less than or equal to 30% and class I symptoms of HF have class I indications for prophylactic ICD implantation according to the 2008 published guidelines.[25]

## CLINICAL TRIALS IN PATIENTS WITH NONISCHEMIC CARDIOMYOPATHY

Despite its established value in reducing total mortality in patients with ischemic cardiomyopathy, showing a similar benefit of the ICD in nonischemic patients proved to be elusive for several years, until the results of the SCD-HeFT trial were announced. The following sections discuss the highlights from the largest randomized ICD trials in patients with nonischemic heart disease (see **Table 1**).

## AMIOVIRT

The Amiodarone versus Implantable Defibrillator Trial (AMIOVIRT)[16] enrolled 103 patients with nonischemic cardiomyopathy who had an EF less than or equal to 35%, asymptomatic nonsustained VT, and HF symptoms (New York Heart Association classes I through III) and randomized them to receiving an ICD (often with amiodarone) versus receiving amiodarone alone. Although the study was designed to enroll 438 patients, it was stopped prematurely because the mortality rates were similar between the 2 study groups (3-year survival was 88% in the amiodarone group vs 87% in the ICD group, P = .8). In this study, the quality of life was also similar in the 2 study groups.

## CAT

The Cardiomyopathy Trial (CAT)[17] enrolled 104 patients with nonischemic cardiomyopathy who were recently diagnosed (within 9 months) and EF less than or equal to 30% and randomized them into an ICD group vs a control group with no ICD. Here again, the trial showed no difference in cumulative survival between the 2 study groups. The 4-year survival was 86% in the ICD group vs 80% in the control group (P = .554). Thus, this trial as well as the AMIOVIRT[16] trial failed to provide evidence in favor of the use of a prophylactic ICD in the setting of nonischemic cardiomyopathy. The main limitations of these 2 trials,[16,17] however, included their very small size as well as the very low event rates noted in the ICD and control arms, which may have masked a survival benefit for the ICD arm.

## DEFINITE

The Defibrillators in Non-Ischemic Cardiomyopathy Treatment Evaluation (DEFINITE)[18] had a similar design as the AMIOVIRT and the CAT but included a larger number of patients. The DEFINITE enrolled 458 patients with nonischemic cardiomyopathy with an EF less than 36% and with ambient arrhythmia defined as frequent premature ventricular contractions (at least 10 premature beats) or runs of nonsustained VT (at least 1 run of nonsustained VT lasting 3 to 15 beats at a rate >120 beats per minute) on a 24-hour Holter monitor or on telemetry. The enrolled patients had HF symptoms (New York Heart Association classes I through III). However, patients in the New York Heart Association class IV were excluded. Although the DEFINITE showed an 80% relative reduction in the risk of SCD with the use of a prophylactic ICD (P = .006), it failed to reach statistical significance for the primary endpoint of total mortality, although there was a strong trend in this direction (2-year mortality of 7% in the ICD arm vs 14.1% in the control arm, P = .08). Here again, like with the AMIOVIRT[16] and the CAT,[17] the DEFINITE failed to provide a definitive answer as to the benefit of the ICD in reducing total mortality in patients with nonischemic cardiomyopathy. Once more, the event rate that was lower than expected in the overall population may have played a dramatic role in leading to this negative result.

## SCD-HeFT

As discussed earlier, the SCD-HeFT trial,[15] which is the largest of all primary prevention ICD trials, included about 50% of patients with nonischemic HF etiology. The overall study demonstrated a significant reduction in total mortality with the ICD. When the predetermined group of patients with nonischemic cardiomyopathy was examined, there was a 27% relative reduction in total mortality with the ICD compared with the control arm of the study (P = .06). As a result of the SCD-HeFT, patients with nonischemic cardiomyopathy and EF less than or equal to 35% and New York Heart Association class II or III

symptoms of HF now have a class 1 indication for the implantation of a prophylactic ICD.[25]

## CLINICAL TRIALS IN PATIENTS WITH HF WITH LOW EF AND WIDE QRS COMPLEX

The prophylactic use of device therapy based on the presence of left ventricular dysfunction as assessed by a significant reduction in EF took a new dimension over the past several years when the results of clinical trials of cardiac resynchronization therapy (CRT) became available.[19,20] The goal of the prophylactic use of ICD was no longer restricted to reducing total mortality in patients at risk but expanded beyond that to pacing the heart with the goal of affecting its remodeling process and improving HF outcomes. The proposed mechanism of the benefit from CRT is that biventricular pacing corrects at least partially the electric conduction abnormalities of the failing heart, manifested crudely on the surface electrocardiogram as a wide QRS complex (>120 millisecond), thus contributing to myocardial rejuvenation, which may translate into improved HF symptoms and possible decrease in total mortality. The following sections discuss highlights from few of the largest randomized CRT trials in patients with cardiomyopathy and HF (see **Table 1**).

## CARE-HF

The Cardiac Resynchronization–Heart Failure Study (CARE-HF)[19] examined the role of CRT in patients with advanced symptoms of HF (New York Heart Association classes III and IV), low EF (≤35%), and a wide QRS complex on the surface electrocardiogram (>120 millisecond). Patients with borderline QRS width (>120 millisecond but <150 millisecond) had also to meet criteria for cardiac mechanical dyssynchrony obtained from echocardiographic imaging. CARE-HF randomized 813 eligible patients to standard pharmacologic therapy alone versus pharmacologic therapy with CRT. Of note, in this study, CRT was achieved in most patients (98%) through the implantation of a pacing device without defibrillation backup. Aside from its benefits in reducing hospitalizations for HF exacerbation, CARE-HF showed a significant reduction in total mortality in the CRT group compared with the control group at a mean follow-up of 29.4 months (20% vs 30%, P<.002).

## COMPANION

Similarly to the CARE-HF trial, the Comparison of Medical Therapy, Pacing, and Defibrillation in

Heart Failure (COMPANION) trial[20] enrolled 1520 patients with advanced symptoms of HF (New York Heart Association classes III and IV), low EF (≤35%), and a wide QRS complex on the surface electrocardiogram (>120 millisecond). The COMPANION trial compared 3 strategies: (1) optimal pharmacologic therapy alone, (2) optimal pharmacologic therapy with CRT using a pacemaker device, and (3) optimal pharmacologic therapy with CRT using an ICD. Here again, both CRT arms showed a strong reduction in the primary endpoint of death or hospitalization for HF. When total mortality was examined, the patients who underwent CRT with ICD had a significant reduction in total mortality compared with those in the optimal pharmacologic therapy arm (relative reduction of 36%, $P = .003$), whereas the reduction in total mortality in the CRT with pacemaker arm failed to reach statistical significance (relative reduction of 25%, $P = .059$). Based on the results of the CARE-HF[19] and the COMPANION, patients with advanced symptoms of HF (New York Heart Association classes III and IV), low EF (≤35%), and wide QRS complex on surface electrocardiogram (>120 millisecond) have a class 1 indication for having a CRT prophylactic ICD implanted according to the published guidelines.[25]

## MADIT-CRT

The Multicenter Automatic Defibrillator Implantation Trial–Cardiac Resynchronization Therapy (MADIT-CRT)[21] was recently published. Unlike the CARE-HF[19] and the COMPANION,[20] the MADIT-CRT enrolled patients with mild to moderate HF symptoms (New York Heart Association HF classes I and II). The enrolled patients also had to have a low EF (≤30%) and a wide QRS complex (>130 millisecond). A total of 1820 eligible patients were enrolled and randomized to ICD alone versus ICD with CRT. The overall mortality in the MADIT-CRT was similar between the 2 study arms (7.3% in the ICD group vs 6.8% in the CRT defibrillator group, $P = .99$). The CRT group had a 34% reduction, however, in the primary endpoint of death or HF hospitalization ($P = .001$) as well as evidence of reverse remodeling by echocardiographic imaging. Because of these positive findings, the MADIT-CRT may become the basis for emerging indications for CRT in patients with mild symptoms of HF.

## VALUE AND SHORTCOMINGS OF EF IN THE ASSESSMENT OF THE RISK OF SCD

Although the EF has been shown to identify high-risk cardiomyopathy patients (EF≤35%) of both ischemic and nonischemic etiologies in whom ICD therapy confers survival benefit, there remains few shortcomings in the performance of this clinical risk assessment tool. First, although the ICD reduces the risk of death in cardiomyopathy patients, most such patients never experience therapy from their ICD in the form of electrical shock or antitachycardia pacing. It is estimated according to one study[31] that the rate of appropriate ICD therapy in a primary prevention population is on the order of 11 shocks per 100 patient-years. Also, according to the SCD-HeFT trial,[15] less than 25% of patients experience an appropriate therapy from their device. The implication of this experience is that many more patients receive ICD implantations than those who actually need it. Given the nontrivial perioperative and long-term risks of implanting these expensive devices, better clinical identifiers of the risk of lethal ventricular arrhythmias and better fine tuning of the indications for ICD implantations are needed. Second, not every ICD therapy is equivalent to a life saved. In fact, it is estimated that about every 2 to 4 shocks account for one life saved by the ICD. The main reason for this discrepancy stems from the fact that often ventricular arrhythmias are nonsustained (they terminate spontaneously without the need for electrical intervention from the ICD) or are hemodynamically tolerated, therefore not resulting in SCD. Here again, identifying clinical markers that can outperform the EF in identifying the need for ICD are needed but remain thus far elusive. Improving the specificity of device implantation, that is, implanting ICDs only in those patients who will use them, without sacrificing the sensitivity, that is, depriving patients who will have an SCA from the protection of an ICD, remains the Achilles tendon of risk stratification for SCD.

## SUMMARY

ICD therapy has been shown to decrease total mortality in patients with cardiomyopathy with low EF based on both ischemic and nonischemic etiologies except when the time of ICD implantation is immediately after a MI (within 40 days) or cardiac revascularization. As a result, low EF remains the main clinical parameter used in the determination of the need for ICD therapy for the primary prevention of SCD. Because of the shortcomings of EF as a sole risk stratifier for SCD, researchers continue to seek other clinical tools that may better guide the decision to implant ICDs. These tools include but are not limited to cardiac imaging techniques, such as cardiac magnetic resonance imaging, genetic markers, and others. Until the utility of such tools is confirmed and validated in clinical trials, low EF remains, according to the most recently published practice guidelines,[25] the only established criterion for ICD implantation for the primary prevention of SCD.

## REFERENCES

1. Myerburg RJ, Castellanos A. Cardiac arrest and sudden cardiac death. In: Braunwald E, editor. Heart disease: a textbook of cardiovascular medicine. 4th edition. Philadelphia: W.B. Saunders; 1992. p. 756–89.

2. Myerburg RJ, Kessler KM, Castellanos A. Sudden cardiac death. Structure, function, and time-dependence of risk. Circulation 1992;85(Suppl 1): I2–10.

3. Zhang ZJ, Croft JB, Giles WH, et al. Sudden cardiac death in the United States, 1989 to 1998. Circulation 2001;104:2158.

4. Buxton AE, Calkins H, Callans DJ, et al. ACC/AHA/HRS 2006 key data elements and definitions for electrophysiological studies and procedures: a report of the American College of Cardiology/American Heart Association Task Force on Clinical Data Standards (ACC/AHA/HRS Writing Committee to Develop Data Standards on Electrophysiology). Circulation 2006;114:2534.

5. Rea TD, Eisenberg MS, Becker LJ, et al. Temporal trends in sudden cardiac arrest: a 25-year emergency medical services perspective. Circulation 2003;107:2780.

6. Kuck KH, Cappato R, Siebels J, et al, CASH Investigators. Randomized comparison of antiarrhythmic drug therapy with implantable defibrillators in patients resuscitated from cardiac arrest. The Cardiac Arrest Study Hamburg (CASH). Circulation 2000;102:748.

7. Connolly SJ, Gent M, Roberts RS, et al. Canadian Implantable Defibrillator Study (CIDS): a randomized trial of the implantable cardioverter defibrillator against amiodarone. Circulation 2000;101:1297.

8. A comparison of antiarrhythmic-drug therapy with implantable defibrillators in patients resuscitated from near-fatal ventricular arrhythmias. The Antiarrhythmics versus Implantable Defibrillators (AVID) Investigators. N Engl J Med 1997;337:1576.

9. Bigger JT, Coronary Artery Bypass Graft (CABG) Patch Trial Investigators. Prophylactic use of implanted cardiac defibrillators in patients at high risk for ventricular arrhythmias after coronary-artery bypass graft surgery. N Engl J Med 1997;337: 1569–75.

10. Hohnloser SH, Kuck KH, Dorian P, et al. Prophylactic use of an implantable cardioverter-defibrillator after acute myocardial infarction. N Engl J Med 2004; 351:2481.

11. Steinbeck G, Andresen D, Seidl K, et al, IRIS Investigators. Defibrillator implantation early after myocardial infarction. N Engl J Med 2009;361:1427–36.

12. Moss AJ, Hall WJ, Cannom DS, et al, Multicenter Automatic Defibrillator Implantation Trial Investigators. Improved survival with an implanted defibrillator in patients with coronary disease at high risk for ventricular arrhythmia. N Engl J Med 1996;335: 1933.

13. Buxton AE, Lee KL, Fisher JD, et al. A randomized study of the prevention of sudden death in patients with coronary artery disease. Multicenter Unsustained Tachycardia Trial Investigators. N Engl J Med 1999;341:1882.

14. Moss AJ, Zareba W, Hall WJ, et al. Prophylactic implantation of a defibrillator in patients with myocardial infarction and reduced ejection fraction. N Engl J Med 2002;346:877.

15. Bardy GH, Lee KL, Mark DB, et al. Amiodarone or an implantable cardioverter-defibrillator for congestive heart failure. N Engl J Med 2005;352:225.

16. Strickberger SA, Hummel JD, Bartlett TG, et al. Amiodarone versus implantable cardioverter-defibrillator: randomized trial in patients with nonischemic dilated cardiomyopathy and asymptomatic nonsustained ventricular tachycardia—AMIOVIRT. J Am Coll Cardiol 2003;41:1707.

17. Bansch D, Antz M, Boczor S, et al. Primary prevention of sudden cardiac death in idiopathic dilated cardiomyopathy: the Cardiomyopathy Trial (CAT). Circulation 2002;105:1453.

18. Kadish A, Dyer A, Daubert JP, et al. Prophylactic defibrillator implantation in patients with nonischemic dilated cardiomyopathy. N Engl J Med 2004; 350:2151.

19. Cleland JG, Daubert JC, Erdmann E, et al. The effect of cardiac resynchronization on morbidity and mortality in heart failure. N Engl J Med 2005;352: 1539.

20. Bristow MR, Saxon LA, Boehmer J, et al. Cardiac-resynchronization therapy with or without an implantable defibrillator in advanced chronic heart failure. N Engl J Med 2004;350:2140.

21. Moss AJ, Hall WJ, Cannom DS, et al, MADIT-CRT Trial Investigators. Cardiac-resynchronization therapy for the prevention of heart-failure events. N Engl J Med 2009;361:1329–38.

22. Costantini O, Hohnloser SH, Kirk MM, et al, ABCD Trial Investigators. The ABCD (Alternans Before Cardioverter Defibrillator) Trial: strategies using T-wave alternans to improve efficiency of sudden cardiac death prevention. J Am Coll Cardiol 2009;53:471–9.

23. Chow T, Kereiakes DJ, Onufer J, et al, MASTER Trial Investigators. Does microvolt T-wave alternans testing predict ventricular tachyarrhythmias in patients with ischemic cardiomyopathy and prophylactic defibrillators? The MASTER (Microvolt T Wave

Alternans Testing for Risk Stratification of Post-Myocardial Infarction Patients) trial. J Am Coll Cardiol 2008;52:1607–15.

24. La Rovere MT, Bigger JT Jr, Marcus FI, et al. Baroreflex sensitivity and heart-rate variability in prediction of total cardiac mortality after myocardial infarction. ATRAMI (Autonomic Tone and Reflexes After Myocardial Infarction) Investigators. Lancet 1998;351:478–84.

25. Epstein AE, DiMarco JP, Ellenbogen KA, et al. ACC/AHA/HRS 2008 guidelines for device-based therapy of cardiac rhythm abnormalities: a report of the American College of Cardiology/American Heart Association Task Force on Practice Guidelines (Writing Committee to Revise the ACC/AHA/NASPE 2002 Guideline Update for Implantation of Cardiac Pacemakers and Antiarrhythmia Devices): developed in collaboration with the American Association for Thoracic Surgery and Society of Thoracic Surgeons. Circulation 2008;117:e350.

26. Berger CJ, Murabito JM, Evans JC, et al. Prognosis after first myocardial infarction. Comparison of Q-wave and non-Q-wave myocardial infarction in the Framingham Heart Study. JAMA 1992;268:1545.

27. A randomized trial of propranolol in patients with acute myocardial infarction. I. Mortality results. JAMA 1982;247:1707–14.

28. Domanski MJ, Exner DV, Borkowf CB, et al. Effect of angiotensin converting enzyme inhibition on sudden cardiac death in patients following acute myocardial infarction. J Am Coll Cardiol 1999;33:598.

29. Pfeffer MA, McMurray JJ, Velazquez EJ, et al. Valsartan, captopril, or both in myocardial infarction complicated by heart failure, left ventricular dysfunction, or both. N Engl J Med 2003;349:1893.

30. Solomon SD, Zelenkofske S, McMurray JJ, et al. Sudden death in patients with myocardial infarction and left ventricular dysfunction, heart failure, or both. N Engl J Med 2005;352:2581.

31. Otmani A, Trinquart L, Marijon E, et al, EVADEF investigators. Rates and predictors of appropriate implantable cardioverter-defibrillator therapy delivery: results from the EVADEF cohort study. Am Heart J 2009;158:230–7, e1.

# Secondary Prevention in Heart Failure

Melissa R. Robinson, MD, Andrew E. Epstein, MD, FHRS,
David J. Callans, MD, FHRS*

## KEYWORDS

- Sudden cardiac death • Secondary prevention
- Antiarrhythmic therapy • Defibrillator therapy

Despite advances in pharmacologic and interventional therapies for heart failure, sudden cardiac death (SCD) remains a common cause of death in patients with advanced structural heart disease. Recent statistics show that 5.7 million Americans have congestive heart failure and that nearly 300,000 die annually due to complications of heart failure.[1] For SCD survivors, prevention of recurrent events is paramount for survival. This article deals with the current therapy options for SCD survivors with congestive heart failure.

## DEFINITIONS

Sudden cardiac death is variably defined as death of cardiac origin occurring unexpectedly within 1 hour of the onset of new symptoms or death that is unwitnessed and unexpected, unless a specific noncardiac cause of death is confirmed.[2] Despite the simplicity of this definition, adjudication of SCD events in clinical study can be difficult.[3] Within the context of a trial, categorical terms such as arrhythmic death versus pump failure have generally been favored; however, it is often the case that multiple processes may have contributed to a "sudden" death event. Some investigators have advocated for a more descriptive classification scheme, including details surrounding death events in clinical trials, perhaps as a method to strengthen comparisons between various trials.[4,5]

As the definition of SCD remains controversial, the precise meaning behind the term "SCD survivor" can generate even more confusion. Within the context of this discussion and the trials discussed, SCD survivors have experienced sustained ventricular arrhythmias either requiring defibrillation or cardioversion in the case of symptomatic ventricular tachycardia (VT).

## PRESENTATION

SCD may be a first presentation of cardiomyopathy or occur in the course of established disease. Harbingers may include worsening heart failure, new or progressive angina, or syncope. Furthermore, sudden death in congestive heart failure may be bradycardic and not related to VT or ventricular fibrillation (VF). The following focuses on efforts to prevent SCD presumed to be caused by ventricular arrhythmias.

In the modern area of primary prevention, implantable cardioverter-defibrillators (ICDs) have become first-line therapy for patients with severe structural heart disease in the absence of a prior aborted SCD event (as discussed elsewhere in this issue). As such, aborted SCD in heart failure patients may also present as ICD therapy, either shocks or antitachycardia pacing. The assumption

Conflicts of interest: Melissa Robinson, MD. none. Andrew Epstein, MD: Advisor Relationships: St Jude Medical, Data and Safety Monitoring Board/Event Committee: Boston Scientific, Medtronic/Cryocath, St Jude Medical, Fellowship Support: Boston Scientific, Medtronic, St Jude Medical, Research Grants: Biotronik, Boston Scientific, Cameron Health, Medtronic, St Jude Medical, Honoraria: Biotronik, Boston Scientific, Medtronic, St Jude Medical. David J. Callans, MD: Fellowship Support: Boston Scientific, Medtronic, St Jude Medical, Honoraria: Biotronik, Boston Scientific, Medtronic, St Jude Medical.
Electrophysiology Section, Division of Cardiovascular Medicine, Hospital of the University of Pennsylvania, 9 Founders Pavilion, 3400 Spruce Street, Philadelphia, PA 19104, USA
* Corresponding author.
E-mail address: david.callans@uphs.upenn.edu

Heart Failure Clin 7 (2011) 185–194
doi:10.1016/j.hfc.2010.12.002
1551-7136/11/$ – see front matter © 2011 Elsevier Inc. All rights reserved.

that ICD therapy is equivalent to an aborted sudden death episode has been a source of significant controversy in the literature, especially in the era of antitachycardia pacing.[6] Some episodes of sustained VT are clearly associated with minimal or no symptoms. In addition, other episodes, even VF or polymorphic VT, may have been self-limited, but may trigger ICD therapy before they can terminate.

The equivalence of ICD therapy, even for documented ventricular arrhythmias, with an aborted SCD episode was challenged by an elegant secondary analysis by Ellenbogen and colleagues of the Defibrillators in Nonischemic Cardiomyopathy Treatment Evaluation (DEFINITE) study.[7,8] In this primary prophylaxis trial, SCD was dramatically reduced with ICD therapy (hazard ratio 0.20, P = .006) in nonischemic patients. Of interest, however, the number of appropriate ICD shocks far outweighed the number of sudden death episodes in the control arm, although the risk for life-threatening ventricular arrhythmia would be assumed to be equal between these groups. When syncopal episodes and sudden death in the control group were combined, this was equivalent to the ICD shock rate in the defibrillator arm. These data suggest that many ventricular arrhythmias that may even cause syncope can be long enough to trigger ICD detection and lead to therapy, and yet may have stopped on their own.[8] Supraventricular tachycardias, especially atrial fibrillation with rapid ventricular rates, are also common in the heart failure population, and may lead to ICD therapy. Device programming, especially antitachycardia pacing, is quite variable in clinical practice and may result in differing patient groups being labeled as sudden death survivors.

In addition to those with syncope or aborted SCD discussed here, patients who present with tolerated VT may represent a unique subset, albeit one with still significant residual risk of sudden death. Early studies have examined the prognostic differences between tolerated VT and sudden death, and the results are perhaps not surprising. In a study by Saxon and colleagues,[9] comparing survival in patients with cardiac arrest versus tolerated VT, the 4-year survival from sudden death and total mortality was 59% ± 11% versus 87% ± 6% and 45% ± 10% versus 67% ± 8%, respectively (P<.05 for both comparisons). This and other early studies identified predictors for mortality such as presentation with VT/VF early after myocardial infarction, severe left ventricular dysfunction, and symptomatic heart failure as additional prognosticators.[10,11] Although these studies were conducted in an era of markedly

different treatment strategies for congestive heart failure, they nonetheless underscore the significant mortality risk in patients who present even with tolerated ventricular arrhythmias. As such, these patients should be considered under the banner of secondary prophylaxis as well.[12]

## ANTIARRHYTHMIC THERAPY

The enthusiasm for antiarrhythmic therapy for patients with ventricular arrhythmias in the setting of structural heart disease has diminished dramatically in the last 2 decades. The initial wave of this disenchantment was provided by primary prevention trials demonstrating that membrane active agents dramatically increased the risk of total mortality.[13,14] Although this was considered at the time to be agent specific, or potentially ameliorated by the concurrent use of β-blockers, more recent trials in patients with atrial and ventricular arrhythmias have increased the level of concern.[15,16] More importantly, secondary prevention trials with direct comparison of ICD and pharmacologic therapy have consistently demonstrated that ICD therapy is superior (see later discussion). There is a general consensus that treatment with amiodarone may be appropriate for patients who are too ill to qualify for or refuse defibrillator implantation. This conventional wisdom was questioned slightly by the finding that amiodarone did not have a protective effect compared with placebo in the Sudden Cardiac Death in Heart Failure Trial (SCD-HeFT).[17]

Today, the more common use of antiarrhythmic therapy is to prevent ICD shocks. There are some data demonstrating that membrane active agents provide benefit, even when added to background optimal pharmacologic therapy for heart failure. Pacifico and colleagues[18] studied the effect of sotalol in patients who had previously received ICD shock in a placebo-controlled study. There were 4 deaths in the sotalol group, compared with 7 in the control group (P not significant). Treatment with sotalol significantly reduced recurrent ICD shocks (1.43 ± 3.53 shocks per year vs 3.89 ± 10.65 in the placebo group; P = .008); this effect did not differ significantly based on left ventricular ejection fraction (LVEF) (stratified at 30%). In the Optimal Pharmacologic Therapy in Cardioverter Defibrillator Patients (OPTIC) Trial, 412 patients with recent ICD implantation (within 21 days, for indications similar to those in the Antiarrhythmics vs Implantable Defibrillators [AVID] trial)[19] were randomized to β-blocker therapy alone, sotalol alone, or amiodarone plus β-blocker. Over 1 year of follow-up, shocks occurred in 38.5% of patients in the β-blocker treatment group;

amiodarone reduced the risk for ICD shocks compared with both β-blocker alone and sotalol (hazard ratio [HR] 0.44, *P* = .001). There was a trend for sotalol to reduce shocks compared with β-blocker alone (HR 0.61, *P* = .055). Adverse effects resulting in drug discontinuation were seen in 23.5% of patients treated with sotalol, 18.2% with amiodarone, and 5.3% with β-blockers.[20]

Although not approved for use in the treatment of ventricular arrhythmias, dronedarone significantly reduced the risk of arrhythmic death in the ATHENA (A Trial With Dronedarone to Prevent Hospitalization or Death in Patients With Atrial Fibrillation) study (HR 0.55, *P* = .01) in patients with atrial fibrillation and at least one risk factor for cardiac death versus placebo.[21] These results must be balanced with the data from the ANDROMEDA (European Trial of Dronedarone in Moderate to Severe Congestive Heart Failure) study, which demonstrated an increase in all-cause mortality in patients with severe heart failure who were prophylactically treated with dronedarone versus placebo (HR 2.13, *P* = .03).[22] Taken together, antiarrhythmic drug therapy for secondary prophylaxis of SCD has proved to be disappointing.

## DEFIBRILLATOR THERAPY

The original description of ICD use in a human patient was for recurrent SCD.[23] Indeed, to receive one, survival of not one but two cardiac arrests was required. As the therapy matured and physician demand increased, survival of a single sudden death event became an acceptable indication for implantation. It is remarkable that, in the context of modern acceptance and regulatory approval of devices and drugs, no randomized trial was done for over a decade, and then only with great controversy.[24–26]

### Early Trials

In contrast to its widespread acceptance into clinical practice today, the implantable ICD was highly controversial at the time of its first clinical description. Despite the bleak prognosis faced by survivors of cardiac arrest, the ICD was criticized as bringing pain and suffering without reliable prolongation of life.[27] The now universal acceptance that an implantable ICD can detect and treat a life-threatening ventricular arrhythmia was not immediately appreciated. As implantation techniques improved, abolishing the necessity of a thoracotomy, the application of this technology to a wider patient population became inevitable.[28] This expansion was largely driven by numerous nonrandomized reports suggesting improved

survival with ICD therapy for secondary prophylaxis.[29–32]

### Secondary Prevention Trials

Brave clinical investigators embarked on several randomized trials in an effort to assess the true benefit of ICD therapy in the sudden cardiac arrest survivor. There are 4 trials that provide the bulk of the evidence base supporting ICD therapy for secondary prevention: the AVID trial mentioned previously, the Canadian Implantable Defibrillator Study (CIDS), and the Cardiac Arrest Study Hamburg (CASH) (**Table 1**), which were preceded by a smaller Dutch study. As each study enrolled patients who had survived a cardiac arrest or potentially fatal ventricular arrhythmia, a control group receiving no additional therapy was deemed unethical. Therefore, patients enrolled in the ICD arms of these trials were universally compared with antiarrhythmic therapy.

### The Dutch study

The first, albeit smallest, of the randomized trials to evaluate ICD therapy in SCD was the Dutch study.[33] Conceived in 1989, this trial randomized 60 cardiac arrest survivors with remote myocardial infarctions to ICD implantation or conventional therapy, consisting of the antiarrhythmic therapy guided by programmed electrical stimulation. Of the 29 patients who received an ICD, there were only 4 deaths (13%) versus 11 (35%) in the antiarrhythmic arm by an intention to treat analysis over a mean follow-up of 27 months. Twenty of 31 patients randomized to drug therapy continued to have inducible arrhythmias and therefore went on to further therapy (map-guided VT surgery in 6 patients, of whom 1 died, 1 had cardiac transplantation, and 1 had an ICD implantation) or ICD implantation in 14 patients, 3 of whom died during follow-up. Of the remaining 11 who received drug therapy alone, 2 died in the hospital before being retested, 5 subsequently died, and 1 survived cardiac arrest. Therefore, 16 patients who initially received conventional drugs ended up with an ICD, and 3 subsequently died to give a mortality of 11 (35%) in the drug group versus 13% for the ICD group.

Critics of this trial noted its small numbers, therefore limiting the statistical significance of even its impressive mortality differences, and the large crossover rate to ICD. In addition, class I agents or sotalol were used in all but 2 patients in the drug therapy arm. Though appropriate for the time of the study, the limited use of amiodarone may have diminished the possible efficacy of the antiarrhythmic arm.[34] Despite this, the Dutch study provided the first randomized data

**Table 1**
**Major clinical trials of defibrillator therapy for secondary prevention of sudden cardiac death**

|  | AVID[19] | CASH[39] | CIDS[37] |
|---|---|---|---|
| N = | 1016 | 288[a] | 659 |
| Study design | Multicenter RCT of amiodarone or sotalol vs ICD | Multicenter RCT of amiodarone or metoprolol vs ICD[a] | Multicenter RCT of amiodarone vs ICD |
| Eligibility | Near-fatal VT/VF, sustained VT with syncope or sustained VT with LVEF ≤0.40 and symptoms | Resuscitated cardiac arrest from VT/VF | VF, out-of-hospital defibrillation, symptomatic VT or syncope with VT induced at EPS |
| Male | 79% | 80% | 85% |
| LVEF (%) | 32 ± 13 | 45 ± 18 | 34 ± 14 |
| CAD | 82% | 75% | 83% |
| NYHA class ≥III | 9% | 19% | 11% |
| Mean follow-up (mo) | 18.2 | 57 | 35.4 |
| Deaths (rate) |  |  |  |
| Amiodarone | 122 (16.5%) | 84 (9.3%)[a] | 98 (10.2%) |
| ICD | 80 (10%) | 36 (7.7%) | 83 (8.3%) |
| Sudden arrhythmic deaths (rate) |  |  |  |
| Amiodarone | 55 (7.4%) | 62 (6.9%)[a] | 43 (4.5%) |
| ICD | 24 (3%) | 13 (2.8%) | 30 (3.0%) |
| Relative risk of death (CI) | 0.66 (0.51, 0.85) | 0.82 (0.60, 1.11) | 0.85 (0.67, 1.10) |

*Abbreviations:* AVID, Antiarrhythmics Versus Implantable Defibrillator study; CAD, coronary artery disease; CASH, Cardiac Arrest Study Hamburg; CIDS, Canadian Implantable Defibrillator Study; CA, cardiac arrest; CI, 95% confidence interval; EPS, electrophysiologic study; ICD, implantable cardioverter-defibrillator; LVEF, left ventricular ejection fraction; NYHA, New York Heart Association; RCT, randomized controlled trial; VF, ventricular fibrillation; VT, ventricular tachycardia.

[a] Includes ICD, Amiodarone, and Metoprolol arms only. Excludes propafenone arm. Outcomes are for ICD versus Combined Amiodarone/Metoprolol group.

suggesting a significant mortality benefit in cardiac arrest survivors with structural heart disease. This study was followed by the publication of the largest and most influential secondary prophylaxis trial, AVID.

## AVID (Antiarrhythmics Vs Implantable Defibrillators trial)

The AVID trial was the largest and the first of the 3 main studies.[19] The trial was designed as a randomized comparison of ICD therapy versus a class III antiarrhythmic in patients with an either prior cardiac arrest or symptomatic VT and an ejection fraction of 40% or less. A total of 1013 patients were randomized between 1993 and 1997. The mean ejection fraction was 31% ± 13%, with 80% of patients having a history of coronary artery disease and two-thirds a history of myocardial infarction. Slightly over half of the patients had a history of congestive heart failure,

with most of these being New York Heart Association functional class I or II.

The vast majority of patients in the antiarrhythmic arm received amiodarone, with only 3% discharged from the index hospitalization on sotalol. The trial was stopped prematurely by the Data Safety and Monitoring Board when analysis indicated that survival benefit afforded by ICDs exceeded the statistical boundary for early termination. After a mean follow-up of 18 ± 12 months, mortality was 15.8% in the ICD group and 24% in the antiarrhythmic group (P<.02), corresponding to a 27% relative reduction in mortality at 2 years. This benefit was shown despite a large crossover from the amiodarone group to ICD of 18.4%, perhaps masking an even more significant benefit to ICD therapy. Approximately one-third of the patients in the ICD group were taking antiarrhythmics at the termination of the study as well.

Subsequent subgroup analysis evaluated the influence of LVEF on ICD survival benefit, with interesting results. Despite the overall benefit from ICD implantation in this population, those patients with LVEF of 35% or greater did not derive a survival benefit from implantation of a defibrillator at 1- or 2-year follow-up.[35] The reasons for this finding in a secondary prophylaxis cohort are not entirely clear, but do not seem to be due to cross-over, which was relatively low in patients with higher ejection fractions.

The AVID trial has been criticized for a few important reasons. Of importance, the use of β-blockers in the ICD and antiarrhythmic arms was significantly different (39.4% vs 10.1% at 24 months) and certainly lower than the current standard of care for heart failure patients. In addition, the reduction in mortality afforded by the ICD amounted to only an additional 2.7-month increase in life expectancy at 3 years, and this came at a marginal cost efficacy of $66,677 per life-year saved.[36] However, this sort of analysis cannot account for the artificially short follow-up of a clinical trial, especially one that is terminated early. ICD therapy can be expected to provide continued benefit over the lifetime of the device.

### CIDS (Canadian Implantable Defibrillator Study)
The CIDS enrolled patients with not only cardiac arrest or symptomatic ventricular arrhythmias, but also included patients with structural heart disease and unexplained syncope with subsequently documented or inducible ventricular arrhythmias.[37] A total of 659 patients were enrolled between 1990 and 1997, randomized to either ICD or amiodarone. The patient population was similar to AVID, with the majority being males having coronary artery disease and a mean LVEF of 34%. Over a mean follow-up of 3 years, there were 98 deaths in the amiodarone group compared with 83 in the ICD group, leading to an all-cause annual mortality rate of 10.2% versus 8.3% (P = .14) and a total mortality rate of 27% versus 23.3%. However, the result was not statistically significant (P = .07), due to the smaller trial size and limited power. One criticism of this study was the relatively higher use of β-blockers in the ICD group (42% vs 17%), which could bias results toward false protection of ICDs as was also seen in AVID. Nonetheless, the results were consistent with what was already shown in AVID and later confirmed by the CASH study.

One particular strength of the CIDS trial lies in the long-term follow-up data collected from one of the enrolling centers, reported separately as a substudy. In these 120 patients followed for a mean of 5.6 ± 2.6 years, mortality in the ICD group was 27% compared with 47% in the amiodarone group (P = .0213).[38] This benefit also

appeared to be increasing over time. The presence of coronary artery disease was also found to increase the risk of death.

### CASH (Cardiac Arrest Study Hamburg)
The CASH trial randomized patients with symptomatic ventricular arrhythmias to either ICD therapy, metoprolol, amiodarone, or propafenone.[39] Original enrollment began in 1987; however, interim analysis showed an increased mortality in the propafenone arm and therefore this therapy was discontinued in 1992. The study concluded in 1995 after a full 2-year follow-up in each of the 288 patients assigned to the nonpropafenone groups. All patients in CASH had survived cardiac arrest with documented VT or VF, with 90% having structural heart disease. Coronary artery disease accounted for three-quarters of the substrate.

Compared with the combined metoprolol and amiodarone groups, ICD implantation was associated with a nonsignificant 23% reduction in mortality (P = .08) over a mean follow-up of 57 ± 34 months. Overall mortality was 36.4% (95% confidence interval [CI] 26.9%–46.6%) in the ICD group and 44.4% (95% CI 37.2%–51.8%) in the combined metoprolol/amiodarone group. Perhaps as a testimony to improving therapy for congestive heart failure and coronary artery disease overall, the 20% 2-year all-cause mortality rate seen in the "control" groups was far lower than the 40% mortality rate the investigators used to calculate the original trial sample size; therefore, the trial ended up underpowered, to show a potentially significant benefit in the ICD arm.

Given their similarities, the AVID, CIDS, and CASH trials led to a well-executed meta-analysis, which added to the enthusiasm for secondary prophylaxis ICD use.[40] Combining the AVID, CASH, and amiodarone/ICD arms of CIDS, the meta-analysis looked at event rates in 1866 patients. The HR for total mortality with an ICD versus amiodarone therapy was 0.73 (95% CI 0.60–0.87, P<.0001). Again, an incremental separation in the risk for death occurred, with an estimated prolongation of life of 2.1 months at 3 years in the ICD arm over the amiodarone group, and 4.4 months at 6 years. This nonlinear improvement over time has been shown in a subsequent analysis, including both secondary and primary prophylaxis trials, and has given weight to the evidence that ICD therapy is life preserving.[41]

AVID, CIDS, and CASH provided the initial clinical trial evidence that advocated the use of ICDs for prevention of sudden death. The consistent benefit observed with ICD therapy in the 3 trials was an important milestone in the continued development of the ICD, and validated what many electrophysiologists were already practicing. The argument then changed from whether or not ICD therapy prolonged life to by how much and in whom.[42] The next phase of evidence-based practice related to ICD therapy was introduced with the prophylactic ICD trials over the next decade.

## Other Trials

Further nonrandomized trials have strengthened the body of evidence supporting the use of ICD therapy for secondary prophylaxis of SCD.

### Swiss study
In a single-center study using programmed stimulation to predict response to antiarrhythmic therapy, ICDs were found to offer a mortality benefit over amiodarone therapy.[43] Eighty-four patients with VT in the setting of healed myocardial infarction underwent amiodarone loading after baseline programmed stimulation. A second electrophysiologic study was then performed and patients were assigned therapy based on the results of this test. Patients in whom VT was no longer inducible or if the index VT slowed and became hemodynamically stable ("amiodarone predicted responders," n = 43) received amiodarone; nonresponders (n = 41) received ICD therapy. Over a mean follow-up period of 63 ± 30 months, total mortality was greater in the amiodarone group than in the ICD group (42 vs 15%, $P$ = .02).

### AVID registry
In a similar manner, a retrospective multivariable analysis of the entire AVID registry (3559 patients originally screened for AVID, but not randomized) demonstrated that prognosis was determined predominantly by the severity of structural heart disease and the presence of heart failure. Overall in the registry, ICD therapy was protective (HR, 0.51; $P$<.001).[44] This effect was independent of the severity of the original arrhythmia presentation. The presenting ventricular arrhythmia in the AVID Registry was classified according to type, with a category for reversible or transient causes of ventricular arrhythmia. These arrhythmias are associated with acute infarction, electrolyte imbalance, illicit drug use, or antiarrhythmic drug reaction. Of interest, 2-year survival rates in this group were similar to those in the total cohort,[45] despite a higher use of β-blockers and revascularization in this cohort, and may have been worsened by a relatively lower ICD implantation rate.

## Are Shocks Harmful?

Despite the fact that ICDs are designed to deliver therapy for ventricular arrhythmias and have been shown to improve survival, the therapy itself has been associated with a negative impact on survival. Daubert and colleagues[46] observed in the Multicenter Automatic Implantable Defibrillator Implantation Trial II (MADIT-II) that the delivery of inappropriate shocks constituted 31.2% of all shock episodes, and importantly, patients with inappropriate shocks had a greater likelihood of death in follow-up (HR 2.29, $P$ = .025). Further concern for the prognostic importance of ICD shocks in patients with heart failure was provided by Poole and colleagues[47] in the examination of both appropriate and inappropriate shocks in the SCD-HeFT trial. Over a median follow-up of 46 months, 33.2% of patients received at least one ICD shock. After adjustment for baseline variables, the delivery of appropriate compared with no shocks was associated with an increased risk of death from all causes (HR 5.68, $P$<.001). As ventricular arrhythmias may represent a "final common pathway" of nonarrhythmic death (VF in the setting of overwhelming ischemia or terminal heart failure), a separate analysis was performed in patients who survived at least 24 hours after appropriate ICD shock; the increased risk of death remained in this subset (HR 2.99, $P$<.001). The delivery of inappropriate as compared with no inappropriate shocks was associated with an increased risk of death (HR 1.98, $P$ = .002), and for patients who received both appropriate and inappropriate shocks, the HR for all-cause mortality was a remarkable 11.27 ($P$<.001). Progressive heart failure was the most common cause of death in patients who received ICD shocks.

In view of these risks, future research should be directed to decrease the risk of recurrent episodes: secondary prophylaxis within the previously implanted ICD population. One such strategy is catheter ablation for VT (also discussed in another article elsewhere in this issue). The Substrate Mapping and Ablation in Sinus Rhythm to Halt Ventricular Tachycardia (SMASH VT) trial showed that in patients undergoing ICD implantation for secondary prevention (resuscitated VT or VF), preemptory VT ablation decreased the risk of receiving an appropriate shock by 65% ($P$ = .007).[48] Similar results were observed in the recently published Ventricular Tachycardia Ablation in Addition to Implantable Defibrillators in Coronary Heart Disease (VTACH) trial that enrolled only patients with stable VT.[49] At 2-year follow-up, the VT recurrence rate was decreased from 71% to 53% (HR 0.61, $P$ = .045) and VT storm rate from 30% to 25% (HR 0.73, $P$ = .395) with catheter ablation. Although ablation cannot substitute for ICD implantation, its use as adjunctive therapy may afford patients further improvement in survival over and above that provided by an ICD alone by decreasing the occurrence of shocks.

## Device Management After Therapy

Another important aspect of secondary prophylaxis involves management of a defibrillator event in a primary or secondary prophylaxis device patient. As a primary evaluation, new ischemia and electrolyte disturbances should be addressed. Neurohormonal blockade should also be maximized. Antiarrhythmic drugs have been discussed earlier and remain the most common treatment. In addition, device programming and device selection are now reviewed.

Device programming can have a significant impact on the number and type of defibrillator interventions. In an early safety and feasibility study, Wathen and colleagues[50] showed antitachycardia pacing (ATP) to be safe and effective for terminating fast VT (188–250 bpm) in patients with coronary artery disease. The follow-up, randomized trial entitled PainFREE Rx II compared this standardized empirical ATP strategy for fast VT with shock. These investigators also employed a longer detection time (18/24 intervals) than many prior studies. About half of the patients were secondary prophylaxis patients. Although mortality was unchanged between the 2 strategies, in the one-third of ventricular arrhythmia events falling in the fast VT zone, shocks were needed 28% of the time in the ATP group versus 64% in the shock-only arm.[51] This empiric programming strategy has been shown to be noninferior to physician-tailored therapy and to extend to primary prophylaxis patients as well.[52,53]

Although the majority of patients in the ICD benefit studies were implanted with single-chamber devices, the bulk of devices implanted in clinical practice have been dual chamber, even in the absence of a current bradycardic pacing indication. The effect of dual-chamber pacing on outcome in defibrillator patients was evaluated in the Dual Chamber and VVI Implantable Defibrillator (DAVID) trial.[54] New dual-chamber ICD patients randomized to DDDR 70 bpm (resulting in about 60% right ventricular [RV] pacing) versus VVI back-up pacing at 40 bpm had an HR of 1.61 (CI, 1.06–2.44; $P<03$) for the combined end point of death or hospitalization for new or worsened heart failure at 12 months. Both the DAVID II and Intrinsic RV trials showed that the avoidance of RV pacing through atrial-based pacing or prolonging atrioventricular delays mediates these differences.[55,56]

The role of cardiac resynchronization therapy (CRT) specifically for secondary prevention in heart failure patients remains uncertain. Despite demonstrating significant improvements in heart failure symptoms and death, CRT has not been convincingly shown to decrease ventricular arrhythmias or ICD interventions. In the Multi-center InSync Randomized Clinical Evaluation (MIRACLE) ICD trial, patients with symptomatic heart failure, wide QRS and a then contemporary indication for ICD implantation, symptomatic ventricular arrhythmias or inducibility at electrophysiologic study, were randomized to an ICD with CRT off (control) versus an ICD with CRT turned on.[57] There was no overall survival difference in the study; however, the primary end points of quality of life score, 6-minute walk, and functional class were all improved. Although the number of patients experiencing appropriate ICD events was not different between the CRT and control groups, the number of events experienced by these patients was markedly higher in the controls over the 6-month trial period (155 shocks in 26 patients in the control group vs 88 shocks in 24 patients in the CRT arm; 618 ATP events in 32 controls vs 219 in 32 CRT patients). This finding has not, however, been reproducible in other studies.[58]

## Guidelines

The most recent guidelines for the implantation of cardiac devices specifically define indications for secondary prophylaxis devices.[59] Class 1 indications for ICD implantation include individuals who are survivors of cardiac arrest due to VF or hemodynamically unstable sustained VT after evaluation to define the cause of the event and to exclude completely reversible causes. In addition, ICD therapy is indicated with patients with structural heart disease and spontaneous sustained VT whether hemodynamically stable or unstable. The further challenge for the future is to increase adherence to guidelines, as ICD implantation in the community is not always provided.[60]

## SUMMARY

Patients with heart failure remain at risk for death due to arrhythmic and other cardiac causes in addition to comorbidities. Clinical trials have clearly shown that for those fortunate enough to have been resuscitated from a sustained life-threatening ventricular arrhythmia, device implantation improved survival. Although antiarrhythmic therapy has been disappointing in this population, there may be a role for antiarrhythmics in preventing recurrent ventricular arrhythmias after ICD implantation. Of importance, for those with heart failure and a wide QRS the benefit of ICD implantation is closely related to the application of biventricular pacing, which itself has a salutary benefit in decreasing mortality. Despite the clear benefits of ICD therapy in patients with heart failure, not only does the general population remain underserved,[61] but so also do special populations including women and minorities.[62,63] Further research is necessary to more precisely define individuals who will and will not benefit from ICD therapy, focusing on not only special populations (the elderly and those with renal failure) but also those who have been underserved in the past (women and minorities).

## REFERENCES

1. American Heart Association. Heart disease and stroke statistics. 2009. Available at: http://circ.ahajournals.org/cgi/content/full/119/3/480. Accessed January 23, 2009.

2. Pratt CM, Greenway PS, Schoenfeld MH, et al. Exploration of the precision of classifying sudden cardiac death. Implications for the interpretation of clinical trials. Circulation 1996;93(3):519–24.

3. Hinkle LE Jr, Thaler HT. Clinical classification of cardiac deaths. Circulation 1982;65(3):457–64.

4. Epstein AE, Carlson MD, Fogoros RN, et al. Classification of death in antiarrhythmia trials. J Am Coll Cardiol 1996;27(2):433–42.

5. Boehmer JP, Carlson MD, De Marco T, et al. Adjudication of mortality events in a heart failure-arrhythmia trial by a multiparameter descriptive method: comparison with methods used in heart failure trials and methods used in arrhythmia trials. J Interv Card Electrophysiol 2008;23(2):101–10.

6. Kim SG, Fogoros RN, Furman S, et al. Standardized reporting of ICD patient outcome: the report of a North American Society of Pacing and Electrophysiology Policy Conference, February 9–10, 1993. Pacing Clin Electrophysiol 1993;16(7 Pt 1):1358–62.

7. Kadish A, Dyer A, Daubert JP, et al. Prophylactic defibrillator implantation in patients with nonischemic dilated cardiomyopathy. N Engl J Med 2004; 350(21):2151–8.

8. Ellenbogen KA, Levine JH, Berger RD, et al. Are implantable cardioverter defibrillator shocks a surrogate for sudden cardiac death in patients with nonischemic cardiomyopathy? Circulation 2006;113(6):776–82.

9. Saxon LA, Uretz EF, Denes P. Significance of the clinical presentation in ventricular tachycardia/fibrillation. Am Heart J 1989;118(4):695–701.

10. Brugada P, Talajic M, Smeets J, et al. The value of the clinical history to assess prognosis of patients with ventricular tachycardia or ventricular fibrillation after myocardial infarction. Eur Heart J 1989;10(8):747–52.

11. Willems AR, Tijssen JG, van Capelle FJ, et al. Determinants of prognosis in symptomatic ventricular tachycardia or ventricular fibrillation late after myocardial infarction. The Dutch Ventricular Tachycardia Study Group of the Interuniversity Cardiology Institute of The Netherlands. J Am Coll Cardiol 1990; 16(3):521–30.

12. Callans DJ. Patients with hemodynamically tolerated ventricular tachycardia require implantable cardioverter defibrillators. Circulation 2007;116(10):1196–203.

13. Echt DS, Liebson PR, Mitchell LB, et al. Mortality and morbidity in patients receiving encainide, flecainide, or placebo. The Cardiac Arrhythmia Suppression Trial. N Engl J Med 1991;324(12):781–8.

14. Waldo AL, Camm AJ, deRuyter H, et al. Effect of d-sotalol on mortality in patients with left ventricular dysfunction after recent and remote myocardial infarction. The SWORD Investigators. Survival With Oral d-Sotalol. Lancet 1996;348(9019):7–12.

15. Corley SD, Epstein AE, DiMarco JP, et al. Relationships between sinus rhythm, treatment, and survival in the Atrial Fibrillation Follow-Up Investigation of Rhythm Management (AFFIRM) Study. Circulation 2004;109(12):1509–13.

16. Wyse DG, Waldo AL, DiMarco JP, et al. A comparison of rate control and rhythm control in patients with atrial fibrillation. N Engl J Med 2002; 347(23):1825–33.

17. Bardy GH, Lee KL, Mark DB, et al. Amiodarone or an implantable cardioverter-defibrillator for congestive heart failure. N Engl J Med 2005;352(3):225–37.

18. Pacifico A, Hohnloser SH, Williams JH, et al. Prevention of implantable-defibrillator shocks by treatment with sotalol. d,l-Sotalol Implantable Cardioverter-Defibrillator Study Group. N Engl J Med 1999; 340(24):1855–62.

19. A comparison of antiarrhythmic-drug therapy with implantable defibrillators in patients resuscitated from near-fatal ventricular arrhythmias. The Antiarrhythmics versus Implantable Defibrillators (AVID) Investigators. N Engl J Med 1997;337(22):1576–83.

20. Connolly SJ, Dorian P, Roberts RS, et al. Comparison of beta-blockers, amiodarone plus beta-blockers, or sotalol for prevention of shocks from implantable cardioverter defibrillators: the OPTIC Study: a randomized trial. JAMA 2006;295(2):165–71.

21. Hohnloser SH, Crijns HJ, van Eickels M, et al. Effect of dronedarone on cardiovascular events in atrial fibrillation. N Engl J Med 2009;360(7):668–78.

22. Kober L, Torp-Pedersen C, McMurray JJ, et al. Increased mortality after dronedarone therapy for severe heart failure. N Engl J Med 2008;358(25):2678–87.

23. Mirowski M, Reid PR, Mower MM, et al. Termination of malignant ventricular arrhythmias with an

implanted automatic defibrillator in human beings. N Engl J Med 1980;303(6):322–4.

24. Epstein AE. AVID necessity. Pacing Clin Electrophysiol 1993;16(9):1773–5.

25. Mower MM. AVID necessity. Pacing Clin Electrophysiol 1994;17(2):258–60, author reply 262–56.

26. Singer I. AVID necessity. Pacing Clin Electrophysiol 1994;17(2):260–2, author reply 262–6.

27. Lown B, Axelrod P. Implanted standby defibrillators. Circulation 1972;46(4):637–9.

28. Lehmann MH, Steinman RT, Schuger CD, et al. The automatic implantable cardioverter defibrillator as antiarrhythmic treatment modality of choice for survivors of cardiac arrest unrelated to acute myocardial infarction. Am J Cardiol 1988;62(10 Pt 1):803–5.

29. Mirowski M, Reid PR, Winkle RA, et al. Mortality in patients with implanted automatic defibrillators. Ann Intern Med 1983;98(5 Pt 1):585–8.

30. Winkle RA, Mead RH, Ruder MA, et al. Long-term outcome with the automatic implantable cardioverter-defibrillator. J Am Coll Cardiol 1989;13(6):1353–61.

31. Palatianos GM, Thurer RJ, Cooper DK, et al. The implantable cardioverter-defibrillator: clinical results. Pacing Clin Electrophysiol 1991;14(2 Pt 2):297–301.

32. Saksena S, Poczobutt-Johanos M, Castle LW, et al. Long-term multicenter experience with a second-generation implantable pacemaker-defibrillator in patients with malignant ventricular tachyarrhythmias. The Guardian Multicenter Investigators Group. J Am Coll Cardiol 1992;19(3):490–9.

33. Wever EF, Hauer RN, van Capelle FL, et al. Randomized study of implantable defibrillator as first-choice therapy versus conventional strategy in postinfarct sudden death survivors. Circulation 1995;91(8):2195–203.

34. Zipes DP. Are implantable cardioverter-defibrillators better than conventional antiarrhythmic drugs for survivors of cardiac arrest? Circulation 1995;91(8):2115–7.

35. Domanski MJ, Sakseena S, Epstein AE, et al. Relative effectiveness of the implantable cardioverter-defibrillator and antiarrhythmic drugs in patients with varying degrees of left ventricular dysfunction who have survived malignant ventricular arrhythmias. AVID Investigators. Antiarrhythmics Versus Implantable Defibrillators. J Am Coll Cardiol 1999;34(4):1090–5.

36. Larsen G, Hallstrom A, McAnulty J, et al. Cost-effectiveness of the implantable cardioverter-defibrillator versus antiarrhythmic drugs in survivors of serious ventricular tachyarrhythmias: results of the Antiarrhythmics Versus Implantable Defibrillators (AVID) economic analysis substudy. Circulation 2002;105(17):2049–57.

37. Connolly SJ, Gent M, Roberts RS, et al. Canadian implantable defibrillator study (CIDS): a randomized trial of the implantable cardioverter defibrillator against amiodarone. Circulation 2000;101(11):1297–302.

38. Bokhari F, Newman D, Greene M, et al. Long-term comparison of the implantable cardioverter defibrillator versus amiodarone: eleven-year follow-up of a subset of patients in the Canadian Implantable Defibrillator Study (CIDS). Circulation 2004;110(2):112–6.

39. Kuck KH, Cappato R, Siebels J, et al. Randomized comparison of antiarrhythmic drug therapy with implantable defibrillators in patients resuscitated from cardiac arrest: the Cardiac Arrest Study Hamburg (CASH). Circulation 2000;102(7):748–54.

40. Connolly SJ, Hallstrom AP, Cappato R, et al. Meta-analysis of the implantable cardioverter defibrillator secondary prevention trials. AVID, CASH and CIDS studies. Antiarrhythmics vs Implantable Defibrillator study. Cardiac Arrest Study Hamburg. Canadian Implantable Defibrillator Study. Eur Heart J 2000;21(24):2071–8.

41. Salukhe TV, Dimopoulos K, Sutton R, et al. Life-years gained from defibrillator implantation: markedly nonlinear increase during 3 years of follow-up and its implications. Circulation 2004;109(15):1848–53.

42. Josephson M, Nisam S. Prospective trials of implantable cardioverter defibrillators versus drugs: are they addressing the right question? Am J Cardiol 1996;77(10):859–63.

43. Schlapfer J, Rapp F, Kappenberger L, et al. Electrophysiologically guided amiodarone therapy versus the implantable cardioverter-defibrillator for sustained ventricular tachyarrhythmias after myocardial infarction: results of long-term follow-up. J Am Coll Cardiol 2002;39(11):1813–9.

44. Pinski SL, Yao Q, Epstein AE, et al. Determinants of outcome in patients with sustained ventricular tachyarrhythmias: the antiarrhythmics versus implantable defibrillators (AVID) study registry. Am Heart J 2000;139(5):804–13.

45. Anderson JL, Hallstrom AP, Epstein AE, et al. Design and results of the antiarrhythmics vs implantable defibrillators (AVID) registry. The AVID Investigators. Circulation 1999;99(13):1692–9.

46. Daubert JP, Zareba W, Cannom DS, et al. Inappropriate implantable cardioverter-defibrillator shocks in MADIT II: frequency, mechanisms, predictors, and survival impact. J Am Coll Cardiol 2008;51(14):1357–65.

47. Poole JE, Johnson GW, Hellkamp AS, et al. Prognostic importance of defibrillator shocks in patients with heart failure. N Engl J Med 2008;359(10):1009–17.

48. Reddy VY, Reynolds MR, Neuzil P, et al. Prophylactic catheter ablation for the prevention of defibrillator therapy. N Engl J Med 2007;357(26):2657–65.

49. Kuck KH, Schaumann A, Eckardt L, et al. Catheter ablation of stable ventricular tachycardia before

defibrillator implantation in patients with coronary heart disease (VTACH): a multicentre randomised controlled trial. Lancet 2010;375(9708):31–40.

50. Wathen MS, Sweeney MO, DeGroot PJ, et al. Shock reduction using antitachycardia pacing for spontaneous rapid ventricular tachycardia in patients with coronary artery disease. Circulation 2001;104(7):796–801.

51. Wathen MS, DeGroot PJ, Sweeney MO, et al. Prospective randomized multicenter trial of empirical antitachycardia pacing versus shocks for spontaneous rapid ventricular tachycardia in patients with implantable cardioverter-defibrillators: pacing Fast Ventricular Tachycardia Reduces Shock Therapies (PainFREE Rx II) trial results. Circulation 2004;110(17):2591–6.

52. Wilkoff BL, Ousdigian KT, Sterns LD, et al. A comparison of empiric to physician-tailored programming of implantable cardioverter-defibrillators: results from the prospective randomized multicenter EMPIRIC trial. J Am Coll Cardiol 2006;48(2):330–9.

53. Wilkoff BL, Williamson BD, Stern RS, et al. Strategic programming of detection and therapy parameters in implantable cardioverter-defibrillators reduces shocks in primary prevention patients: results from the PREPARE (Primary Prevention Parameters Evaluation) study. J Am Coll Cardiol 2008;52(7):541–50.

54. Wilkoff BL, Cook JR, Epstein AE, et al. Dual-chamber pacing or ventricular backup pacing in patients with an implantable defibrillator: the Dual Chamber and VVI Implantable Defibrillator (DAVID) Trial. JAMA 2002;288(24):3115–23.

55. Wilkoff BL, Kudenchuk PJ, Buxton AE, et al. The DAVID (Dual Chamber and VVI Implantable Defibrillator) II trial. J Am Coll Cardiol 2009;53(10):872–80.

56. Olshansky B, Day JD, Moore S, et al. Is dual-chamber programming inferior to single-chamber programming in an implantable cardioverter-defibrillator? results of the INTRINSIC RV (Inhibition of Unnecessary RV Pacing With AVSH in ICDs) study. Circulation 2007;115(1):9–16.

57. Young JB, Abraham WT, Smith AL, et al. Combined cardiac resynchronization and implantable cardioversion defibrillation in advanced chronic heart failure: the MIRACLE ICD Trial. JAMA 2003;289(20):2685–94.

58. Lin G, Rea RF, Hammill SC, et al. Effect of cardiac resynchronisation therapy on occurrence of ventricular arrhythmia in patients with implantable cardioverter defibrillators undergoing upgrade to cardiac resynchronisation therapy devices. Heart 2008;94(2):186–90.

59. Epstein AE, DiMarco JP, Ellenbogen KA, et al. ACC/AHA/HRS 2008 Guidelines for Device-Based Therapy of Cardiac Rhythm Abnormalities: a report of the American College of Cardiology/American Heart Association Task Force on Practice Guidelines (Writing Committee to Revise the ACC/AHA/NASPE 2002 Guideline Update for Implantation of Cardiac Pacemakers and Antiarrhythmia Devices) developed in collaboration with the American Association for Thoracic Surgery and Society of Thoracic Surgeons. J Am Coll Cardiol 2008;51(21):e1–62.

60. Mehra MR, Yancy CW, Albert NM, et al. Evidence of clinical practice heterogeneity in the use of implantable cardioverter-defibrillators in heart failure and post-myocardial infarction left ventricular dysfunction: findings from IMPROVE HF. Heart Rhythm 2009;6(12):1727–34.

61. Voigt A, Ezzeddine R, Barrington W, et al. Utilization of implantable cardioverter-defibrillators in survivors of cardiac arrest in the United States from 1996 to 2001. J Am Coll Cardiol 2004;44(4):855–8.

62. Curtis LH, Al-Khatib SM, Shea AM, et al. Sex differences in the use of implantable cardioverter-defibrillators for primary and secondary prevention of sudden cardiac death. JAMA 2007;298(13):1517–24.

63. Hernandez AF, Fonarow GC, Liang L, et al. Sex and racial differences in the use of implantable cardioverter-defibrillators among patients hospitalized with heart failure. JAMA 2007;298(13):1525–32.

# Role of Antiarrhythmic Drugs: Frequent Implantable Cardioverter-Defibrillator Shocks, Risk of Proarrhythmia, and New Drug Therapy

Christopher Droogan, DO[a,b,c,*], Chinmay Patel, MD[d],
Gan-Xin Yan, MD, PhD[b,c,d], Peter R. Kowey, MD[b,c,d]

**KEYWORDS**

- Implantable cardioverter-defibrillator
- Ventricular arrhythmia • Antiarrhythmic drug therapy
- Adjuvant therapy • ICD shocks

Implantable cardioverter-defibrillators (ICDs) have revolutionized the care of patients with ischemic and nonischemic cardiomyopathy.[1,2] The primitive ICD introduced in the 1980s by Mirowski and colleagues has become much more sophisticated with programming capabilities, atrial and ventricular leads, antitachycardia pacing (ATP) algorithms, biventricular pacing, and cardioverting and defibrillating shocks.[1,3] Similarly, indications for ICD implantation are expanding as well.[4] Due to mortality benefits, assessment for eligibility of an ICD implantation is considered one of the integral parts of management of patients with cardiomyopathy.[1,2] Consequently, the number of ICD implantations has increased significantly in the last decade with a concurrent decrease in the use of stand-alone antiarrhythmic drugs for ventricular arrhythmic indications.[5–7]

The ICD prevents sudden cardiac death (SCD) by terminating the episodes of ventricular tachycardia (VT) or ventricular fibrillation (VF), delivering ATP therapy or an ICD shock. Therefore, patients with an ICD typically receive 1 or more ICD therapies for spontaneous arrhythmias following implantation.[1,8] Despite the technological evolution of ICD systems, more than 20% of the shocks delivered are caused by supraventricular arrhythmias and are categorized as inappropriate.[9–11] ICD shocks are physically and emotionally painful, and most patients dread

---

Funding Source: None.

Disclosure: None.

[a] Department of Cardiology, Main Line Health Heart Center and Lankenau Hospital, 100 Lancaster Avenue, MOBE 356, Wynnewood, PA 19096, USA

[b] Department of Pharmacology, Jefferson Medical College, Thomas Jefferson University Hospital, 111 South 11th Street, Philadelphia, PA 19107, USA

[c] Department of Cardiology, Lankenau Institute for Medical Research, 100 Lancaster Avenue, MOBE 558, Wynnewood, PA 19096, USA

[d] Department of Cardiology, Main Line Health Heart Center and Lankenau Hospital, 100 Lancaster Avenue, MOBE 558, Wynnewood, PA 19096, USA

* Corresponding author. Department of Cardiology, Main Line Health Heart Center and Lankenau Hospital, 100 Lancaster Avenue, MOBE 356, Wynnewood, PA 19096.

E-mail address: drooganc@mlhs.org

Heart Failure Clin 7 (2011) 195–205

doi:10.1016/j.hfc.2010.12.003

**Table 1**
**Clinical trials summarizing benefits of adjuvant antiarrhythmic drug therapy**

| Study | Drug/Dose | N per Group | Follow-up | Primary End Point | Secondary End Point |
|---|---|---|---|---|---|
| Pacifico et al[20] | Sotalol (207 ± 55 mg) vs placebo | 151 | 12 mo | All-cause death or all-cause ICD shock<br>Sotalol: 44%[a] (HR = 0.52)<br>Placebo: 56% | Mean frequency of shocks due to any cause<br>Sotalol: 1.43 ± 3.53[a]<br>Placebo: 3.89 ± 10.65 |
| Kuhlkamp et al[21] | Sotalol (80–400 mg) vs placebo | ≈46 | 12 mo | Recurrence of VT/VF<br>Sotalol: 32.6%[a]<br>Placebo: 53.2% | Total mortality same across the groups |
| Seidl et al[24] | Metoprolol (104 ± 37 mg) vs sotalol (242 ± 109 mg) | 35 | 26 ± 16 mo | Appropriate ICD therapy<br>VT treated by ATP<br>Metoprolol: 20%[a]<br>Sotalol: 49%<br>Fast VT/VF treated by ICD shocks<br>Metoprolol: 20%[a]<br>Sotalol: 54% | Total mortality<br>Metoprolol: 3 deaths<br>Sotalol: 6 deaths<br>Actuarial survival rate not different between the 2 groups |
| Kettering et al[23] | Metoprolol (108 ± 44 mg) vs sotalol (319 ± 91 mg) | 50 | 727 d | Recurrent VT/VF requiring ICD therapy<br>Metoprolol: 66%<br>Sotalol: 60%<br>Event free survival not different between groups | Total mortality<br>Metoprolol: 8 deaths<br>Sotalol: 6 deaths<br>not different between the 2 groups |

| Study | Drugs compared | Patients | Duration | Frequency of appropriate ICD shocks and ATP | Appropriate ICD therapy |
|---|---|---|---|---|---|
| Singer et al[26] | AZ 35, 75, or 125 mg vs placebo | ≈35–46 | 374 d | Placebo: 36<br>35-mg AZ: 10[a]<br>75-mg AZ: 12[a]<br>125-mg AZ: 9[a] per patient-year (HR = 0.31) | — |
| Dorian et al[27] SHIELD | AZ 75 and 125 mg vs placebo | ≈199–214 | 1 y | All-cause shock and ATP<br>75-mg AZ (HR = 0.43)[a]<br>125-mg AZ (HR = 0.53)[a] as compared with placebo<br>All-cause shock<br>Tread toward reduction in treatment group | Appropriate ICD therapy<br>75-mg AZ (HR = 0.52)[a]<br>125-mg AZ (HR = 0.38)[a] as compared with placebo |
| Connolly et al[29] OPTIC | β-Blocker vs sotalol vs amiodarone plus β-blocker | ≈134–138 | 1 y | All-cause ICD shock<br>β-blocker: 38.5%<br>Sotalol: 24.3%<br>Amiodarone plus β-blocker: 10.3%[a] (HR = 0.27 vs β-blocker, HR = 0.43 vs sotalol) | — |

*Abbreviations:* AZ, azimilide; HR, hazard ratio; OPTIC, Optimal Pharmacologic Therapy in Cardioverter Defibrillator Patients; SHIELD, Shock Inhibition Evaluation with Azimilide.

[a] Significant *P* value.

*Data from* Patel C, Yan GX, Kocovic D, et al. Should catheter ablation be the preferred therapy for reducing ICD shocks?: ventricular tachycardia ablation versus drugs for preventing ICD shocks: role of adjuvant antiarrhythmic drug therapy. Circ Arrhythm Electrophysiol 2009;2:707.

future shocks.[12] Many patients experience symptoms such as dizziness, palpitations, nervousness, flushing, or even syncope before receiving an ICD shock.[13] A higher incidence of depression and poor quality of life has been reported in patients who have received 1 or more ICD shocks, and adverse psychological outcomes directly correlate to the number of ICD shocks.[14–16]

Several antiarrhythmic drugs have been shown to reduce ICD therapies including shocks. More than 70% of patients end up receiving adjuvant antiarrhythmic drug therapy for this indication.[17,18] This finding was best exemplified in the device arm of the Antiarrythmics Versus Implantable Defibrillator (AVID) trial.[19] About 18% of patients in the ICD arm of the AVID trial had to be started on adjuvant antiarrhythmic drug therapy (amiodarone 42%, sotalol 21%, and mexiletine 20%) to reduce frequent ICD shocks and prevent recurrent ventricular arrhythmia.[19] Adjuvant antiarrhythmic drug therapy in these crossover patients reduced the 1-year arrhythmia event rate from 90% to 64%. Potential benefits, pitfalls, need for caution, and the clinical trials of adjuvant antiarrhythmic drugs in ICD-implanted patients are discussed in this review.

## CLINICAL TRIALS SUPPORTING THE EFFICACY OF ADJUVANT ANTIARRHYTHMIC DRUG THERAPY

Major clinical trials establishing the role of adjuvant antiarrhythmic drugs and their principal outcomes are listed in **Table 1**. Most patients enrolled in these trials received an ICD for secondary prevention of SCD or for a documented episode of VT/VF.

Sotalol was one of the first antiarrhythmic drugs tested for such an indication by Pacifico and colleagues.[20] In this double-blind, prospective, multicenter trial, 302 patients with ICDs were randomized to receive either 160 to 320 mg of D,L-sotalol (n = 151) or matching placebo (n = 151) and were followed up for 12 months. In this study, compared with placebo, treatment with sotalol led to a 48% risk reduction of all-cause mortality and delivery of first shock for any reason (**Fig. 1**). When ICD shock was categorized as appropriate versus inappropriate, there was a 64% risk reduction for all-cause death or first inappropriate shock and a 44% risk reduction for all-cause death or first appropriate shock. The results remained unchanged when stratified by left ventricular ejection fraction or concomitant use of β-blockers. The mean frequency of all-cause shock was 1.43 ± 3.53 in the sotalol group compared with 3.89 ± 10.65 in the control group. Rate of discontinuation of the drug was about 33% at 1 year in the sotalol and placebo groups. Patients receiving sotalol were more likely to have bradycardia and QT prolongation, but only 1 episode of torsades de pointes (TdP) was reported. Similar efficacy of sotalol was reported in another small-scale study of 46 patients.[21] Similar to sotalol, dofetilide, a pure rapidly activating delayed rectifier potassium current blocker, was shown to be effective in increasing the median time to first all-cause ICD shocks in a study by

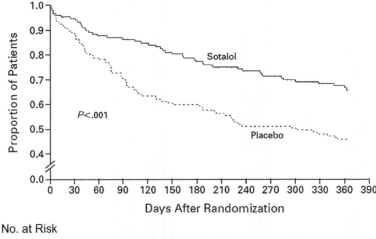

No. at Risk

| | | | | | | | | | | | | | |
|---|---|---|---|---|---|---|---|---|---|---|---|---|---|
| Placebo | 151 | 129 | 114 | 101 | 90 | 84 | 84 | 77 | 70 | 70 | 69 | 65 | 49 |
| Sotalol | 151 | 136 | 123 | 119 | 115 | 109 | 104 | 101 | 99 | 95 | 91 | 90 | 70 |

**Fig. 1.** The Kaplan-Meier time-to-event curves for combined end point of all-cause death or all-cause shock in the control and sotalol groups. Treatment with sotalol reduced the relative risk of combined end point by 48%. (*Reproduced from* Pacifico A, Hohnloser SH, Williams JH, et al. Prevention of implantable-defibrillator shocks by treatment with sotalol. d,l-Sotalol Implantable Cardioverter-Defibrillator Study Group. N Engl J Med 1999;340:1858; with permission.)

O'Toole and colleagues.[22] However, dofetilide administration was associated with a high incidence of TdP in this study.

Although most of the patients with ICDs receive β-blockers as part of a comprehensive medical regimen, it is worth underscoring the importance of beta-adrenergic blockade in the prevention of ICD shocks. Simple β-blockers have been shown to be at least equally or more effective than sotalol in the prevention of ICD shocks. In a small prospective trial of 100 patients with an existing ICD, Kettering and colleagues[23] showed that metoprolol was as effective as sotalol in preventing VT/VF and the resultant ICD interventions. Similarly, in a post hoc analysis of 691 patients with ischemic cardiomyopathy in the Multicenter Automatic Defibrillator Implantation Trial II (MADIT-II), patients who received higher doses of metoprolol, atenolol, and carvedilol had a 52% relative risk reduction for recurrent VT/VF requiring ICD therapy as compared with patients who did not take β-blockers. Superior efficacy of metoprolol to sotalol was demonstrated in a small prospective study of 70 patients with ICD.[24] The probability of reaching a combined end point of symptomatic recurrence of fast VT or VF or death was significantly lower at 1 and 2 years in the metoprolol group (83% and 74%, respectively) as compared with the sotalol group (47% and 38%, respectively, $P = .004$). ICD interventions in the form of ATP and shocks were significantly lower in the metoprolol compared with the sotalol arm.

Azimilide is a novel class III drug that blocks both the rapid and slow components of the delayed rectifier cardiac potassium current and is effective in a variety of supraventricular arrhythmias.[25] Recent clinical trials have demonstrated its role in the prevention of ICD shocks. In a dose-range pilot study of 172 patients with an ICD, Singer and colleagues[26] demonstrated that azimilide reduced the relative risk of appropriate ICD therapy (shocks and ATP) by 69% at all administered doses (35 mg, 75 mg, or 125 mg) as compared with placebo at 1-year follow-up. Azimilide did not have adverse effects on left ventricular function, resting heart rate, defibrillation threshold (DFT) or pacing threshold.

The efficacy of azimilide was further investigated by Dorian and colleagues[27] in the large prospective double-blind trial Shock Inhibition Evaluation with Azimilide (SHIELD) conducted in 633 ICD recipients. The 2 primary end points of this trial were (1) all-cause shocks plus symptomatic tachyarrhythmias terminated by ATP and (2) all-cause shocks. A single secondary end point was all appropriate ICD therapies. Azimilide was tested in 75 and 125 mg doses. At a median follow-up

period of 1 year, azimilide significantly reduced the first primary end point of all-cause shocks plus symptomatic arrhythmia terminated by ATP in both doses as compared with placebo (hazard ratio [HR], 0.43 for 75-mg dose; HR, 0.53 for 125-mg dose) (**Fig. 2**). There was no statistically significant difference in efficacy between the 2 doses, and there was a trend toward a reduction in the primary end point of all-cause shock alone with both doses of azimilide.

The secondary end point of all appropriate ICD therapies (shocks or ATP) was reduced by both 75 and 125 mg/d dosages of azimilide (HR = 0.52 and 0.38 with $P = .017$ and $P<.001$, respectively, see **Fig. 2**) with a trend toward a more significant effect at the 125 mg dose. Additional analysis revealed that treatment with azimilide led to a significant decrease in the incidence of all ICD interventions and all-cause shocks with an increased interevent interval, suggesting a possible benefit in the treatment of electric storm. This result was confirmed by subsequent analysis of the SHIELD data by Dorian and colleagues[28] who showed that treatment with 75 and 125 mg/d dosages of azimilide reduced the risk of electric storm by 37% and 55%, respectively, as compared with placebo. These beneficial effects of azimilide translated into reduced emergency department visits and hospitalizations.

Azimilide was well tolerated as an addition to conventional therapy. About 86% of the patients were on concomitant β-blocker therapy, suggesting that the benefits of azimilide were over and above traditional therapy. The overall incidence of adverse events and rates of early discontinuation (35%–36%) were similar to placebo.[26,27,29] Azimilide therapy led to a dose-dependent prolongation of the QT interval; however, TdP was reported in 5 patients without any consequences[27] One patient had severe but reversible neutropenia with 75 mg of azimilide.[27] In the context of these data, azimilide is the first drug submitted to the Food and Drug Administration for use with an ICD and is currently under review to be used for this indication.

When compared with other antiarrhythmic drugs, amiodarone remains one of the most commonly used, especially in patients with advanced cardiomyopathy, because of its established efficacy and cardiac safety profile. The OPTIC (Optimal Pharmacological Therapy in Cardioverter Defibrillator Patients) study investigated the efficacy of β-blocker, sotalol, and β-blocker plus amiodarone in the prevention of ICD shocks.[29] The OPTIC investigators randomized 412 patients with ICD to receive β-blocker alone, sotalol alone, and amiodarone plus β-blocker,

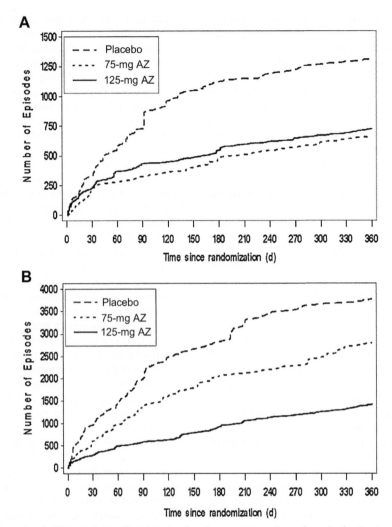

**Fig. 2.** (*A*) Effect of azimilide (AZ) on all-cause shocks plus symptomatic tachyarrhythmias terminated by ATP. Treatment with 75 and 125 mg/d dosages of AZ significantly reduced the risk of all-cause shocks and symptomatic tachyarrhythmia by 57% and 47%, respectively. (*B*) Effect of AZ on all appropriate ICD therapies. Treatment with 75 and 125 mg/d dosages of AZ significantly reduced the risk of all appropriate ICD therapies by 48% and 62%, respectively. (*Reproduced from* Dorian P, Borggrefe M, Al-Khalidi HR, et al. Placebo-controlled, randomized clinical trial of azimilide for prevention of ventricular tachyarrhythmias in patients with an implantable cardioverter defibrillator. Circulation 2004;110:3646–54; with permission.)

and the patients were followed up for 1 year. The results showed that the patients treated with sotalol or amiodarone had a reduced risk of shock by 56% compared with β-blocker alone. In addition, amiodarone plus β-blocker was more effective than β-blocker alone (HR = 0.27, *P*<.001) or sotalol alone (HR = 0.43, *P* = .02) in preventing both appropriate and inappropriate ICD shocks (**Fig. 3**). Mortality was not significantly different among the 3 groups, and no cases of TdP were reported. Rates of study drug discontinuation at 1 year were 18.2% for amiodarone, 23.5% for sotalol, and 5.3% for β-blocker alone groups. Adverse pulmonary, thyroid, and bradycardic

events were more common with amiodarone treatment.

Similar to its congener amiodarone, dronedarone was effective in reducing the rate of appropriate ICD intervention during a 30-day follow-up in a small study.[30]

## BENEFITS OF ADJUVANT ANTIARRHYTHMIC DRUG THERAPY

Clearly, antiarrhythmic drugs reduce the incidence of both appropriate as well as inappropriate ICD therapies (both ATP and shock) by more than half.[20,27,29] Such a reduction in ICD shocks would

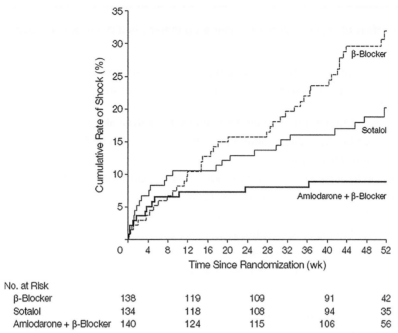

**Fig. 3.** Cumulative risk of shock in all 3 treatment groups. Amiodarone plus β-blocker significantly reduced the risk of shock compared with β-blocker alone (HR = 0.27, P<.001) and sotalol alone (HR = 0.43, P = .02). (*Reproduced from* Connolly SJ, Dorian P, Roberts RS, et al. Comparison of beta-blockers, amiodarone plus beta-blockers, or sotalol for prevention of shocks from implantable cardioverter defibrillators: the OPTIC Study: a randomized trial. JAMA 2006;295:165–71; with permission.)

be expected to decrease emergency department visits and the rate of hospitalization.[27,28] A decrease in the number of ICD discharges also prolongs the battery life of the device.[31] As such, antiarrhythmic drug therapy results in an overall improvement in the quality of life of ICD-implanted patients. Additionally, most antiarrhythmic drugs tend to prolong the tachycardia cycle length and may render the tachycardia more hemodynamically stable and thus amenable to termination with ATP.[32] Some antiarrhythmic drugs may reduce the DFT and facilitate defibrillation of VT/VF as discussed later.

About 10% to 30% of patients with an ICD develop electric storm, defined as 3 or more episodes of hemodynamically destabilizing VT/VF occurring in a 24-hour period. Development of electric storm is associated with increased morbidity and a 40% 3-month mortality.[33–35] Although recent clinical trials have suggested catheter ablation techniques as first line therapy for electric storm, antiarrhythmic drugs still remain the cornerstone of therapy for electric storm. Reversal of precipitating factors, optimization of β-blocker therapy, and addition of intravenous amiodarone followed by oral maintenance dosing are required in most cases to abort and prevent recurrent ventricular arrhythmia.[33,36] As outlined earlier, the investigational agent azimilide has been shown to reduce the risk of electric storm

by 37% to 55%.[37] The principal advantages of adjuvant antiarrhythmic drug therapy are summarized in **Table 1**.

## DRUG-DEVICE INTERACTION

A great deal of caution needs to be exercised when a new antiarrhythmic drug is administered in a patient with an implanted device. Potential adverse drug-device interactions are listed in **Box 1**.

One of the most important drug-device interactions is a drug-induced increase in defibrillation and pacing thresholds leading to failure of treatment of life-threatening arrhythmia. Although most antiarrhythmic drugs increase the DFT, some may lower it. In a substudy of 94 patients from the OPTIC trial, amiodarone plus β-blocker therapy led to a small but statistically significant increase (1.29 J) in DFT after 8 to 13 weeks of therapy.[38] In contrast, treatment with sotalol and β-blocker was associated with a decrease in DFT by 0.89 J and 1.67 J, respectively. Careful testing of DFTs should be performed in all patients, with special attention to those who have monophasic waveform ICDs, with an epicardial lead system,[39] with a high DFT at baseline, and who are treated with high-dose[40] long-term amiodarone.[41–44]

Azimilide has been shown to have minimal effects on the DFT or pacing thresholds in patients

---

**Box 1**
**Benefits and pitfalls of adjuvant antiarrhythmic drug therapy in ICD-implanted patients**

Pros

    Decrease in appropriate ICD shocks due to suppression of recurrent VT/VF

    Decrease in inappropriate ICD shocks due to reduced frequency and better rate control of supraventricular rhythm

    Slowing of rate of tachycardia, leading to improved hemodynamic tolerance

    Slowing of rate of tachycardia, facilitating successful termination by ATP

    Prolongation of ICD battery life

    Decrease in the frequency of symptomatic nonsustained ventricular arrhythmias

    Prevention and better treatment of electric storm

    Improved quality of life and sense of well-being

    Reduced DFT, facilitating easier defibrillation

    Improved control of maximal sinus rate

    Reduced rate of recurrent ICD-related hospitalizations

Cons

    Interference in ICD function due to

        increase in DFT

        increase in pacing threshold

    Interference in accurate arrhythmia detection due to

        slowing of rate of VT

        decrease in amplitude of electrocardiogram interfering with sensing

        limited effectiveness of rate stability criterion

Adverse effects

    Cardiac

        Bradyarrhythmia

        TdP

        Impairment of myocardial function

    Extracardiac toxicity

*Data from* Patel C, Yan GX, Kocovic D, et al. Should catheter ablation be the preferred therapy for reducing ICD shocks?: ventricular tachycardia ablation versus drugs for preventing ICD shocks: role of adjuvant antiarrhythmic drug therapy. Circ Arrhythm Electrophysiol 2009;2:706.

---

with an ICD.[26,45] Similarly, dronedarone has been shown to have no effect on defibrillation safety margin or pacing thresholds at its therapeutic or higher dose.[30,46]

Antiarrhythmic drugs usually prolong the cycle length of VT, which improves hemodynamic tolerability and effectiveness of ATP in most situations. The downside is that drugs such as amiodarone and sotalol may slow the tachycardia rate to such a degree that it becomes lower than that of the programmed tachycardia detection rate of the ICD leading to failure to sense VT.[47] Appropriate adjustments in the detection algorithm are necessary when adjuvant antiarrhythmic drugs are instituted. Antiarrhythmic drugs, especially class IC agents, may also affect the morphology of the QRS complex and thus affect the morphology sensing and rhythm stability criterion leading to incorrect rhythm interpretation by the ICD and resultant inappropriate treatment.[48]

Drug-induced proarrhythmia, especially TdP, is rare but a serious problem when drugs with Class III effects, such as azimilide, sotalol, dofetilide, and amiodarone, are used, especially in patients with compromised repolarization reserve.[49] Extracardiac side effects of antiarrhythmic drugs such as amiodarone are a limitation to their long-term use. This limitation may be less of an issue with new drugs such as dronedarone or azimilide.[46]

## EXPERT OPINION

In conclusion, adjuvant antiarrhythmic drug therapy should be considered an integral part of the management of patients with an ICD. Unanswered questions are (1) which patients should receive adjuvant antiarrhytmic drug therapy? (2) when to start the therapy? (3) what drugs to administer? (4) when to consider catheter-based ablation techniques?

Most clinical trials outlined earlier enrolled patients for whom the ICD was implanted for secondary prevention of SCD. Similar evidence in patients who have received the ICD for primary prevention is lacking. Such patients seem to have fewer device activations.[50,51] In the context of a lower-risk population, adjuvant antiarrhythmic drug therapy should be started only if 1 or more ICD shocks have been delivered, with the expectation that well-designed therapy can reduce ICD shocks and improve the quality of life. The timing of antiarrhythmic drug therapy in patients should always be based on best physician judgment and patient preference.

It is important to note that no drug has achieved approval for the prevention of ICD shocks, and no data are available to support the early prophylactic use of drugs. Although starting antiarrhythmic drug therapy before an ICD shock is delivered might be valuable, it should be kept in mind that antiarrhythmic drug therapy itself carries substantial risk.

When patients need an antiarrhythmic drug because of frequent ICD shocks, the weight of evidence supports optimizing β-blocker therapy. If β-blockers are ineffective or poorly tolerated, amiodarone, azimilide, or sotalol may provide benefit. Any antiarrhythmic drug prescribed to treat serious ventricular arrhythmias, including those that have triggered an ICD shock, should be administered under observation not only to observe for toxicity but also to gauge efficacy. If proarrhythmia occurs, it tends to manifest during the early stages of therapy as drug concentrations approach steady state.

Catheter-based mapping and ablation techniques have been considered a last resort treatment in patients with recurrent VT that is refractory to adjuvant drug therapy.[52] Although recent clinical trials support the role of catheter ablation techniques as a first line treatment for prevention of recurrent ICD therapies including electric storm, these techniques are invasive and their results are operator dependent.[53–55] Data supporting the use of catheter ablation therapy are limited and do not address issues such as quality of life and cost. The authors believe that antiarrhythmic drugs remain the first line therapeutic agents for the prevention of ICD shocks in most patients.[56]

## REFERENCES

1. DiMarco JP. Implantable cardioverter-defibrillators. N Engl J Med 2003;349:1836–47.
2. Reiffel JA. Drug and drug-device therapy in heart failure patients in the post-COMET and SCD-HeFT era. J Cardiovasc Pharmacol Ther 2005;10(Suppl 1): S45–58.
3. Mirowski M, Reid PR, Mower MM, et al. Termination of malignant ventricular arrhythmias with an implanted automatic defibrillator in human beings. N Engl J Med 1980;303:322–4.
4. Epstein AE, DiMarco JP, Ellenbogen KA, et al. ACC/AHA/HRS 2008 Guidelines for Device-Based Therapy of Cardiac Rhythm Abnormalities: a report of the American College of Cardiology/American Heart Association Task Force on Practice Guidelines (Writing Committee to Revise the ACC/AHA/NASPE 2002 Guideline Update for Implantation of Cardiac Pacemakers and Antiarrhythmia Devices): developed in collaboration with the American Association for Thoracic Surgery and Society of Thoracic Surgeons. Circulation 2008;117:e350–408.
5. Al-Khatib SM, LaPointe NM, Curtis LH, et al. Outpatient prescribing of antiarrhythmic drugs from 1995 to 2000. Am J Cardiol 2003;91:91–4.
6. Hine LK, Gross TP, Kennedy DL. Outpatient antiarrhythmic drug use from 1970 through 1986. Arch Intern Med 1989;149:1524–7.
7. Zhan C, Baine WB, Sedrakyan A, et al. Cardiac device implantation in the United States from 1997 through 2004: a population-based analysis. J Gen Intern Med 2008;23(Suppl 1):13–9.
8. Patel C, Yan GX, Kocovic D, et al. Should catheter ablation be the preferred therapy for reducing ICD shocks?: ventricular tachycardia ablation versus drugs for preventing ICD shocks: role of adjuvant antiarrhythmic drug therapy. Circ Arrhythm Electrophysiol 2009;2:705–11.
9. Dorian P, Philippon F, Thibault B, et al. Randomized controlled study of detection enhancements versus rate-only detection to prevent inappropriate therapy in a dual-chamber implantable cardioverter-defibrillator. Heart Rhythm 2004;1:540–7.
10. Nanthakumar K, Paquette M, Newman D, et al. Inappropriate therapy from atrial fibrillation and sinus tachycardia in automated implantable cardioverter defibrillators. Am Heart J 2000;139:797–803.

11. Rosenqvist M, Beyer T, Block M, et al. Adverse events with transvenous implantable cardioverter-defibrillators: a prospective multicenter study. European 7219 Jewel ICD investigators. Circulation 1998;98:663–70.

12. Ahmad M, Bloomstein L, Roelke M, et al. Patients' attitudes toward implanted defibrillator shocks. Pacing Clin Electrophysiol 2000;23:934–8.

13. Pelletier D, Gallagher R, Mitten-Lewis S, et al. Australian implantable cardiac defibrillator recipients: quality-of-life issues. Int J Nurs Pract 2002;8:68–74.

14. Dougherty CM. Psychological reactions and family adjustment in shock versus no shock groups after implantation of internal cardioverter defibrillator. Heart Lung 1995;24:281–91.

15. Heller SS, Ormont MA, Lidagoster L, et al. Psychosocial outcome after ICD implantation: a current perspective. Pacing Clin Electrophysiol 1998;21:1207–15.

16. Sola CL, Bostwick JM. Implantable cardioverter-defibrillators, induced anxiety, and quality of life. Mayo Clin Proc 2005;80:232–7.

17. Greene HL. Interactions between pharmacologic and nonpharmacologic antiarrhythmic therapy. Am J Cardiol 1996;78:61–6.

18. Movsowitz C, Marchlinski FE. Interactions between implantable cardioverter-defibrillators and class III agents. Am J Cardiol 1998;82:41I–8I.

19. Steinberg JS, Martins J, Sadanandan S, et al. Antiarrhythmic drug use in the implantable defibrillator arm of the Antiarrhythmics Versus Implantable Defibrillators (AVID) Study. Am Heart J 2001;142:520–9.

20. Pacifico A, Hohnloser SH, Williams JH, et al. Prevention of implantable-defibrillator shocks by treatment with sotalol. d, l-Sotalol Implantable Cardioverter-Defibrillator Study Group. N Engl J Med 1999;340:1855–62.

21. Kuhlkamp V, Mewis C, Mermi J, et al. Suppression of sustained ventricular tachyarrhythmias: a comparison of d, l-sotalol with no antiarrhythmic drug treatment. J Am Coll Cardiol 1999;33:46–52.

22. O'Toole M, O'Neill G, Kluger J, et al. Efficacy and safety of oral dofetilide in patients with an implantable defibrillator: a multi-center study. Circulation 1999;100:I–794.

23. Kettering K, Mewis C, Dornberger V, et al. Efficacy of metoprolol and sotalol in the prevention of recurrences of sustained ventricular tachyarrhythmias in patients with an implantable cardioverter defibrillator. Pacing Clin Electrophysiol 2002;25:1571–6.

24. Seidl K, Hauer B, Schwick NG, et al. Comparison of metoprolol and sotalol in preventing ventricular tachyarrhythmias after the implantation of a cardioverter/defibrillator. Am J Cardiol 1998;82:744–8.

25. Connolly SJ, Schnell DJ, Page RL, et al. Dose-response relations of azimilide in the management of symptomatic, recurrent, atrial fibrillation. Am J Cardiol 2001;88:974–9.

26. Singer I, Al-Khalidi H, Niazi I, et al. Azimilide decreases recurrent ventricular tachyarrhythmias in patients with implantable cardioverter defibrillators. J Am Coll Cardiol 2004;43:39–43.

27. Dorian P, Borggrefe M, Al-Khalidi HR, et al. Placebo-controlled, randomized clinical trial of azimilide for prevention of ventricular tachyarrhythmias in patients with an implantable cardioverter defibrillator. Circulation 2004;110:3646–54.

28. Dorian P, Al-Khalidi HR, Hohnloser SH, et al. Azimilide reduces emergency department visits and hospitalizations in patients with an implantable cardioverter-defibrillator in a placebo-controlled clinical trial. J Am Coll Cardiol 2008;52:1076–83.

29. Connolly SJ, Dorian P, Roberts RS, et al. Comparison of beta-blockers, amiodarone plus beta-blockers, or sotalol for prevention of shocks from implantable cardioverter defibrillators: the OPTIC Study: a randomized trial. JAMA 2006;295:165–71.

30. Kowey PR, Singh BN. Dronedarone in patients with implantable defibrillators. Heart Rhythm 2004: 25th Annual Scientific Sessions of the Heart Rhythm Society, late-breaking clinical trials oral presentation, San Francisco (CA), May 19–22, 2004.

31. Dorian P. Combination ICD and drug treatments-best options. Resuscitation 2000;45:S3–6.

32. Mazur A, Anderson ME, Bonney S, et al. Pause-dependent polymorphic ventricular tachycardia during long-term treatment with dofetilide: a placebo-controlled, implantable cardioverter-defibrillator-based evaluation. J Am Coll Cardiol 2001;37:1100–5.

33. Credner SC, Klingenheben T, Mauss O, et al. Electrical storm in patients with transvenous implantable cardioverter-defibrillators: incidence, management and prognostic implications. J Am Coll Cardiol 1998;32:1909–15.

34. Exner DV, Pinski SL, Wyse DG, et al. Electrical storm presages nonsudden death: the antiarrhythmics versus implantable defibrillators (AVID) trial. Circulation 2001;103:2066–71.

35. Villacastin J, Almendral J, Arenal A, et al. Incidence and clinical significance of multiple consecutive, appropriate, high-energy discharges in patients with implanted cardioverter-defibrillators. Circulation 1996;93:753–62.

36. Greene M, Newman D, Geist M, et al. Is electrical storm in ICD patients the sign of a dying heart? Outcome of patients with clusters of ventricular tachyarrhythmias. Europace 2000;2:263–9.

37. Hohnloser SH, Al-Khalidi HR, Pratt CM, et al. Electrical storm in patients with an implantable defibrillator: incidence, features, and preventive therapy: insights from a randomized trial. Eur Heart J 2006;27:3027–32.

38. Hohnloser SH, Dorian P, Roberts R, et al. Effect of amiodarone and sotalol on ventricular defibrillation

threshold: the Optimal Pharmacological Therapy in Cardioverter Defibrillator Patients (OPTIC) trial. Circulation 2006;114:104–9.

39. Kuhlkamp V, Mewis C, Suchalla R, et al. Effect of amiodarone and sotalol on the defibrillation threshold in comparison to patients without antiarrhythmic drug treatment. Int J Cardiol 1999;69: 271–9.

40. Zhou L, Chen BP, Kluger J, et al. Effects of amiodarone and its active metabolite desethylamiodarone on the ventricular defibrillation threshold. J Am Coll Cardiol 1998;31:1672–8.

41. Wood MA, Ellenbogen KA. Follow-up defibrillator testing for antiarrhythmic drugs: probability and uncertainty. Circulation 2006;114:98–100.

42. Epstein AE, Ellenbogen KA, Kirk KA, et al. Clinical characteristics and outcome of patients with high defibrillation thresholds. A multicenter study. Circulation 1992;86:1206–16.

43. Fain ES, Lee JT, Winkle RA. Effects of acute intravenous and chronic oral amiodarone on defibrillation energy requirements. Am Heart J 1987;114: 8–17.

44. Pelosi F Jr, Oral H, Kim MH, et al. Effect of chronic amiodarone therapy on defibrillation energy requirements in humans. J Cardiovasc Electrophysiol 2000; 11:736–40.

45. Qi XQ, Newman D, Dorian P. Azimilide decreases defibrillation voltage requirements and increases spatial organization during ventricular fibrillation. J Interv Card Electrophysiol 1999;3:61–7.

46. Patel C, Yan GX, Kowey PR. Droendarone. Circulation 2009;120:636–44.

47. Bansch D, Castrucci M, Bocker D, et al. Ventricular tachycardias above the initially programmed tachycardia detection interval in patients with implantable cardioverter-defibrillators: incidence, prediction and significance. J Am Coll Cardiol 2000;36:557–65.

48. Rajawat YS, Patel VV, Gerstenfeld EP, et al. Advantages and pitfalls of combining device-based and pharmacologic therapies for the treatment of ventricular arrhythmias: observations from a tertiary referral center. Pacing Clin Electrophysiol 2004;27: 1670–81.

49. Wolbrette DL. Risk of proarrhythmia with class III antiarrhythmic agents: sex-based differences and other issues. Am J Cardiol 2003;91:39D–44D.

50. Bardy GH, Lee KL, Mark DB, et al. Amiodarone or an implantable cardioverter-defibrillator for congestive heart failure. N Engl J Med 2005;352:225–37.

51. Kadish A, Dyer A, Daubert JP, et al. Prophylactic defibrillator implantation in patients with nonischemic dilated cardiomyopathy. N Engl J Med 2004; 350:2151–8.

52. Morady F. Radio-frequency ablation as treatment for cardiac arrhythmias. N Engl J Med 1999;340: 534–44.

53. Carbucicchio C, Santamaria M, Trevisi N, et al. Catheter ablation for the treatment of electrical storm in patients with implantable cardioverter-defibrillators: short- and long-term outcomes in a prospective single-center study. Circulation 2008;117:462–9.

54. Reddy VY, Reynolds MR, Neuzil P, et al. Prophylactic catheter ablation for the prevention of defibrillator therapy. N Engl J Med 2007;357:2657–65.

55. Weinstock J, Wang PJ, Homoud MK, et al. Clinical results with catheter ablation: AV junction, atrial fibrillation and ventricular tachycardia. J Interv Card Electrophysiol 2003;9:275–88.

56. Estes NA III. Ablation after ICD implantation–bridging the gap between promise and practice. N Engl J Med 2007;357:2717–9.

# The Role of Ventricular Tachycardia Ablation in the Reduction of Implantable Defibrillator Shocks

Ganesh Venkataraman, MD*, S. Adam Strickberger, MD

## KEYWORDS
- Ventricular tachycardia • Cardiac ablation
- Defibrillator • ICD shocks

Implantable defibrillator (ICD) shocks can be a life-saving therapy for patients with malignant ventricular arrhythmias. However, electrical storm and frequent ICD shocks are associated with increased mortality and morbidity, and a decreased quality of life. Attempts to prevent ICD shocks have included pharmacologic and nonpharmacologic approaches. β-blockers and antiarrhythmic agents have been shown to reduce ICD shocks. ICD programming features such as antitachycardia pacing (ATP) may also reduce ICD shocks. Despite these techniques, some patients have recurrent ventricular tachycardia (VT) and ICD shocks. In this situation, ablation of VT can be helpful. The purpose of this review is to discuss the role of VT ablation in reducing ICD shocks.

## FREQUENCY AND EFFECT OF ICD SHOCKS

More than 200,000 patients with heart failure have received an ICD to reduce their risk of sudden cardiac death (SCD) since 2005.[1] Approximately 30% of patients who receive an ICD for primary prevention of SCD receive an appropriate shock for VT or ventricular fibrillation (VF) within 3 years of implantation.[2,3] Nearly 45% of patients who are treated with an ICD for secondary prevention of SCD receive an appropriate shock within 1 year.[4]

Electrical storm, defined as 3 or more appropriate ICD therapies within a 24-hour period for VT or VF, often results in multiple ICD shocks. Among patients with an ischemic cardiomyopathy who were treated with an ICD for primary prevention of SCD, the incidence of electrical storm was 4%.[5] In patients treated with an ICD for secondary prevention of SCD, the incidence of electrical storm was nearly 20%. VT was responsible for the electrical storm in 86% of these patients.[6]

Electrical storm and frequent ICD shocks may adversely affect patient outcomes. Multiple ICD shocks may cause myocardial injury and fibrosis, worsening left ventricular ejection fraction (LVEF), and heart failure.[7] In addition, ICD shocks may cause acute hospitalization, premature battery depletion, pain, anxiety, and a diminished quality of life. In patients treated with an ICD, there is a strong association between electrical storm and cardiovascular mortality.[5,6] In patients with heart failure, a single ICD shock is associated with a 2- to 5-fold increase in mortality.[2]

## PHARMACOLOGIC ATTEMPTS TO REDUCE ICD SHOCKS

Pharmacologic agents can be used to prevent ICD shocks. Standard heart failure therapy with β-blockers and angiotensin-converting enzyme

This work was not supported by external funding.

Washington Electrophysiology, and Cardiovascular Research Institute, Washington Hospital Center, 106 Irving Street, NW, South #204, Washington, DC 20010-2975, USA

* Corresponding author.

*E-mail address:* Ganesh.S.Venkataraman@medstar.net

inhibitors has been shown to reduce the incidence of SCD.[8] In a subgroup analysis of MADIT-II (Multicenter Automatic Defibrillator Implantation Trial-II), a significant reduction in VT and VF was noted in patients taking large doses of β-blockers.[9]

Antiarrhythmic drug therapy can be used to treat patients with an initial ICD shock for VT. A multicenter trial[10] randomized 302 patients with an ICD to either sotalol or placebo, and reported that sotalol significantly reduced the incidence of ICD shocks. A more recent study[11] randomized 412 patients with an ICD to 3 different drug regimens, and found that amiodarone in addition to β-blockers was more effective than sotalol or a β-blocker alone in reducing the frequency of ICD shocks. However, this drug combination was discontinued significantly more often, in approximately 20% of patients.

## ICD PROGRAMMING FEATURES TO REDUCE ICD SHOCKS

Several ICD features are designed to reduce the number of ICD shocks for VT or VF. Algorithms that discriminate between supraventricular tachycardia and VT have had modest success in decreasing ICD shocks, whereas a prolonged tachycardia detection interval significantly reduced appropriate ICD shocks during the first year of follow-up.[12,13] ATP may terminate VT. Numerous studies have reported that ATP terminates 70% to 80% of VT up to 250 beats per minute, with a 2% to 4% risk of accelerating the VT or causing it to degenerate to VF.[14–16] Patients treated with an ICD, in whom VT is terminated with ATP therapy, have an improved survival compared with patients who require an ICD shock.[17]

## VT: METHODS OF MAPPING AND ABLATION

In the setting of structural heart disease, reentry is the most common mechanism for sustained monomorphic VT. Reentry requires a discrete, protected zone of slow conduction within a region of dense scar. The exit site of the circuit is consistently located at the border zone of the scar. Concealed entrainment and substrate mapping are helpful techniques to map and ablate reentrant VT.

Concealed entrainment defines a critical isthmus of the VT circuit. A hemodynamically stable VT is required to map with concealed entrainment. An adequate ablation end point requires that the tachycardia is reproducibly inducible. When pacing with ventricular capture during VT results in a QRS complex that is identical in all electrocardiogram (ECG) leads to the QRS morphology of the VT, then concealed entrainment

has been shown (**Fig. 1**). Target sites for ablation may include any site with concealed entrainment, with or without diastolic potentials and/or continuous electrograms, sites where the pacing stimulus-QRS duration is equal to that of the local electrogram-QRS duration, and where the pacing stimulus-QRS duration is 70% or less of the tachycardia cycle length.[18,19] When the clinical VT is either hemodynamically unstable or not reproducibly inducible, substrate mapping can be used. By delineating areas of scar and normal myocardium based on voltage mapping, border zones as well as a potential critical isthmus can be identified and targeted empirically during VT ablation.[20] Three-dimensional electroanatomic mapping systems allow for creation of voltage-based substrate maps, and can assist in the ablation of VT (**Fig. 2**).[21]

Because most patients with sustained monomorphic VT have coronary artery disease (CAD) and infarct-related scar, the bulk of the literature regarding VT ablation involves patients with a history of previous myocardial infarction. In the first series of 15 patients with VT and a history of previous myocardial infarction, VT ablation was found to be safe, with an 80% success rate.[22] In a later series of 52 patients with VT and a history of previous myocardial infarction, VT ablation was associated with a similar success rate, but because of the moderate success and high recurrence rates, the investigators concluded that VT ablation was largely adjunctive to antiarrhythmic agents and ICDs in this population. Moreover, the procedure-related mortality was 2%.[23] More recently, a multicenter series of 231 patients with recurrent monomorphic VT and previous myocardial infarction, showed that VT ablation when using a saline-cooled irrigated catheter combined with an electroanatomic mapping system was associated with a 53% freedom from recurrent VT at 6 months. with a procedure-related mortality of 3%.[24]

VT ablation has been extended to treatment of patients with various forms of nonischemic cardiomyopathy. Sustained monomorphic VT is an uncommon clinical finding in patients with dilated nonischemic cardiomyopathy: there are limited data regarding catheter ablation in this patient population. The largest series includes 28 patients with dilated cardiomyopathy and recurrent sustained monomorphic VT, and showed a 54% success rate with VT ablation.[25] Patients with arrhythmogenic right ventricular dysplasia (ARVD) often present with VT and ICD shocks. A series of 24 patients with ARVD undergoing catheter ablation for treatment of VT found an acute success rate of 77%, but was associated with an

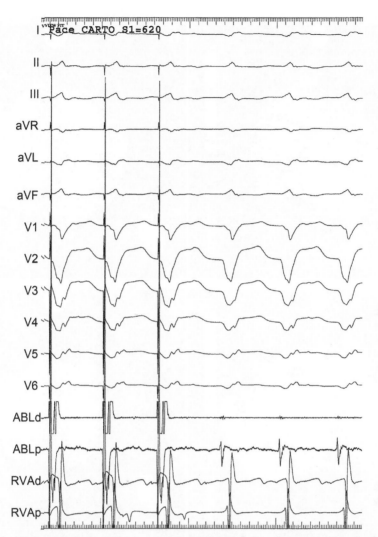

**Fig. 1.** Concealed entrainment during VT at successful ablation site. From top to bottom, the following recordings are displayed: a standard 12-lead ECG (leads I–V6), the distal and proximal ablation electrode pairs (ABLd and ABLp, respectively), and the distal and proximal right ventricular apical electrode pairs (RVAd and RVAp, respectively). Pacing during VT resulted in a paced 12-lead ECG QRS morphology that is identical to the 12-lead ECG QRS morphology during VT. The postpacing interval is nearly identical to the tachycardia cycle length. The stimulus-QRS interval is 0 milliseconds, and is equal to the electrogram-QRS interval during VT. A short stimulus-QRS interval is a marker of a good target site. Ablation at this site resulted in termination of VT.

85% recurrence rate.[26] There are limited data on catheter ablation of VT associated with Chagas disease. The largest series of 31 patients with a history of sustained VT and Chagas disease undergoing VT ablation reported a 70% success rate.[27]

Generally, VT ablation is performed with an endocardial approach with radiofrequency (RF) energy. However, in some patients, an epicardial approach may be necessary for successful ablation of VT.[28] In a series of 28 patients with dilated cardiomyopathy, 25% of the patients required an epicardial approach to achieve success ablation

of VT.[25] Intracoronary mapping with antiarrhythmic drugs and intracoronary infusion of ethanol for ablation of VT has also been used, although rarely.[29]

Traditionally, VT mapping and ablation have been performed with 4-mm-tip catheters, using standard temperature-controlled RF ablation. Larger 8- and 10-mm-tip catheters allow for larger lesion sizes, but compromise electrogram precision. An irrigated saline-cooled 3.5-mm-tip catheter allows for precise mapping afforded with smaller electrodes, larger lesions, and an improved acute success rate.[30,31]

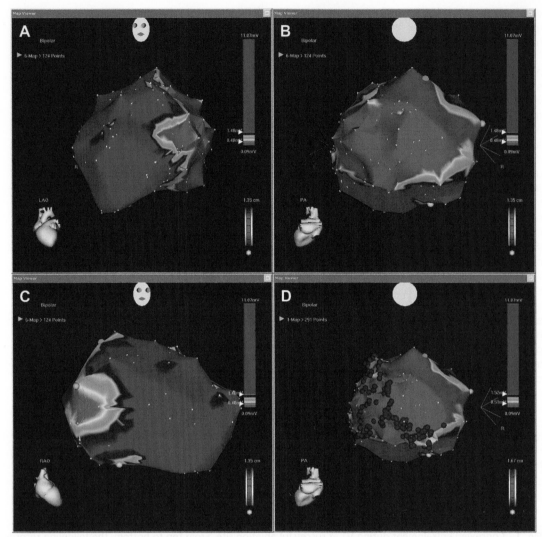

**Fig. 2.** (*A–D*) Voltage-guided substrate mapping and ablation of VT. (*A*) LAO view. (*B*) Posterior view. (*C*) RAO view. (*D*) Posterior view with ablation points marked with red dots. Ablation was performed in the left ventricle at the border zones between the large posterior scar (*red*) and healthy viable myocardium (*purple*), as well as within the posterior scar. LAO, left anterior oblique; RAO, right anterior oblique.

## ROLE OF VT ABLATION TO REDUCE ICD SHOCKS

RF ablation of VT is recommended in patients with frequent ICD shocks or electrical storm.[32] In the first study of patients with coronary disease and an ICD with frequent shocks, VT ablation had a reasonable success rate, significantly reduced ICD therapies, and was associated with an improved quality of life.[33] In that study of 21 patients, VT was successfully ablated in 76% of patients, with a reduction of ICD shocks from 60 per month to 0.1 per month at 1 year of follow-up. If the VT was hemodynamically stable and reproducibly inducible, the success rate

was approximately 90%.[33] In patients with an ICD who had recurrent VT or VF, VT ablation also led to an improved quality of life compared with treatment with amiodarone.[34]

In a prospective series of 95 patients with drug-refractory electrical storm and frequent ICD shocks, VT ablation acutely suppressed electrical storm in all patients. In 85% of patients, the clinical VT was not inducible after ablation. Although most of these patients had coronary disease, this study included a significant number of patients with non-ischemic dilated cardiomyopathy and ARVD. Ten patients required an epicardial approach for VT ablation. Successful VT ablation in patients in whom VT resulted in electrical storm was associated with significant improvement in cardiac mortality.[35]

Although most ICD shocks are caused by VT, VF and VF storm remain a significant cause of ICD shocks. In some patients, unifocal premature ventricular contractions (PVC) that originate in the Purkinje system trigger or induce VF.[36] In patients with idiopathic VF, PVC ablation is associated with long-term elimination of VF.[37]

VT ablation may also be considered in patients undergoing ICD implantation who have not yet received an ICD shock. The role of prophylactic VT ablation as an adjunct to ICD therapy was evaluated in the Substrate Mapping and Ablation in Sinus Rhythm to Halt Ventricular Tachycardia (SMASH-VT) trial and VTACH (Ventricular Tachycardia before Defibrillator Implantation in Patients with Coronary Heart Disease) trials.[38,39] In SMASH-VT, 128 patients with previous myocardial infarction, undergoing ICD implantation for either a primary or secondary prevention indication, were randomized to either an ICD alone or an ICD plus VT ablation. The group who underwent VT ablation in addition to ICD implantation had a significantly decreased number of ICD shocks compared with those patients who received ICD therapy alone. In VTACH, 110 patients with previous myocardial infarction, stable VT, and reduced LVEF were randomized either to a VT ablation and an ICD, or to an ICD. The primary end point (time to first recurrence of VT or VF) was significantly prolonged in patients also treated with VT ablation. Neither study reported a mortality benefit.

## ROLE OF VT ABLATION IN PATIENT MANAGEMENT: A SUGGESTED ALGORITHM

An approach to the management of patients with VT is presented in **Fig. 3**. In a patient with a history of sustained VT who is planning to undergo ICD implantation, it seems reasonable to perform VT ablation as an adjunct to ICD at the time of implant. For primary prevention of SCD, it seems reasonable to proceed with ICD implantation alone.

VT ablation should be considered a reasonable alternative to antiarrhythmic medications in patients who receive an initial ICD shock for VT. In patients with frequent episodes of VT despite antiarrhythmic medications, VT ablation is clearly indicated. ATP therapy should be activated in all patients undergoing ICD implantation. In certain high-risk groups, such as patients with severe atherosclerotic disease of the aorta and iliac arteries, mechanical aortic and/or mitral valves, left ventricular assist devices, and/or a history of left ventricular thrombus, attempts should be

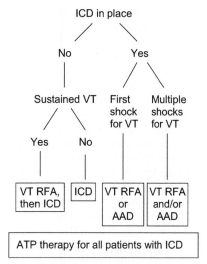

**Fig. 3.** Algorithm for management of the patient with VT and ICD shocks. AAD, antiarrhythmic drug; RFA, radiofrequency ablation.

made to maximize medical therapy before consideration of VT ablation.

## SUMMARY

Patients with an ICD receive appropriate ICD shocks for VT, and less frequently for VF. Frequent ICD shocks can have adverse cardiac affects, lead to increased pain, anxiety, and a decreased quality of life, and possibly increase mortality. Pharmacologic attempts at reducing ICD shocks have had modest results, with frequent discontinuation because of side effects.

VT ablation is an effective tool to reduce the frequency of VT and ICD shocks. This benefit has been seen in patients with ischemic and non-ischemic cardiomyopathy. Based on available evidence, VT ablation is a reasonable treatment option in patients with frequent ICD shocks caused by VT. VT ablation may also be considered in patients with an initial ICD shock or as a prophylactic treatment at the time of ICD placement in patients with a history of sustained VT.

## REFERENCES

1. Mishkin JD, Saxonhouse SJ, Woo GW, et al. Appropriate evaluation and treatment of heart failure patients after implantable cardioverter-defibrillator discharge: time to go beyond the initial shock. J Am Coll Cardiol 2009;54(22):1993–2000.
2. Poole JE, Johnson GW, Hellkamp AS, et al. Prognostic importance of defibrillator shocks in patients with heart failure. N Engl J Med 2008;359(10):1009–17.

3. Moss AJ, Greenberg H, Case RB, et al. Multicenter Automatic Defibrillator Implantation Trial-II (MADIT-II) Research Group. Long-term clinical course of patients after termination of ventricular tachyarrhythmia by an implanted defibrillator. Circulation 2004;110(25):3760–5.

4. The Antiarrhythmics versus Implantable Defibrillators (AVID) Investigators. A comparison of antiarrhythmic-drug therapy with implantable defibrillators in patients resuscitated from near-fatal ventricular arrhythmias. N Engl J Med 1997;337(22):1576–83.

5. Sesselberg HW, Moss AJ, McNitt S, et al. MADIT-II Research Group. Ventricular arrhythmia storms in postinfarction patients with implantable defibrillators for primary prevention indications: a MADIT-II sub-study. Heart Rhythm 2007;4(11):1395–402.

6. Exner DV, Pinski SL, Wyse DG, et al. Electrical storm presages nonsudden death: the antiarrhythmics versus implantable defibrillators (AVID) trial. Circulation 2001;103(16):2066–71.

7. Hurst TM, Hinrichs M, Breidenbach C, et al. Detection of myocardial injury during transvenous implantation of automatic cardioverter-defibrillators. J Am Coll Cardiol 1999;34(2):402–8.

8. Domanski MJ, Exner DV, Borkowf CB, et al. Effect of angiotensin converting enzyme inhibition on sudden cardiac death in patients following acute myocardial infarction. A meta-analysis of randomized clinical trials. J Am Coll Cardiol 1999;33(3):598–604.

9. Brodine WN, Tung RT, Lee JK, et al. MADIT-II Research Group. Effects of beta-blockers on implantable cardioverter defibrillator therapy and survival in the patients with ischemic cardiomyopathy (from the Multicenter Automatic Defibrillator Implantation Trial-II). Am J Cardiol 2005;96(5):691–5.

10. Pacifico A, Hohnloser SH, Williams JH, et al. Prevention of implantable-defibrillator shocks by treatment with sotalol. d, l-Sotalol Implantable Cardioverter-Defibrillator Study Group. N Engl J Med 1999; 340(24):1855–62.

11. Connolly SJ, Dorian P, Roberts RS, et al. Optimal Pharmacological Therapy in Cardioverter Defibrillator Patients (OPTIC) Investigators. Comparison of beta-blockers, amiodarone plus beta-blockers, or sotalol for prevention of shocks from implantable cardioverter defibrillators: the OPTIC Study: a randomized trial. JAMA 2006;295(2):165–71.

12. Klein GJ, Gillberg JM, Tang A, et al. Worldwide Wave Investigators. Improving SVT discrimination in single-chamber ICDs: a new electrogram morphology-based algorithm. J Cardiovasc Electrophysiol 2006;17(12):1310–9.

13. Wilkoff BL, Williamson BD, Stern RS, et al. PREPARE Study Investigators. Strategic programming of detection and therapy parameters in implantable cardioverter-defibrillators reduces shocks in primary prevention patients: results from the PREPARE (Primary Prevention Parameters Evaluation) study. J Am Coll Cardiol 2008;52(7):541–50.

14. Peinado R, Almendral J, Rius T, et al. Randomized, prospective comparison of four burst pacing algorithms for spontaneous ventricular tachycardia. Am J Cardiol 1998;82(11):1422–5, A8–9.

15. Wathen MS, Sweeney MO, DeGroot PJ, et al. Pain-FREE Investigators. Shock reduction using antitachycardia pacing for spontaneous rapid ventricular tachycardia in patients with coronary artery disease. Circulation 2001;104(7):796–801.

16. Wathen MS, DeGroot PJ, Sweeney MO, et al. Pain-FREE Rx II Investigators. Prospective randomized multicenter trial of empirical antitachycardia pacing versus shocks for spontaneous rapid ventricular tachycardia in patients with implantable cardioverter-defibrillators: Pacing Fast Ventricular Tachycardia Reduces Shock Therapies (PainFREE Rx II) trial results. Circulation 2004;110(17):2591–6.

17. Sweeney MO, Sherfesee L, Degroot PJ, et al. Differences in effects of electrical therapy type for ventricular arrhythmias on mortality in implantable cardioverter-defibrillator patients. Heart Rhythm 2010;7(3):353–60.

18. Morady F, Kadish A, Rosenheck S, et al. Concealed entrainment as a guide for catheter ablation of ventricular tachycardia in patients with prior myocardial infarction. J Am Coll Cardiol 1991; 17(3):678–89.

19. Stevenson WG, Khan H, Sager P, et al. Identification of reentry circuit sites during catheter mapping and radiofrequency ablation of ventricular tachycardia late after myocardial infarction. Circulation 1993;88: 1647–70.

20. Hsia HH, Lin D, Sauer WH, et al. Anatomic characterization of endocardial substrate for hemodynamically stable reentrant ventricular tachycardia: identification of endocardial conducting channels. Heart Rhythm 2006;3(5):503–12.

21. Strickberger SA, Knight BP, Michaud GF, et al. Mapping and ablation of ventricular tachycardia guided by virtual electrograms using a noncontact, computerized mapping system. J Am Coll Cardiol 2000;35(2):414–21.

22. Morady F, Harvey M, Kalbfleisch SJ, et al. Radiofrequency catheter ablation of ventricular tachycardia in patients with coronary artery disease. Circulation 1993;87(2):363–72.

23. Stevenson WG, Friedman PL, Kocovic D, et al. Radiofrequency catheter ablation of ventricular tachycardia after myocardial infarction. Circulation 1998; 98(4):308–14.

24. Stevenson WG, Wilber DJ, Natale A, et al. Multicenter Thermocool VT Ablation Trial Investigators. Irrigated radiofrequency catheter ablation guided by electroanatomic mapping for recurrent ventricular tachycardia after myocardial infarction: the

Multicenter Thermocool Ventricular Tachycardia Ablation Trial. Circulation 2008;118(25):2773–82.

25. Soejima K, Stevenson WG, Sapp JL, et al. Endocardial and epicardial radiofrequency ablation of ventricular tachycardia associated with dilated cardiomyopathy: the importance of low-voltage scars. J Am Coll Cardiol 2004;43(10):1834–42.

26. Dalal D, Jain R, Tandri H, et al. Long-term efficacy of catheter ablation of ventricular tachycardia in patients with arrhythmogenic right ventricular dysplasia/cardiomyopathy. J Am Coll Cardiol 2007; 50(5):432–40.

27. Távora MZ, Mehta N, Silva RM, et al. Characteristics and identification of sites of chagasic ventricular tachycardia by endocardial mapping. Arq Bras Cardiol 1999;72(4):451–74.

28. Sosa E, Scanavacca M, D'Avila A, et al. Endocardial and epicardial ablation guided by nonsurgical transthoracic epicardial mapping to treat recurrent ventricular tachycardia. J Cardiovasc Electrophysiol 1998;9(3):229–39.

29. Brugada P, de Swart H, Smeets JL, et al. Transcoronary chemical ablation of ventricular tachycardia. Circulation 1989;79:475–82.

30. Calkins H, Epstein A, Packer D, et al. Catheter ablation of ventricular tachycardia in patients with structural heart disease using cooled radiofrequency energy: results of a prospective multicenter study. Cooled RF Multi Center Investigators Group. J Am Coll Cardiol 2000;35(7):1905–14.

31. Soejima K, Delacretaz E, Suzuki M, et al. Saline-cooled versus standard radiofrequency catheter ablation for infarct-related ventricular tachycardias. Circulation 2001;103(14):1858–62.

32. Aliot EM, Stevenson WG, Almendral-Garrote JM, et al. EHRA/HRS Expert Consensus on Catheter Ablation of Ventricular Arrhythmias: developed in a partnership with the European Heart Rhythm Association (EHRA), a Registered Branch of the European Society of Cardiology (ESC), and the Heart Rhythm Society (HRS); in collaboration with the American College of Cardiology (ACC) and the American Heart Association (AHA). Heart Rhythm 2009;6(6):886–933.

33. Strickberger SA, Man KC, Daoud EG, et al. A prospective evaluation of catheter ablation of ventricular tachycardia as adjuvant therapy in patients with coronary artery disease and an implantable cardioverter-defibrillator. Circulation 1997;96(5):1525–31.

34. Calkins H, Bigger JT Jr, Ackerman SJ, et al. Cost-effectiveness of catheter ablation in patients with ventricular tachycardia. Circulation 2000;101(3): 280–8.

35. Carbucicchio C, Santamaria M, Trevisi N, et al. Catheter ablation for the treatment of electrical storm in patients with implantable cardioverter-defibrillators: short- and long-term outcomes in a prospective single-center study. Circulation 2008;117(4):462–9.

36. Haïssaguerre M, Shoda M, Jaïs P, et al. Mapping and ablation of idiopathic ventricular fibrillation. Circulation 2002;106(8):962–7.

37. Knecht S, Sacher F, Wright M, et al. Long-term follow-up of idiopathic ventricular fibrillation ablation: a multicenter study. J Am Coll Cardiol 2009;54(6): 522–8.

38. Reddy VY, Reynolds MR, Neuzil P, et al. Prophylactic catheter ablation for the prevention of defibrillator therapy. N Engl J Med 2007;357(26):2657–65.

39. Kuck KH, Schaumann A, Eckardt L, et al. VTACH study group. Catheter ablation of stable ventricular tachycardia before defibrillator implantation in patients with coronary heart disease (VTACH): a multicentre randomised controlled trial. Lancet 2010; 375(9708):31–40.

# Device Features for Managing Patients with Heart Failure

Niraj Varma, MA, DM, FRCP*, Bruce Wilkoff, MD, FHRS

**KEYWORDS**

• Heart failure • Monitoring • Follow-up • Remote monitoring

Hospitalizations for acute decompensated heart failure (ADHF) have more than doubled in the past 20 years and continue to increase.[1] More than 75% of patients with ADHF have a previous history of heart failure, which has significant sequelae for patient morbidity. Patients with preserved left ventricular systolic function have a slightly lower in-hospital mortality (2.9%) than those with a left ventricular ejection fraction of less than 40% (3.9%). However, 3-month mortalities are similar for both groups (9.5% vs 9.8%, respectively). Rehospitalization rates remain as high as 30% for patients with both preserved and decreased left ventricular systolic function, and rehospitalization is an independent predictor of 1-year mortality, especially in elderly patients.[2,3] In addition, patients with ADHF are at greater risk for death and morbidity than those with stable chronic heart failure,[4] which has fiscal repercussions for health care services. In 2006, more than $30 billion were spent on heart failure care, of which almost 60% was related to in-hospital care.

The development of ADHF is complex. It involves several processes, which may include hemodynamic, neurohumoral, electrophysiological, and vascular abnormalities that converge to manifest with fluid congestion. Elevation of ventricular diastolic pressures with worsening dilatation and remodeling, development of functional mitral regurgitation, decreased coronary perfusion, and the development of renal insufficiency may contribute singly or in combination. After hospitalization, management is directed to identification and correction of precipitating factors and comorbidities, and management of fluid overload, arrhythmias, and any conduction system problems. Repeated cycles of ADHF each may result in myocardial injury, ultimately leading to progressive chronic heart failure. Thus, a history of repeated episodes of decompensation requiring hospitalization despite best medical therapy portends a poorer prognosis. Therapeutic interventions aimed at interrupting this sequence of events are potentially valuable. This strategy may be possible because, in most cases, pathophysiologic processes progress over days to weeks before clinical presentation with a fluid-overloaded state. However, the initial inciting events may vary and therefore early detection remains challenging.

## DEVICES

Implantable devices may permit identification of upstream factors triggering heart failure deterioration.

A large number of patients with heart failure receive implants in response to widening indications.[5] For example, prophylactic implantable cardioverter defibrillators (ICDs) and cardiac resynchronization therapy devices (CRTs) are implanted in populations vulnerable to not only arrhythmias but also ADHF. Examination of stored information regarding atrial and ventricular arrhythmias and device function may facilitate diagnosis and direct appropriate treatment. These data are routinely quantified in device diagnostics. Additional features may also report conditions (eg,

Cardiac Pacing and Electrophysiology, Department of Cardiovascular Medicine, Cleveland Clinic, 9500 Euclid Avenue, Cleveland, OH 44195, USA
* Corresponding author.
*E-mail address:* varman@ccf.org

fluid overload) that reflect the stability of patients with heart failure. The following cases illustrate these points.

## Case 1

This middle-aged man had a long-standing history of ischemic cardiomyopathy and left bundle branch block treated with a CRT. He had had several bouts of atrial fibrillation requiring cardioversion and then had been maintained on dofetilide. The patient had felt lassitude and worsening shortness of breath in the face of unchanged daily weights or worsening edema for several weeks. However, he contacted providers late only when fluid congestion started to occur.

At outpatient evaluation, he was found to have both atrial fibrillation and congestive heart failure and was admitted for treatment with diuretics. Device interrogation showed several notable features (**Fig. 1**). The patient had developed atrial fibrillation before development of heart failure symptoms. Rapid ventricular conduction during atrial fibrillation sometimes led to loss of biventricular pacing. Device-retrieved data recorded reduced patient activity and progressive fluid accumulation. He was treated with diuretics and cardioverted. He subsequently relapsed, with similar episodes of ADHF precipitated by atrial fibrillation, and underwent ablative therapy for atrial fibrillation. His condition stabilized.

## Case 2

This patient with ischemic cardiomyopathy and underlying conduction system disorder (QRS duration >120 ms) had been treated with a prophylactic dual-chamber ICD. He had remained very stable (New York Heart Association [NYHA] II) for several years but then presented with shortness of breath, weight gain, and edema. In the outpatient clinic, he was found to be having atrial fibrillation. His electrocardiogram showed continuous right ventricular pacing (**Fig. 2A**). Device interrogation indicated that atrial fibrillation had developed 50 days earlier and had persisted (see **Fig. 2B**). In this case (in contrast to Case 1), average ventricular rate did not change but the percentage of ventricular pacing increased from 0% to greater than 50%, because atrioventricular nodal conduction diminished during atrial fibrillation causing loss of intrinsic conduction and initiation of back up ventricular pacing. Patient activity diminished. An asymptomatic episode of ventricular tachycardia (VT) occurred during atrial fibrillation and was treated successfully with anti-tachycardia pacing (see **Fig. 2C**).

These two cases illustrate how stored device data may direct diagnosis and treatment of heart failure precipitants. Although both patients presented with fatigue, shortness of breath, and fluid congestion, these symptoms had resulted from different processes and could be resolved through attention to several parameters tracked over time and accurately quantified with device diagnostics. In particular, these included asymptomatic events, such as atrial fibrillation, occurrence of right ventricular pacing, or lack of biventricular pacing. These examples showed the interplay of several factors that contributed to heart failure decompensation and the length of time taken from an inciting event to clinical presentation.

## ATRIAL FIBRILLATION

Atrial fibrillation in patients with heart failure may be associated with increased morbidity and mortality,[6,7] and is likely multifactorial, involving increased risk of heart failure and stroke, and possibly facilitation of ventricular arrhythmias. Atrial fibrillation may precipitate ADHF by adversely affecting ventricular hemodynamics. In the illustrated patients, atrial fibrillation exerted very separate effects and on the function of the implanted devices. In Case 1 with a CRT, atrial fibrillation was associated with periods of rapid conduction, which resulted in withdrawal of ventricular pacing. In Case 2, atrial fibrillation reduced ventricular conduction, an effect of a concealed conduction block in the atrioventricular node, and engaged ventricular back up pacing from the dual chamber cardioverter defibrillator.

## RIGHT VENTRICULAR PACING

Unnecessary right ventricular pacing (RVP), even when atrioventricular synchrony was preserved, increased hospitalization for heart failure and worsened mortality.[8] These effects were manifestations of the deleterious effects of ventricular desynchronization promoted by RVP. The mechanism likely involves electrical partitioning of the left ventricle into early- and late-activated areas generating mechanical inefficiencies, with redistribution of mechanical work, perfusion, and oxygen demand. This process initiates adverse remodeling, particularly in late-activated areas (ie, the inferolateral basal left ventricle).[9] Greater left ventricular activation delay correlates with development of left ventricular dysfunction and heart failure hospitalizations. Delays are accentuated with wider baseline QRS durations during intrinsic conduction, as in Case 2.[10] Thus, RVP during left ventricular dysfunction with preexisting left bundle

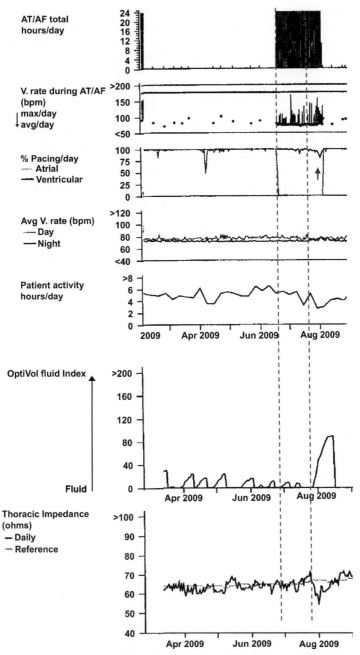

**Fig. 1.** Device diagnostic data from interrogation. An episode of persistent atrial fibrillation (atrial fibrillation hours per day) is illustrated. Note initiation toward the end of June (*first vertical blue dashed line*) marked by withdrawal of atrial pacing, although presentation with clinical decompensation occurred 6 weeks later in August. A steeper rate of deterioration in parameters is marked by the second vertical blue dashed line in the 2 to 3 weeks preceding hospitalization. These instances were characterized by longer bursts of accelerated ventricular rates, greater loss of biventricular pacing to approximately 80% (*arrow*), diminished patient activity, and progressively increasing intrathoracic impedance (Optivol fluid index). This index is derived from the difference between the daily and reference intrathoracic impedance (*bottom graph*) and may reflect accumulation of fluid in the thorax. Prompt resolution in all these parameters occurred after treatment of atrial fibrillation. (*From* Varma N. Automatic remote monitoring of implantable cardiac devices in heart failure: the TRUST trial. Journal of Innovations in Cardiac Rhythm Management 2010;1:22–9; with permission.)

branch block had severe clinical effects (increased mortality and hospitalization).[11] Increased electrical dispersion may contribute to the occurrence of increased ventricular arrhythmia in this group.[12,13] If pacing is necessary in patients with heart failure, it may be best performed through atrial pacing without right ventricular stimulation, thus avoiding deleterious effects of RVP. This effect was shown in the Dual Chamber and VVI Implantable Defibrillator (DAVID) II and Inhibition of Unnecessary RV Pacing With AVSH in ICDs (INTRINSIC) studies.[14,15] Algorithms designed to minimize right ventricular paced burden[16] reduced the incidence of heart failure hospitalizations in patients with depressed left ventricular function. In Case 2, the patient was treated with anticoagulation, dofetilide, cardioversion, and reprogramming to ensure atrial pacing permitting intrinsic

conduction. Development of permanent atrial fibrillation, committing this patient to right ventricular apical pacing, would merit upgrade to CRT, especially if the patient redevelops NYHA functional class III symptoms.[5]

## CRT

CRT has a significant clinical effect in patients with congestive heart failure and intraventricular conduction delay. Incidence of heart failure hospitalization and mortality are reduced and this effect is incremental to best medical therapy.[17] Improved patient status requires maintenance of pacing. The performance of the left ventricular lead may vary. In some devices, left ventricular pacing thresholds may be self-monitored at regular intervals and stimulus auto-adjusted accordingly. Recent studies

**A**

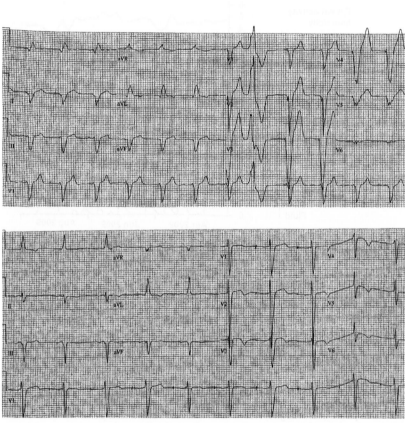

**Fig. 2.** (*A*) Electrocardiogram at presentation (*top*) shows atrial fibrillation and continuous pacing from the right ventricular pacing electrode. Electrocardiogram at resolution (*bottom*), after treatment of atrial fibrillation and commencement of anti-arrhythmic therapy. Atrial pacing is present, permitting intrinsic conduction, which occurs with a wide QRS configuration. (*B*) Device diagnostic data from interrogation. This illustration shows initiation of persistent atrial fibrillation in mid-October, loss of atrial pacing, and increased burden of right ventricular pacing (absent before atrial fibrillation). The patient presented almost 2 months after atrial fibrillation started, after progressive clinical deterioration recorded by "patient activity" (*bottom*). One episode of ventricular tachycardia is seen just before presentation (*top*). (*C*) Dual tachycardia. An episode of ventricular tachycardia occurring during persistent atrial fibrillation results in successful antitachycardia pacing therapy and return to atrial fibrillation with sensed ventricular conduction.

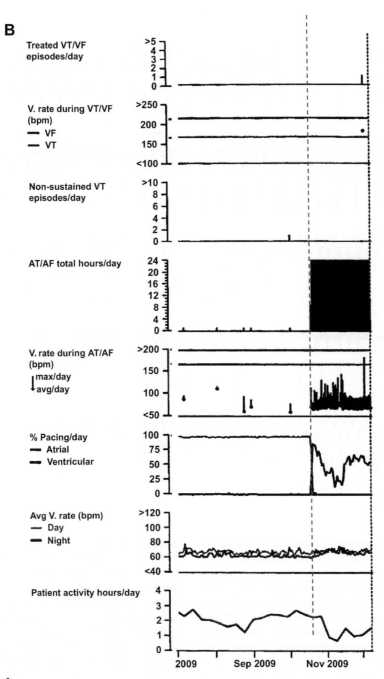

**B**

Treated VT/VF episodes/day

V. rate during VT/VF (bpm)
— VF
— VT

Non-sustained VT episodes/day

AT/AF total hours/day

V. rate during AT/AF (bpm)
↑max/day
↓avg/day

% Pacing/day
— Atrial
— Ventricular

Avg V. rate (bpm)
— Day
— Night

Patient activity hours/day

2009      Sep 2009      Nov 2009

**Fig. 2.** (*continued*)

indicate that diminution of pacing to less than 92% (because of atrial fibrillation or significant ventricular ectopy) may cause loss of beneficial effect.[18] Thus, atrial fibrillation with a rapid ventricular response in Case 1 promoted loss of biventricular stimulation, which may have been a significant contributor to ADHF. Different manufacturers use several mechanisms to promote continuous CRT delivery under these conditions. For example, each right ventricular sensed event may trigger a paced response immediately (within 10 ms) in one or both ventricles, depending on how ventricular pacing is programmed. During atrial tachyarrhythmias, the device may be programmed to increase pacing rate in concert with the patient's ventricular response (Conducted AF Response,

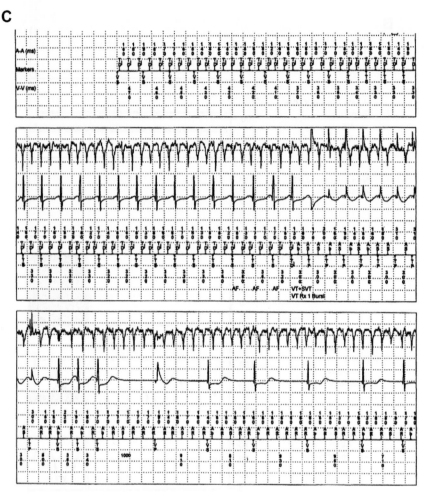

**Fig. 2.** (*continued*)

Medtronic, Minneapolis, Minnesota). This function regularizes the ventricular rate through adjusting the pacing escape interval after each ventricular event. The escape interval increases or decreases depending on whether the preceding events were paced or sensed. Through dynamically matching the patient's own response, the device can increase the percentage of ventricular pacing with minimal increase in daily average heart rate. Another feature designed to preserve CRT delivery during premature ventricular contractions or rapid 1:1 sinus rhythm is atrial tracking recovery. If the device recognizes a sensing pattern suitable for intervention, it temporarily shortens post ventricular atrial refractory period to regain atrial tracking.

The response to CRT may be affected by programmed atrioventricular or interventricular delay. No uniform method of optimizing these intervals exists. In practice, they may be assigned arbitrarily (nominal setting), through Doppler echocardiography measurements of mitral inflow or aortic outflow velocities, or using calculations based on intracardiac electrograms. Intervals optimized with these techniques may differ between atrial sensing and pacing in the same individual. In one study comparing these techniques, the optimal atrioventricular interval varied markedly among patients.[19] Arbitrarily assigned values or those determined by the Ritter method (ie, representing a large proportion of clinical practice) were found to have significant limitations. An electrogram-based method that has the goal of achieving fusion between intrinsic activation through preserved right bundle branch fibers and left ventricular paced wavefronts was associated with superior left ventricular hemodynamic improvement in acute studies.[19] This technique may avoid extensive perturbation of right ventricular and septal activation.[20] Development of dynamic automatic optimization that accommodate changing degrees of atrioventricular nodal conduction and atrial pacing may enhance CRT effect.

These conditions illustrate that heart failure is a dynamic process and patients who undergo CRT require close attention and optimization.[21] A mechanism of early notification of loss of CRT paced effect (which is usually asymptomatic) through remote monitoring may provide information for preemptive intervention (discussed later). Interest has been shown in expanding indications of CRT, an important heart failure therapy, to other groups. CRT prevented ADHF in NYHA class 1 and II patients with left ventricular conduction delay.[22] However, CRT had no beneficial effect in patients with narrow QRS duration.[23] In these patients, when intermittent ventricular pacing is required, the threshold of right ventricular paced burden and characteristics of ventricular dyssynchrony meriting CRT upgrade remains unclear. Guidelines consider CRT as reasonable in patients with LVEF of 35% or less, with NYHA functional class III or ambulatory class IV symptoms, who are receiving optimal recommended medical therapy and have frequent dependence on ventricular pacing.[5]

## VENTRICULAR ARRHYTHMIA

Atrial fibrillation may facilitate ventricular arrhythmias either directly from tachycardia-induced changes in ventricular refractoriness or indirectly because of hemodynamic alterations, ischemia, or neurohumoral activation, which facilitate induction in these patients. The irregular rhythm of atrial fibrillation may cause short-long-short sequences, which are potentially proarrhythmic. In one study, 20% of patients that had ventricular tachycardia/ ventricular fibrillation (VT/VF) events during follow-up had at least one dual tachycardia episode. Prompt termination of atrial tachyarrhythmia significantly delayed the time to the next episode of VT/VF.[24] Increased electrical dispersion may contribute to the increased ventricular arrhythmia incidence observed in patients committed to right ventricular pacing.[12,13] In Case 2, VT was successfully treated with pacing, but further episodes may have warranted shock therapy. This possibility is important because emerging data indicate that shock delivery may have deleterious long-term consequences.[25,26] Early recognition of nonsustained runs presaging shock therapy may provide an opportunity to improve patient outcomes.[27]

## FLUID DETECTION

Heart failure precipitants (atrial fibrillation and pacing in these cases) act to converge on the common pathway of fluid congestion, causing patients to present with dyspnea or peripheral edema. However, these symptoms and signs usually appear late in the development of ADHF. Logic suggests that a mechanism for early detection of excess fluid or elevated cardiac filling pressures before evidence of edema or pulmonary congestion may provide an opportunity for early preemptive therapy. Hence, guidelines (American College of Cardiology/American Heart Association/Heart Failure Society of America[28]) recommend that patients obtain a scale and follow their weight at home after hospitalization for a heart failure. However, trials have shown this technique of self-reported body weight to have variable success.[29–32] Some implantable devices (LATITUDE, Boston Scientific, Natick, MA, USA) enable blood pressure (and weight) data to be transmitted weekly. A confounding issue is that changes in body weight may not be reliable over time because of changing nonfluid contributions.

Device-based monitoring may be more effective. Decreased electrical impedance between the right ventricular lead and a device may indicate increases in lung water secondary to fluid overload. Intrathoracic impedance measured this way in **Fig. 1** showed an interesting trend. In a trial, impedance correlated inversely with pulmonary capillary wedge pressures in hospitalized patients[33] and began decreasing approximately 2 weeks before hospitalization for ADHF. Because fluid sensors report consequences of hemodynamic deterioration, monitors designed specifically for primary detection of hemodynamic deviation itself may enable earlier detection of ADHF. For example, in the COMPASS-HF trial, 274 patients with class III or IV heart failure were implanted with a lead to measure pulmonary artery pressure. Use of these data tended to reduce heart failure hospitalizations.[34] A new miniature fully implantable device permits wireless monitoring of pulmonary artery pressure curves.[35] Direct left atrial pressure monitoring with a novel implantable device in ambulatory patients with heart failure was well tolerated, feasible, and accurate during short-term follow-up.[36] Impedance vectors using a left ventricular lead may improve monitoring capability.[37]

These sensors merit testing in clinical trials.[38] To be effective, they must have a high predictive value for ADHF requiring hospitalization, and also enable implementation of a treatment algorithm that may prevent hospitalization. In this regard, preliminary data are modest. For example, fluid sensors showed 60% sensitivity with 60% positive predictive value for detecting hospitalization. The false-positive rate was 38%.[39] The sensor is vulnerable to confounding factors, such as pneumonia, atrial fibrillation, and pocket edema.

Results are awaited from large prospective randomized outcome trials assessing the effect on patients with heart failure managed with versus without information on intrathoracic impedance. Application of stand-alone technology as long-term management to a large number of patients with heart failure in whom conventional devices are not currently indicated remains unclear.

## HEART RATE VARIABILITY

Heart rate variability (HRV) reflects degree of vagal cardiac autonomic control and may be derived from implantable devices (although this was not available in illustrated cases). Reduced variability indicates vagal withdrawal and an autonomic balance. The absolute value of standard deviation of 5-minute median atrial–atrial intervals (SDAAM) and its change over time are important markers of clinical stability.[40] Continuously measured SDAAM increased with CRT, indicating a significant change in autonomic control of the heart. Devices with implanted leads facilitate HRV calculations through continuous measurements of atrial-to-atrial depolarization intervals during a predominance of sinus rhythm. In one study of 288 patients with class III–IV heart failure, decreased HRV was observed 16 days before clinical decompensation.[41] The measure cannot be derived during atrial fibrillation or if atrial pacing is required for more than 80% of the 24 hours. Continuous, device-based heart rate variability (measured via direct patient contact or remotely [see later discussion]) may enable identification of future clinical decompensation, but this requires prospective evaluation of change-detection algorithms.

## DEVICE-BASED REMOTE MONITORING: EARLY DETECTION

Preemptive treatment of ADHF hinges on early evaluation of parameter deviation from baseline values. Problem detection using an implanted device without concomitant physician notification is ineffective for enabling early therapeutic intervention, as shown in the illustrated cases. This issue is an inherent limitation associated with asymptomatic events characteristic of most of the trigger factors for ADHF. Valuable diagnostic data remain concealed for extended periods and are available only on interrogation, such as when patients present with ADHF or for routine follow-up. Intensive patient surveillance with increased frequency of face-to-face encounters between physicians and patients is generally not feasible, and in any case, no monitoring occurs between hospital visits (ie, most of the time). A mechanism for performing intensive device surveillance without overburdening device clinics is desirable; this role may be fulfilled through remote monitoring. Available technologies are in various developmental phases and have different capabilities and modes of operation.[42–44]

Wand-based systems require patient-driven communication via telephone connections to monitoring facilities.[42,44] This process requires patients to operate some form of programmer at home and coordinate with clinic personnel to ensure communication and transmission. These systems are cumbersome, time consuming (which challenges compliance), and likely to overlook asymptomatic events, thus yielding late detection.[45] In contrast, an automatic transmission mechanism fully independent of patient or physician interaction has considerable advantages. This technology uses automatic (cellular- or landline-based) data transmissions, which may be reviewed securely via the Internet. A low-power radiofrequency transmitter integrated within the pulse generator wirelessly transmits stored data on a daily basis to a mobile transceiver (typically placed bedside at night). The communicator relays this wirelessly or via landline to a service center, which generates customized summary trends, charts, parameters, and electrograms. The physician may review these reports online via secure Internet access. Service center processing and data upload on the Web page are automatic, bypassing the potential delays (and errors) associated with manual processing. Thus, daily patient monitoring occurs between scheduled face-to-face device interrogations.

The system also fulfils the role of a monitoring tool because it is continuously (and not intermittently) active. Critical event data may be transmitted immediately and flagged for attention. Automatic alerts can occur for silent but potentially dangerous events (with no patient or nurse involvement), such as device/lead failure, onset of asymptomatic arrhythmia, or acute deviation of a monitored parameter from chronic trends. This feature allows for early notification, enabling prompt clinical intervention if necessary. Technology reliability and early notification ability of this type of communication system (Home Monitoring, Biotronik, Berlin, Germany) have been excellent.[43]

Remote monitoring holds several promises. Automatic technology was tested prospectively in patients with ICDs in the Lumos-T Reduces Routine Office Device Follow-Up (TRUST) trial.[46] Its application allowed an approximately 50% reduction in face-to-face scheduled and unscheduled hospital evaluations.[47] The balance of hospital visits shifted from scheduled in-person evaluations (which were largely nonactionable) to exception-based care. This reduction was accomplished safely without detrimental effect in patient morbidity or mortality. Despite fewer face-to-face encounters, the system permitted earlier detection and physician evaluation (median <2 days) of cardiac or device problems, even when asymptomatic,[48] including advent of arrhythmias or departure from established trended values. Continuous monitoring did not lead to data overload; the median number of event notifications in 1 year of follow-up was fewer than 2 per patient, indicating that daily interrogation did not lead to distracting data.[49,50] With this system, Web-based programming (ie, not requiring patient attendance and device reprogramming) provides immediate flexibility in customizing received data according to patient need.

TRUST showed that remote monitoring may be used for efficient management of a large patient volume with implanted devices by reducing unnecessary routine evaluation yet, performing intensive surveillance and acting as an early detection mechanism to enable earlier evaluations of patients when necessary. These characteristics are suited to managing patients with heart failure. The ability to self-declare out-of-range asymptomatic events is critical to allow timely intervention. For instance, in the illustrated figures, notification of atrial fibrillation, loss of CRT, increase in right ventricular paced burden, incidence of ventricular arrhythmia, and deviation of fluid sensor index all occurred asymptomatically before presentation of heart failure. All would have triggered immediate event notifications if the implanted devices had been equipped with an automatic remote monitoring mechanism, and would have enabled early therapy to preempt ADHF. Alternatively, following physicians may have reviewed and quantified trended data in these higher-risk patients and identified important deviations of single or combined trends.[51] Minimizing inappropriate therapy through early identification of atrial arrhythmias and nonsustained ventricular arrhythmias,[27,43] and maximizing appropriate therapy through evaluating efficacy of drugs and other treatments, are important potential benefits of remote monitoring. A decrease in patient follow-up visits and early identification of problems that could, if managed expeditiously, prevent patient morbidity and hospitalization have major ramifications for health care budgets.

## FUTURE DIRECTION

Device-based physiologic information and diagnostics support the concept that several interdependent cardiovascular factors may change several days to weeks before patients present with volume overload necessitating hospitalization. Aside from arrhythmias and paced burden shifts, intrathoracic impedance, vagal withdrawal, and intracardiac hemodynamic changes may occur weeks before hospitalization. A combined risk score incorporating all of these individual factors may improve predictive value for prompt rapid preemptive therapy to prevent volume accumulation. The need for intensive and comprehensive monitoring, data management, and early notification for out-of-bounds parameters may be served through remote monitoring equipped with the capacity to automatic archive. This idea is undergoing prospective evaluation in ongoing trials.[52]

Access to Internet-based information systems provides a framework for multidisciplinary communication and collaboration, such as among electrophysiologists monitoring device function (eg, arrhythmias, paced burden) and heart failure experts, to assess diagnostic information regarding heart failure. Information sharing and multidisciplinary effort improved patient care when applied to a CRT optimization clinic.[21] This practice may be facilitated through remote monitoring interfacing with electronic medical records, thus placing all relevant data in a single central database accessible to all treating physicians. Thus, remote monitoring represents a milestone, with considerable ramifications for management of heart failure populations, especially as heart failure sensors are incorporated into existing device technology.

## REFERENCES

1. Rosamond W, Flegal K, Friday G, et al. Heart disease and stroke statistics—2007 update: a report from the American Heart Association Statistics Committee and Stroke Statistics Subcommittee. Circulation 2007;115(5):e69–171.
2. Pulignano G, Del Sindaco D, Tavazzi L, et al. Clinical features and outcomes of elderly outpatients with heart failure followed up in hospital cardiology units: data from a large nationwide cardiology database (IN-CHF Registry). Am Heart J 2002;143(1):45–55.
3. Blackledge HM, Tomlinson J, Squire IB. Prognosis for patients newly admitted to hospital with heart failure: survival trends in 12 220 index admissions in Leicestershire 1993–2001. Heart 2003;89(6): 615–20.
4. Fonarow GC, Adams KF Jr, Abraham WT, et al. Risk stratification for in-hospital mortality in acutely decompensated heart failure: classification and regression tree analysis. JAMA 2005;293(5):572–80.

5. Epstein AE, DiMarco JP, Ellenbogen KA, et al. ACC/AHA/HRS 2008 Guidelines for Device-Based Therapy of Cardiac Rhythm Abnormalities: a report of the American College of Cardiology/American Heart Association Task Force on Practice Guidelines (Writing Committee to Revise the ACC/AHA/NASPE 2002 Guideline Update for Implantation of Cardiac Pacemakers and Antiarrhythmia Devices) developed in collaboration with the American Association for Thoracic Surgery and Society of Thoracic Surgeons. J Am Coll Cardiol 2008;51(21):e1–62.

6. Ehrlich JR, Hohnloser SH. Milestones in the management of atrial fibrillation. Heart Rhythm 2009; 6(11 Suppl):S62–7.

7. Bunch TJ, Day JD, Olshansky B, et al. Newly detected atrial fibrillation in patients with an implantable cardioverter-defibrillator is a strong risk marker of increased mortality. Heart Rhythm 2009;6(1):2–8.

8. Wilkoff BL, Cook JR, Epstein AE, et al. Dual-chamber pacing or ventricular backup pacing in patients with an implantable defibrillator: the Dual Chamber and VVI Implantable Defibrillator (DAVID) Trial. JAMA 2002;288(24):3115–23.

9. Spragg DD, Akar FG, Helm RH, et al. Abnormal conduction and repolarization in late-activated myocardium of dyssynchronously contracting hearts. Cardiovasc Res 2005;67(1):77–86.

10. Varma N. Left ventricular conduction delays induced by right ventricular apical pacing: effect of left ventricular dysfunction and bundle branch block. J Cardiovasc Electrophysiol 2008;19(2):114–22.

11. Hayes JJ, Sharma AD, Love JC, et al. Abnormal conduction increases risk of adverse outcomes from right ventricular pacing. J Am Coll Cardiol 2006;48(8):1628–33.

12. Smit MD, Van Dessel PF, Nieuwland W, et al. Right ventricular pacing and the risk of heart failure in implantable cardioverter-defibrillator patients. Heart Rhythm 2006;3(12):1397–403.

13. Steinberg JS, Fischer A, Wang P, et al. The clinical implications of cumulative right ventricular pacing in the multicenter automatic defibrillator trial II. J Cardiovasc Electrophysiol 2005;16(4):359–65.

14. Wilkoff BL, Kudenchuk PJ, Buxton AE, et al. The DAVID (Dual Chamber and VVI Implantable Defibrillator) II trial. J Am Coll Cardiol 2009;53(10):872–80.

15. Olshansky B, Day JD, Moore S, et al. Is dual-chamber programming inferior to single-chamber programming in an implantable cardioverter-defibrillator? Results of the INTRINSIC RV (Inhibition of Unnecessary RV Pacing With AVSH in ICDs) study. Circulation 2007;115(1):9–16.

16. Sweeney MO, Ellenbogen KA, Miller EH, et al. The Managed Ventricular pacing versus VVI 40 Pacing (MVP) Trial: clinical background, rationale, design, and implementation. J Cardiovasc Electrophysiol 2006;17(12):1295–8.

17. Cleland JG, Daubert JC, Erdmann E, et al. The effect of cardiac resynchronization on morbidity and mortality in heart failure. N Engl J Med 2005; 352(15):1539–49.

18. Koplan BA, Kaplan AJ, Weiner S, et al. Heart failure decompensation and all-cause mortality in relation to percent biventricular pacing in patients with heart failure: is a goal of 100% biventricular pacing necessary? J Am Coll Cardiol 2009;53(4):355–60.

19. Gold MR, Niazi I, Giudici M, et al. A prospective comparison of AV delay programming methods for hemodynamic optimization during cardiac resynchronization therapy. J Cardiovasc Electrophysiol 2007;18(5):490–6.

20. Varma N, Jia P, Ramanathan C, et al. Right ventricular activation in heart failure during right, left and biventricular pacing. JACC Cardiovasc Imaging 2010; 3(6):567–75.

21. Mullens W, Grimm RA, Verga T, et al. Insights from a cardiac resynchronization optimization clinic as part of a heart failure disease management program. J Am Coll Cardiol 2009;53(9):765–73.

22. Moss AJ, Hall WJ, Cannom DS, et al. Cardiac-resynchronization therapy for the prevention of heart-failure events. N Engl J Med 2009;361(14): 1329–38.

23. Beshai JF, Grimm RA, Nagueh SF, et al. Cardiac-resynchronization therapy in heart failure with narrow QRS complexes. N Engl J Med 2007;357(24): 2461–71.

24. Stein KM, Euler DE, Mehra R, et al. Do atrial tachyarrhythmias beget ventricular tachyarrhythmias in defibrillator recipients? J Am Coll Cardiol 2002;40(2): 335–40.

25. Poole JE, Johnson GW, Hellkamp AS, et al. Prognostic importance of defibrillator shocks in patients with heart failure. N Engl J Med 2008;359(10): 1009–17.

26. Sweeney MO, Sherfesee L, Degroot PJ, et al. Differences in effects of electrical therapy type for ventricular arrhythmias on mortality in implantable cardioverter-defibrillator patients. Heart Rhythm 2010;7(3):353–60.

27. Varma N, Johnson MA. Prevalence of cancelled shock therapy and relationship to shock delivery in recipients of implantable cardioverter-defibrillators assessed by remote monitoring. Pacing Clin Electrophysiol 2009;32(Suppl 1):S42–6.

28. Hunt SA, Abraham WT, Chin MH, et al. ACC/AHA 2005 Guideline Update for the Diagnosis and Management of Chronic Heart Failure in the Adult: a report of the American College of Cardiology/American Heart Association Task Force on Practice Guidelines (Writing Committee to Update the 2001 Guidelines for the Evaluation and Management of Heart Failure): developed in collaboration with the American College of Chest Physicians and the

International Society for Heart and Lung Transplantation: endorsed by the Heart Rhythm Society. Circulation 2005;112(12):e154–235.

29. Lewin J, Ledwidge M, O'Loughlin C, et al. Clinical deterioration in established heart failure: what is the value of BNP and weight gain in aiding diagnosis? Eur J Heart Fail 2005;7(6):953–7.

30. Zhang J, Goode KM, Cuddihy PE, et al. Predicting hospitalization due to worsening heart failure using daily weight measurement: analysis of the Trans-European Network-Home-Care Management System (TEN-HMS) study. Eur J Heart Fail 2009; 11(4):420–7.

31. Chaudhry SI, Wang Y, Concato J, et al. Patterns of weight change preceding hospitalization for heart failure. Circulation 2007;116(14):1549–54.

32. Goldberg LR, Piette JD, Walsh MN, et al. Randomized trial of a daily electronic home monitoring system in patients with advanced heart failure: the Weight Monitoring in Heart Failure (WHARF) trial. Am Heart J 2003;146(4):705–12.

33. Yu CM, Wang L, Chau E, et al. Intrathoracic impedance monitoring in patients with heart failure: correlation with fluid status and feasibility of early warning preceding hospitalization. Circulation 2005;112(6): 841–8.

34. Bourge RC, Abraham WT, Adamson PB, et al. Randomized controlled trial of an implantable continuous hemodynamic monitor in patients with advanced heart failure: the COMPASS-HF study. J Am Coll Cardiol 2008;51(11):1073–9.

35. Hoppe UC, Vanderheyden M, Sievert H, et al. Chronic monitoring of pulmonary artery pressure in patients with severe heart failure: multicentre experience of the monitoring Pulmonary Artery Pressure by Implantable device Responding to Ultrasonic Signal (PAPIRUS) II study. Heart 2009;95(13): 1091–7.

36. Ritzema J, Melton IC, Richards AM, et al. Direct left atrial pressure monitoring in ambulatory heart failure patients: initial experience with a new permanent implantable device. Circulation 2007; 116(25):2952–9.

37. Khoury DS, Naware M, Siou J, et al. Ambulatory monitoring of congestive heart failure by multiple bioelectric impedance vectors. J Am Coll Cardiol 2009;53(12):1075–81.

38. Adamson PB, Conti JB, Smith AL, et al. Reducing events in patients with chronic heart failure (REDUC-Ehf) study design: continuous hemodynamic monitoring with an implantable defibrillator. Clin Cardiol 2007;30(11):567–75.

39. Vollmann D, Nagele H, Schauerte P, et al. Clinical utility of intrathoracic impedance monitoring to alert patients with an implanted device of deteriorating chronic heart failure. Eur Heart J 2007;28(15): 1835–40.

40. Adamson PB, Kleckner KJ, VanHout WL, et al. Cardiac resynchronization therapy improves heart rate variability in patients with symptomatic heart failure. Circulation 2003;108(3):266–9.

41. Adamson PB, Smith AL, Abraham WT, et al. Continuous autonomic assessment in patients with symptomatic heart failure: prognostic value of heart rate variability measured by an implanted cardiac resynchronization device. Circulation 2004;110(16):2389–94.

42. Schoenfeld MH, Compton SJ, Mead RH, et al. Remote monitoring of implantable cardioverter defibrillators: a prospective analysis. Pacing Clin Electrophysiol 2004;27(6 Pt 1):757–63.

43. Varma N, Stambler B, Chun S. Detection of atrial fibrillation by implanted devices with wireless data transmission capability. Pacing Clin Electrophysiol 2005;28(Suppl 1):S133–6.

44. Joseph GK, Wilkoff BL, Dresing T, et al. Remote interrogation and monitoring of implantable cardioverter defibrillators. J Interv Card Electrophysiol 2004;11(2):161–6.

45. Crossley GH, Chen J, Choucair W, et al. Clinical benefits of remote versus transtelephonic monitoring of implanted pacemakers. J Am Coll Cardiol 2009; 54(22):2012–9.

46. Varma N. Rationale and design of a prospective study of the efficacy of a remote monitoring system used in implantable cardioverter defibrillator follow-up: the Lumos-T Reduces Routine Office Device Follow-Up Study (TRUST) study. Am Heart J 2007; 154(6):1029–34.

47. Varma N, Michalski J, Epstein AE, et al. Efficacy and safety of automatic remote monitoring for ICD follow-up: the TRUST trial. Circ Arrythm Elecrophysiol 2010;3:428–36.

48. Varma N, Epstein A, Irimpen A, et al. Early detection of ICD events using remote monitoring: the TRUST trial [abstract]. Heart Rhythm 2009;6(5S):S73.

49. Varma N, Epstein A, Irimpen A, et al. Event notifications by remote monitoring systems performing automatic daily checks: load, characteristics and clinical utility. Eur Heart J 2009;30:1909.

50. Theuns DA, Rivero-Ayerza M, Knops P, et al. Analysis of 57,148 transmissions by remote monitoring of implantable cardioverter defibrillators. Pacing Clin Electrophysiol 2009;32(Suppl 1):S63–5.

51. Varma N. Remote monitoring for advisories: automatic early detection of silent lead failure. Pacing Clin Electrophysiol 2009;32(4):525–7.

52. Arya A, Block M, Kautzner J, et al. Influence of Home Monitoring on the clinical status of heart failure patients: design and rationale of the IN-TIME study. Eur J Heart Fail 2008;10(11):1143–8.

# Defibrillators and Cardiac Resynchronization Therapy as a Bridge to Cardiac Transplantation

Ayesha Hasan, MD[a],*, Benjamin Sun, MD[b]

## KEYWORDS

- Implantable cardioverter-defibrillator
- Cardiac resynchronization therapy
- Cardiac transplantation • Ventricular assist device

Despite advances in the treatment and management of refractory heart failure, morbidity and mortality remain alarmingly high. This represents a major public health problem, the prevalence of which has risen over the past decade and whose incidence increases with age. Recent data stress the importance of heart failure stage in predicting mortality, as 5-year survival declines to 20% in stage D patients.[1] Cardiac transplantation is the preferred treatment option in these patients with refractory or end-stage heart failure; median survival has improved to 10 years in posttransplant patients, up to 13 years in those surviving the first year post transplant.[2] Approximately 3200 heart transplants were reported to the International Society for Heart and Lung Transplant (ISHLT) Registry in 2006, representing a small percentage of patients in advanced stages of heart failure. In the past few decades, major accomplishments in the pharmacologic approach to heart failure have targeted neurohormonal mechanisms across all stages of heart failure. Despite the positive impact of medical therapy, the burden of heart failure persists, with disease progression, frequent hospitalizations, and reduced survival.

Mortality in this patient population is related to ventricular tachyarrhythmias and/or pump failure, leading to the introduction of device therapy. Device therapy has been a focus of many landmark trials in the past two decades; implantable cardioverter-defibrillators (ICD) and cardiac resynchronization therapy (CRT) have now been established as the standard of care in selected patients with chronic heart failure. Evidence has clearly shown a survival benefit associated with these devices, alone or in combination, in addition to clinical and morbidity improvement with CRT.[3–9] As guidelines expand for the use of ICD and CRT, the focus turns toward patient selection, to identify the subset of patients who will respond best to CRT or arrhythmia protection from an ICD. Therefore, it is important to review the benefits of ICD and CRT in drug-refractory heart failure, as device therapy is more readily available to qualifying patients, compared with more aggressive therapy such as cardiac transplantation. For those who are "nonresponders" to device therapy, in whom disease continues to progress (whether at a slower rate after device treatment or related to progression of underlying etiology such as ischemia,

[a] Division of Cardiovascular Medicine, Ohio State University Medical Center, 473 West 12th Avenue, 200 DHLRI, Columbus, OH 43201, USA
[b] Minneapolis Heart Institute, Allina Health Systems, 920 East 28th Street, Suite 610, Minneapolis, MN 55407, USA
* Corresponding author.
*E-mail address:* ayesha.hasan@osumc.edu

Heart Failure Clin 7 (2011) 227–239
doi:10.1016/j.hfc.2011.01.001

hypertension, and so forth), device therapy serves as a "bridge" to definitive treatment with cardiac transplantation or permanent mechanical circulatory support.

## IMPLANTABLE CARDIOVERTER-DEFIBRILLATORS IN CHRONIC HEART FAILURE

Sudden cardiac death remains a major cause of mortality in chronic heart failure patients, whether patients are in milder or more advanced stages, leading to significant progress with implantable defibrillators that automatically terminate ventricular fibrillation. Early studies were secondary prevention trials, comparing ICD therapy to antiarrhythmic drug therapy with amiodarone or sotalol in patients who were considered at high risk for sudden cardiac death, defined as a history of documented ventricular arrhythmias, cardiac arrest, or postmyocardial infarction without advanced heart failure symptoms.[10–12] Patient selection has now focused on candidates for primary prevention, or those who are at risk for ventricular arrhythmias, without a documented sustained event. Early primary prevention trials ensured a high-risk population for malignant ventricular arrhythmias by enrolling patients with inducible, nonsuppressible arrhythmias during electrophysiology studies,[3] but later trials have based inclusion on left ventricular (LV) dysfunction and functional status.[4,5] Advances in defibrillator management include enhanced arrhythmia discrimination, "painless" therapy with antitachycardia pacing for ventricular arrhythmias, bradycardia pacing, low-energy cardioversion, high-energy defibrillation, and device algorithms for high defibrillation thresholds (ie, adjusting monophasic waveform tilts and removal or addition of the proximal coil through programming). Implantation is similar to traditional pacemakers, with the majority in the pectoral area, in a subcutaneous or submuscular position, and transvenous leads placed through the subclavian or axillary veins.

### Review of ICD Clinical Trials

The Multicenter Automatic Defibrillator Trials (MADIT I and II) evaluated the prophylactic use of an ICD as primary prevention in high-risk patients with coronary artery disease. MADIT I was the first study, and enrolled 196 patients who were 3 or more weeks postmyocardial infarction with systolic dysfunction (ejection fraction [EF] ≤35%). The patients enrolled were also considered at high risk for malignant ventricular arrhythmias if they had documented arrhythmias, defined as asymptomatic nonsustained ventricular tachycardia (from 3 to 30 beats) and inducible,

nonsuppressible sustained ventricular tachycardia on electrophysiology (EP) study.[3] ICD therapy was compared with conventional medical therapy, including antiarrhythmic drugs at the physician's discretion (usually amiodarone). Patients with defibrillator therapy had a significant reduction in mortality of 54% (hazard ratio [HR] 0.46, 95% confidence interval [CI] 0.26–0.82, $P = .009$), when compared with medical therapy. Critics of this study questioned whether the inclusion of high-risk patients who had refractory arrhythmias on an EP study skewed the benefits of this therapy against the medical therapy group. Other criticisms of the study include the low use of angiotensin-converting enzyme (ACE) inhibitors (55 of 93) and β-blockers (15 of 93) but a high percentage of antiarrhythmic drugs (91 of 93) in the conventional medical therapy arm. As previously mentioned, initial primary and secondary prevention ICD trials did not include patients with symptomatic heart failure despite an ischemic etiology, but MADIT I enrolled patients with New York Heart Association (NYHA) class I to III. Subsequent subgroup analysis revealed ICD prophylaxis predicted survival benefit in higher risk heart failure patients (defined as an EF <26%, heart failure requiring therapy, and QRS ≥120 milliseconds).[13]

Following MADIT I, MADIT II was a much larger trial enrolling 1232 patients and addressed previous criticism by including a lower risk heart failure population without documented ventricular arrhythmias and no requirement for an EP study.[4] The risk of ventricular arrhythmias was based on the patient's history of myocardial infarction and cardiac dysfunction, with a stricter EF criteria (≤30%, compared with 35% in MADIT I). Symptomatically, the majority of these patients had mild to moderate heart failure (NYHA class II–III). MADIT II also compared ICD therapy with a control of conventional medical therapy. The study was terminated early at 20 months' follow-up because of a significant survival benefit in the ICD group, despite higher percentage use of optimal medical therapy (ACE and β-blocker) in both groups compared with MADIT I. Prophylactic ICD implant improved survival with a 31% reduction in all-cause mortality ($P = .016$), which post hoc analysis subsequently found was entirely due to a reduction in sudden cardiac death.[14] Sudden cardiac death occurred in 10% of the conventional medical therapy group versus 3.8% of the ICD group ($P<.01$). Mortality reduction was noted at 9 months postimplantation, compared with the first few months for patients enrolled in MADIT I. The time difference is likely related to the lower risk population and greater amount of patients on optimal medical therapy in MADIT II.

The MADIT trials firmly established the prophylactic use of ICD in ischemic heart failure with risk stratification based on the presence of coronary artery disease and EF. Survival benefit for the prophylactic use of ICD in nonischemic heart failure remained as yet unproven as evaluated in small trials, along with questions regarding amiodarone use in this patient population.[15,16] Both questions would be addressed in The Sudden Cardiac Death Heart Failure Trial (SCD-HeFT), which enrolled both ischemic and nonischemic etiology, symptomatic patients with NYHA class II or III, and EF 35% or less. A total of 2520 patients were randomized to a control of placebo, amiodarone, or shock-only, single-lead ICD with all 3 groups receiving conventional medical therapy. With this design, the study addressed the effect of amiodarone on heart failure mortality and the role of prophylactic ICD in nonischemic heart failure, as 48% had a nonischemic etiology. The primary end point of all-cause mortality was not improved with the addition of amiodarone when compared with standard medical therapy; however, ICD therapy produced a significant 23% relative risk reduction in overall mortality at 5 years, compared with the control of optimal medical therapy. Results of SCD-HeFT represent a milestone in device therapy, as prophylactic ICD was effective in the primary prevention of mortality, regardless of ischemic or nonischemic etiology of heart failure, and documented benefit beyond that of standard medical therapy, in patients with mild to moderate symptoms. It also confirmed that the use of amiodarone to suppress ventricular arrhythmias does not have a favorable survival benefit in these patients.

### Benefit of ICD in Chronic Heart Failure

Clinical trials have shown the efficacy of ICD therapy in reducing all-cause mortality and death due to sudden cardiac arrest in the appropriate patient population. Candidates include most patients with an EF of less than 35%. The goal of such therapy is to prolong survival in patients who are at risk of sudden death, even in milder stages of heart failure when they are not transplant candidates. Before the advent of current evidence–based support for primary prevention, retrospective data in patients listed for transplant revealed the benefit of prophylactic ICD as a bridge to transplantation, through improvement in mortality, which was 13.2% in those with an ICD versus 25.8% in those without ($P$ = .03).[17] Approximately two-thirds of deaths in those on the waiting list were secondary to sudden death in this study, with all occurring in non-ICD patients; absence of an ICD was an independent predictor of all-cause mortality and sudden death

for those on the waitlist. Similar results were also noted in a recent retrospective analysis of patients waiting for ICD implant, with a higher mortality pre-ICD implant (18.8%) compared with post-ICD implant (12.2%) and a higher mortality from sudden death in both groups without an ICD, either waiting for or refusing the device.[18] Limitations to this data are the retrospective nature and small number who refused an ICD (n = 39); regardless, it reinforces mortality risk in heart failure patients who are not yet transplanted and addresses the potential risk of wait time on patient outcomes.

Further support lies in analyses from both MADIT II and SCD-HeFT, which confirmed the survival benefit of prophylactic ICD in patients with heart failure was due solely to a reduction in sudden death.[14,19] In fact, adjudication of cardiac deaths in SCD-HeFT as to ventricular tachyarrhythmia, bradyarrhythmia, heart failure, or other cardiac causes found reduced cardiac mortality (adjusted HR, 0.76; 95% CI, 0.60–0.95) and tachyarrhythmia mortality (adjusted HR, 0.40; 95% CI, 0.27–0.59) compared with the control of medical therapy. There was no impact of ICD on mortality resulting from heart failure or noncardiac causes. The reduction in ventricular tachyarrhythmia mortality with ICD was evident regardless of ischemic or nonischemic etiology, but unexpectedly, the advantage was only evident in NYHA class II functional status, not class III. Possible explanations for this finding include the lower percentage of death from ventricular tachyarrhythmias in the more symptomatic group, compared with mortality from worsening heart failure, which could negate any arrhythmia benefit from an ICD. Right ventricular pacing will often exacerbate LV dysfunction, as demonstrated in both MADIT II and DAVID trials (Dual chamber vs VVI pacing in patients with Implantable Defibrillator trial). In MADIT II, a trend to increased incidence of heart failure hospitalization was found in the ICD group, and in DAVID, increased heart failure hospitalization was associated with a greater percentage of right ventricular (RV) pacing.[4,20] The detrimental effects of right ventricular pacing have led to the premise of LV stimulation in systolic dysfunction, or cardiac resynchronization, which is discussed in further detail in another section.

The timing of ICD implant is not always straightforward, but the benefit increases with time from infarction, as the substrate changes with time because of ventricular remodeling. Results of MADIT II demonstrating the time factor are consistent with DINAMIT and IRIS, both studies revealing no survival benefit soon after myocardial infarction.[21,22] The lack of survival benefit in CABG-Patch also reinforced the antiarrhythmic benefit of revascularization over early use of ICD.[23]

In reviewing the advantages of ICD, it is imperative to emphasize sudden death may still occur in patients, as 3.8% of deaths in the ICD group in MADIT II were classified as such.[14] ICD therapy should not be considered a single intervention, as the effect may vary depending on programming. Multiple programming options exist in terms of antitachycardia pacing, DC cardioversion and vector options, detection algorithms, and discriminators of supraventricular tachycardia (SVT) and ventricular tachyarrhythmias.

### Future of ICD in Heart Failure

Risk stratification is needed in terms of who is most likely to benefit from ICD therapy but also who will not benefit. Mixed results have been found with noninvasive testing, such as T-wave alternans, signal-averaged electrocardiography (ECG), QRS dispersion, and heart rate variability.[24] Retrospective analysis from MADIT II identified a clinical risk score to determine who would benefit from ICD implant; factors included NYHA class more than II, age older than 70 years, QRS greater than 120 milliseconds, blood urea nitrogen greater than 26 mg/dL, and atrial fibrillation.[25] Factors considered very high risk were creatinine 2.5 mg/dL or more and blood urea nitrogen 50 mg/dL or more. Patients who did not gain benefit from ICD had no risk factors, 3 or more risk factors, or had "very high risk" factors; those with 1 or 2 risk factors obtained benefit. When interpreting such risk scores, one must take into account that resynchronization therapy was not used in these primary prevention ICD trials, and higher risk patients are more likely to have considerable issues with heart failure. It has been stipulated that patients with fewer heart failure symptoms are more likely to die from sudden death as opposed to more symptomatic patients, who are more likely to die from worsening heart failure.[26] Regardless, risk stratification needs to be refined to better identify patients who will and will not benefit from ICD implant.

Other issues with ICDs in heart failure patients are inappropriate shocks, which were associated with higher mortality in SCD-HeFT and MADIT II patients.[27,28] Based on these data, methods to reduce not only appropriate but also inappropriate shocks (such as improved SVT discriminators, antitachycardia pacing, and pharmacologic therapy) will potentially benefit patients in terms of survival.

Application of ICD prophylaxis continues to improve in safety profile and effective therapy. Evidence has supported its use to improve patient outcomes with prolonged survival and, therefore, bridge patients to candidacy for advanced therapies such as cardiac transplantation.

## CARDIAC RESYNCHRONIZATION THERAPY IN CHRONIC HEART FAILURE

Resynchronization therapy expands on dual-chamber pacemakers; traditionally, leads are positioned transvenously in right-sided chambers (endocardial placement). CRT incorporates left-sided pacing through coronary sinus cannulation, positioning the lead in a lateral or posterior branch along the epicardial surface of the left ventricle while avoiding diaphragmatic stimulation. The premise of CRT is based on the presence of ventricular dyssynchrony, as evidenced by prolonged QRS duration on surface ECG (ie, left bundle branch block [LBBB]), which is considered electrical evidence of delay in ventricular contraction.[29] In a typical LBBB or wide QRS, delay in contraction may occur at any of 3 levels: (1) atrioventricular, between the left atria and left ventricle, (2) interventricular, between the right and left ventricles, and (3) intraventricular, within the LV segments. Such delays result in a "dyssynchronous" contraction with regional or right to left ventricular delay. The end result is impaired cardiac output from suboptimal LV filling, reduced LV dP/dt, increased LV end-systolic and diastolic volumes, and prolonged mitral regurgitation (MR) often accompanied by diastolic MR. The concept of biventricular pacing involves "resynchronization" of this dyssynchronous contraction, and studies of the acute impact of biventricular pacing showed an increase in LV dP/dt slope and stroke volume,[30] consistent with improved LV systolic function.

Early dual-chamber pacing studies in heart failure have implicated the adverse impact of chronic RV pacing, due to worsening heart failure, suggesting that stimulating univentricular RV pacing exacerbates dyssynchrony in the setting of LV systolic dysfunction.[20] Results from both MADIT II and SCD-HeFT highlighted similar issues in the treatment groups, as patients had a higher incidence of heart failure hospitalization and death related to progressive heart failure, respectively, leading to concerns that this would offset any mortality benefit from ICD in advanced heart failure patients.[4,5] Emerging from these observations, the early CRT trials in the 1990s were based on the premise of resynchronization through simultaneous right and left ventricular pacing, thereby enhancing systolic function. CRT is now the standard of care for moderate to severely symptomatic patients with left ventricular ejection fraction (LVEF) of 35% or less and evidence of dyssynchrony, currently defined by prolonged QRS duration of longer than 120 milliseconds. Early clinical trials focused on clinical primary end points of functional capacity (6-minute walk [6MW] or cardiopulmonary exercise capacity), quality of life (QOL), and NYHA class, but survival and morbidity benefits have been established in more recent trials.[6–9,31] Although clinical end points, such as NYHA class and QOL, are more subjective, they have consistently improved in large studies. Objective measures of improvement include indices of reverse remodeling, or LVEF, LV end-systolic and diastolic volumes, and MR. These measurements have been noted to improve with CRT and subsequently decline with discontinuation of biventricular pacing.[32]

## Review of CRT Clinical Trials

Early CRT trials were small in enrollment but introduced the benefit of biventricular pacing, either acutely in terms of hemodynamics[30] or clinically with improved QOL, exercise capacity, and NYHA functional class.[7,33–35] Epicardial LV leads were implanted in the earliest trials, but transvenous positioning through cannulation of the coronary sinus has been the preferred approach in later trials. The Multicenter InSync Randomized Clinical Evaluation (MIRACLE) trial was the first prospective, randomized double-blind, parallel controlled clinical trial; it was much larger, at 454 patients, and validated the results of previous CRT studies with improvement in clinical end points.[6,36] In addition to the clinical benefit, patients assigned to CRT appeared to have an improvement in heart failure status over controls, with a reduction in heart failure hospitalization (8% vs 15%, $P = .02$) and requirement of intravenous medications (7% vs 15%, $P = .004$) during study follow-up.

Despite the improvement in morbidity associated with CRT in MIRACLE, this trial was not designed to evaluate the impact on mortality. The Comparison of Medical Therapy, Pacing, and Defibrillation in Heart Failure (COMPANION) trial was the first trial designed to evaluate the effects of CRT on mortality and hospitalization in advanced heart failure.[8,31] Treatment groups were CRT alone or CRT combined with ICD (CRT-D) and compared with optimal medical therapy with a primary composite end point of all-cause mortality and all-cause hospitalization. The combined end point was significantly reduced by 20% in both CRT ($P = .008$) and CRT-D ($P = .007$) patients when compared with the control of medical therapy alone. All-cause mortality alone was a secondary end point and was significantly reduced only in the combined treatment group of CRT-D (by 36%, $P<.003$)

when compared with the control. A trend toward mortality reduction was noted in the CRT-only group ($P = .06$); however, it is imperative to note that this study was not designed to compare the treatment groups. Not only did the COMPANION trial confirm previous CRT studies, it was the first to document a survival benefit with combined CRT and ICD therapy in advanced patients. As most heart failure patients who meet criteria for CRT also meet indications for prophylactic ICD, these data support choosing a combined device for prevention of sudden death and to slow disease progression.

Questions regarding the mortality benefit of CRT remained after COMPANION, but were addressed in The Cardiac Resynchronization—Heart Failure (CARE-HF) trial, designed to assess the effects of CRT without a defibrillator in advanced heart failure.[9] CARE-HF was also the first to incorporate echocardiographic evidence of ventricular dyssynchrony in the inclusion criteria (for patients with a QRS between 120 and 150 milliseconds). Echocardiographic evidence of reverse remodeling measured as LVEF, MR, and LV end-systolic volumes was evident with CRT. CRT also achieved survival benefit, with significant reduction in the primary composite end point of all-cause death or cardiovascular hospitalization (HR 0.63, $P<.001$) and the secondary end point of all-cause mortality alone (36% reduction, HR 0.64, $P<.002$). The relative risk reduction in mortality with CRT was similar to CRT-D patients in COMPANION (36%). The CRT-only patients in COMPANION had a trend toward significance in mortality reduction, which could be due to shorter follow-up. Over the 18-month follow-up in CARE-HF, the benefit of CRT increased with duration of therapy, suggesting CRT-only in COMPANION may have reached significance with a longer duration. In this study, heart failure morbidity also improved, as evidenced by a reduction in the combination of all-cause mortality/heart failure hospitalization by 46% and heart failure hospitalization alone by 52% ($P<.001$). Thus, CARE-HF demonstrated the survival benefit of CRT without an ICD in class III and ambulatory class IV heart failure, and verified the morbidity benefit of CRT.

## Recently Published CRT Trials in Chronic Heart Failure

Recent CRT trials have attempted to expand current indications, in terms of QRS duration and functional status, although guidelines have not changed in either category at this time. Echocardiographic parameters, such as tissue Doppler imaging, have shown that inter- and intraventricular dyssynchrony can predict cardiac events in heart failure independent of QRS duration, and have revealed some degree of mechanical dyssynchrony in more than one-third of narrow QRS heart failure patients.[37,38] The Resynchronization Therapy in Normal QRS trial (ReThinQ) based enrollment of narrow QRS (<130 milliseconds) heart failure patients on the echocardiographic evidence of mechanical dyssynchrony in NYHA class III to IV patients, but did not find an improvement in peak oxygen consumption with CRT.[39,40] This trial was a small pilot study of 172 patients with shorter follow-up of 6 months, as compared with many CRT trials. At this time, the use of echocardiographic dyssynchrony in narrow QRS patients is not supported in selecting CRT patients.

A potential for clinical benefit of CRT in milder heart failure has been suggested with reverse remodeling in 2 uncontrolled studies and reduced progression to class III symptoms in a third study, although no major change in functional status was found.[41–43] The 2 most recently published large randomized trials focused on delaying progression of heart failure in less symptomatic patients. The Resynchronization Reverses Remodeling in Systolic Left Ventricular Dysfunction Study (REVERSE) enrolled patients with NYHA class I and II heart failure with LVEF 40% or less and QRS 120 milliseconds or more, and compared medical therapy with

CRT in terms of clinical composite heart failure score.[44,45] Although the percentage "worsened" in the clinical response composite end point was not significantly different in either group, reverse remodeling was significantly improved with CRT along with a reduction in heart failure morbidity (53% relative risk reduction in the time to first heart failure hospitalization, HR 0.47, $P = .03$).

The next clinical trial, Multicenter Automatic Defibrillator Implantation Trial with Cardiac Resynchronization Therapy (MADIT-CRT), evaluated whether CRT would affect the primary composite end point of risk of death and nonfatal heart failure events in mild heart failure.[46] Prophylactic CRT combined with an ICD was compared with ICD only in 1820 patients with EF 30% or less, QRS 130 milliseconds or more, and NYHA class I or II heart failure (ischemic etiology with either functional class, and nonischemic class II only). MADIT-CRT also revealed improvement in ventricular volumes and heart failure morbidity; the significant improvement in the primary end point was driven by the reduction in heart failure events. Both studies emphasize an emerging role for resynchronization therapy to slow disease progression in mild heart failure with wide QRS duration through reverse remodeling, thereby improving heart failure morbidity. Refer to **Table 1** for a summary of CRT trials.

**Table 1**
**Major clinical trials of cardiac resynchronization and enrollment criteria[a]**

| Study (n Randomized) | NYHA Class | QRS | Sinus | ICD? |
|---|---|---|---|---|
| MIRACLE (524) | III, IV | ≥130 | Normal | No |
| MUSTIC SR (58) | III | >150 | Normal | No |
| MUSTIC AF (43) | III | >200 | Atrial fibrillation | No |
| PATH CHF (42) | III, IV | ≥120 | Normal | No |
| CONTAK CD (581) | III, IV | ≥120 | Normal | Yes |
| MIRACLE ICD (362) | III, IV | ≥130 | Normal | Yes |
| PATH CHF II (89) | III, IV | ≥120 | Normal | No |
| COMPANION (1520) | III, IV | ≥120 | Normal | No |
| MIRACLE ICD II (186) | II | ≥130 | Normal | Yes |
| CARE HF (800) | III, IV | ≥120[b] | Normal | No |
| RethinQ (173) | III | <130[c] | Normal | Yes |
| PROSPECT (426) | III, IV | ≥130 | Normal | Yes |
| REVERSE (610) | I, II | ≥120 | Normal | Yes |
| MADIT-CRT (1820) | I, II[d] | ≥130 | Normal | Yes |

[a] Most trials required an ejection fraction (EF) ≤35% and dilated LV dimensions. Exceptions are REVERSE, with an EF ≤40% and MADIT-CRT, EF ≤30%.
[b] Echocardiographic evidence of dyssynchrony if QRS between 120 and 150 milliseconds.
[c] Echocardiographic evidence of dyssynchrony required for enrollment.
[d] NYHA class I: ischemic etiology, NYHA class II: ischemic and nonischemic etiology.

## Benefit and Limitations of CRT and Ventricular Assist Devices in Chronic Heart Failure

CRT and ventricular assist devices (VAD) represent device therapy that has been shown to improve heart failure symptoms and function. In class IV or American College of Cardiology/American Heart Association stage D patients, a large number of VAD implants are performed as a "bridge" to transplantation and/or decision making regarding such candidacy. More importantly, the use of VAD therapy for destination therapy is becoming mainstream and is gaining traction.

From the major landmark trials listed in **Table 1**, the benefit of CRT is well established in terms of clinical parameters, morbidity, and mortality, and is probably related to reverse remodeling, which has also been well documented with significant reduction in MR, LV mass, and ventricular volumes. Before CARE-HF and the mild heart failure studies, meta-analysis of all-cause mortality showed a significant reduction, and data pooled from 6 trials favored fewer heart failure hospitalizations with CRT.[47] In the CRT trials with 6MW as an end point, CRT improved the distance with a weighted mean difference of 28 m (range 16–40 m) in all symptomatic patients and 30 m (range 18–42 m) when limited to NYHA class III or IV. QOL improved in 7 trials by 7.6 points in all CRT patients and 8.4 points in NYHA class III or IV patients. Most patients improve NYHA functional status by at least one class. Major lessons from trial experience with CRT have shown that the survival benefit of CRT is largely attributed to a decrease in progressive heart failure, confirmed in CARE-HF where the mortality benefit was primarily related to a reduction in deaths from worsening heart failure, with a lesser reduction in sudden death.[9] Extrapolation of pooled mortality data from another meta-analysis states that 1 death will be prevented for every 5 patients treated with CRT over 6 years.[48] Perhaps CRT should also be viewed as a "bridge" to transplantation in less severe stages for these described benefits in heart failure progression, as VAD support is a bridge in end-stage patients or in those refractory to therapies like CRT.

As with any therapy for advanced disease, there comes a point when severity of cardiac dysfunction makes response to therapy very unlikely. Studies of CRT in milder heart failure, NYHA class I and II, have promising results of reverse remodeling and reduction in heart failure morbidity, with nearly 50% relative risk reduction of heart failure events or hospitalization in both.[45,46] These findings provide evidence that preventive CRT (±ICD) slows disease progression, and is a promising therapy to improve cardiac function, thus postponing the need for advanced heart failure therapies such as transplant or VAD.

Limitations with resynchronization therapy in heart failure include patient selection and the nonresponder rate. The response rate to CRT varies, usually considered in the range of 60% to 80%; whether one defines CRT response by objective or subjective measures, nonresponders continue to have a decline in their clinical status, require more advanced therapies, and/or expire.

Patients who have no change in imaging profile, such as LVEF and volumes, are also considered nonresponders to biventricular pacing, and interpretation is difficult when a patient improves subjectively in terms of QOL and NYHA class without a change in echocardiographic parameters. However, the natural progression of heart failure is a decline in status; if patients remain stable after resynchronization therapy without the need for advanced therapies, perhaps this should be considered a form of response or efficacy of CRT whereby therapy decelerates progression. In a small study comparing concordance of echocardiographic, clinical, and exercise parameters to assess CRT response, exercise capacity (measured as the maximal oxygen uptake) often correlated with NYHA class improvement when echo parameters did not, suggesting a CRT benefit not detected by imaging.[49]

In those deemed nonresponders, numerous factors contribute, from preprocedure considerations of patient selection (QRS duration, scar burden, comorbidities) to LV lead positioning during implantation, to postprocedural factors such as device programming, loss of LV pacing, and optimization of biventricular pacing parameters.[50] Advocates of CRT optimization, or individually tailoring atrioventricular (AV) and interventricular (VV) delays, maintain that simultaneous CRT is not physiologic, as in normal hearts the activation of the 2 ventricles does not appear to occur simultaneously (epicardial RV depolarization tends to occur a few milliseconds before the LV depolarization).[51] CRT optimization has been shown to improve hemodynamics, diastolic filling, and LVEF when compared with "out of the box" settings and simultaneous biventricular pacing.[50,52–54] Initial studies confirmed immediate benefit through invasive hemodynamic monitoring, but various noninvasive methods have now been evaluated, including multiple echocardiographic parameters, noninvasive cardiac output monitoring, and paced QRS morphology. Device-based algorithms have also been developed based on intracardiac electrograms and surface ECG. AV optimization to maximize LV filling time and cardiac output can be performed by echo-guided methods and may be necessary on a frequent basis. VV optimization is still controversial, based on lack of additional benefit from sequential pacing in 2 recent randomized studies[55,56] and only improved exercise capacity in another.[57] One must also consider the limitation of identifying the most reliable and reproducible echo technique to guide optimization in patients. At this time, VV optimization may not be necessary for all patients after CRT implantation, but could be considered in nonresponders. Studies are ongoing as to whether optimizing pacing delays translates into improved response and long-term outcomes in nonresponders.

The latter deals with postimplant issues, but an essential goal of device therapy is to refine patient selection to reduce the nonresponder rate. This approach not only includes implanting patients in an earlier stage of the disease process but also identifying preimplant prognostic factors. Identifying anatomic locations outside of the traditional endovascular access points for optimal pacing (away from scar via epicardial approach) may be important.

In addition, among patients assigned to a CRT device in CARE-HF, those with persistent moderate or severe MR and/or persistently elevated pro-brain natriuretic peptide did less well than other patients, emphasizing the importance of monitoring for other interventions in a timely manner (optimizing pharmacologic interventions, adjusting device programming, transplant evaluation or mechanical support, palliative care).[58] In this multivariable analysis, pro-brain natriuretic peptide, severity of MR, ischemic etiology, NYHA class IV, and degree of interventricular mechanical delay at baseline all predicted overall long-term mortality in patients, but short-term response with these variables did not predict the reduction in mortality with CRT.

The use of CRT in heart failure patients with secondary moderate to severe MR is controversial. Cabrera-Bueno and colleagues[59] evaluated patients with moderate to severe MR (defined as regurgitant orifice area $\geq$0.2 cm$^2$) pre-CRT implant, and found one-third improved to nonsignificant after 6 months of pacing. However, persistent MR was associated with worse outcomes: higher rates of clinical events (cardiovascular death/heart failure readmission, 46.4% vs 18.7%, $P = .011$), arrhythmic deaths (35.7% vs 14.5%, $P = .034$), and less reverse remodeling (28.5% vs 83.3%, $P<.001$). Once again, these results emphasize the importance of patient selection and who will require more advanced treatment.

At present, patient selection is based on QRS duration on surface ECG, and a large percentage of those enrolled in clinical trials had an LBBB. In terms of QRS pattern, limited data exist regarding right bundle branch block (RBBB) and resynchronization. In a single-center study, patients with RBBB undergoing CRT had the lowest rates of symptomatic and echocardiographic response and the lowest survival free from orthotopic heart transplantation or ventricular assist device placement, when compared with LBBB and paced QRS, despite a QRS of longer than 120 milliseconds in all patients.[60] Patients with LBBB had the best rate of response in all 3 categories, and an intermediate response was found in paced QRS undergoing upgrade.

Current guidelines use surface ECG as electrical evidence of conduction delay; however, standard ECG may not detect all the regional changes in conduction, resulting in normal QRS despite the presence of a dyssynchronous, or mechanically delayed, contraction by other imaging techniques. Focus has turned away from using only the QRS duration as a marker of conduction delay. Mechanical dyssynchrony is present in up to 50% of heart failure patients with a narrow QRS (<120 milliseconds) and absent in up to 20% with wide QRS (>150 milliseconds) meeting current indications.[38,61,62] CARE-HF had strict inclusion criteria, requiring QRS of more than 150 milliseconds or echocardiographic measures of dyssynchrony with QRS between 120 and 149 milliseconds, which could have contributed to the positive results with CRT. However, cardiac dyssynchrony has been difficult to define and measure in the real world setting. It is likely a dynamic process with varying degrees of longitudinal and/or circumferential dyssynchrony present at different times, based on exacerbating factors (ie, rest, stress, ischemia); therefore, the quantity of the different types of dyssynchrony, rather than its actual presence or absence, may contribute more to CRT response. Parameters to measure dyssynchrony in an easily reproducible, nonoperator dependent, less time-consuming manner have not been defined. Uncertainty remains regarding how to measure it, under what physiologic conditions, and frequency of measurements. For these reasons, studies of echocardiographic parameters to predict CRT response and aid in patient selection have not been promising.[63]

Brain natriuretic peptide (BNP) is an important prognostic marker in heart failure patients.[64] Reduction in neurohormonal activity, measured as BNP, has also been seen with long-term CRT.[9,65] Following 6 months of CRT, Sinha and colleagues[66] demonstrated increased BNP after short-term withdrawal of biventricular pacing but subsequent BNP reduction with reinstitution of CRT. BNP could be used to monitor efficacy of CRT, as different levels correlated with different degrees of reverse remodeling and improved exercise capacity. BNP could potentially serve as a prognostic indicator in nonresponders, as a significant increase was associated with poor response after CRT, defined as death, need for transplantation, VAD, or impaired long-term outcome.[67]

VADs have emerged as an established treatment for bridge to transplantation and destination therapy, with regard to clinically significant improvement and survival in end-stage heart failure as compared with medical therapy.[68–72] It is the only therapy that reliably transforms an NYHA class IV patient into a class I/II patient. One-year survival with continuous-flow VADs has now reached 90%.[69] VAD therapy is being employed to improve patients' physiology as a "bridge to candidacy" for cardiac transplantation. Common indications for this include pulmonary hypertension, renal insufficiency, nutritional deficiency, proximity to malignancy, and compliance. Procedural mortality is higher when compared with CRT, and long-term risk is related to infection and thromboembolic complications. CRT is the preferred option in qualifying patients, and is more feasible in terms of cost, ease of implant, and postoperative management,[73] although these therapies are more complementary than comparative. With both procedures, timing of the implant before end-stage disease is critical in order to gain meaningful benefit with device therapy.

Although VAD therapy unloads the left ventricle and decreases the wall tension, malignant arrhythmias remain important. Arrhythmia can be caused by endocardial irritation from suction events or by remaining electrical irritability due to the underlying pathologic process that had led to heart failure. Patients with VAD therapy have better survival with ICD therapy in place. The role of CRT in this patient population has yet to be defined.[72]

### Future of CRT in Chronic Heart Failure

Application of CRT has turned to expanding indications and to refining patient selection and device optimization. The role of CRT is being evaluated in narrow QRS patients, atrial fibrillation, and chronic RV pacing. The efficacy of CRT in mild to moderate heart failure has been further assessed in the Resynchronization/Defibrillation for Ambulatory Heart Failure Trial (RAFT).[74] Current evidence does not support the use of dyssynchrony parameters in narrow QRS heart failure, but symptomatic improvement in previous studies is encouraging. The EchoCRT trial will evaluate the impact of CRT on morbidity and mortality outcomes in narrow QRS patients with NYHA class III/IV symptoms who meet echocardiographic dyssynchrony criteria.[75] The potential effect of device optimization on outcomes and the nonresponder rate is being investigated and randomized clinical trials will continue to determine the application of CRT in various subsets of chronic heart failure.

### SUMMARY

Cardiac transplantation is the gold-standard treatment for end-stage heart failure. However, alternative options must be considered, because of a shortage of donor organs compared with eligible candidates and the mortality risk of waiting for an available organ in end-stage patients. Use of implanted devices is growing rapidly as a treatment option for moderate to severe heart failure, with well-established clinical, mortality, and morbidity benefit. ICDs are the most effective therapy for preventing sudden death and therefore increasing survival. The development of worsening heart failure in defibrillator patients supports biventricular pacing to further improve survival and morbidity in this population. Important steps with both devices are improvement in safety profile, reduction in complications from lead/device malfunction and from surgery, and more effective therapy. For ICDs, this includes improved arrhythmia detection, successful cardioversion, and reduction of inappropriate shocks; new technology also focuses on leads that are easier to extract and subcutaneous devices to avoid venous access. Such advances will serve to improve survival in patients who are appropriate transplant candidates while they accrue time on a waitlist for limited organs. Expanding application of resynchronization is being studied, and emerging data may render CRT (with or without a defibrillator) an option for patients in earlier stages of heart failure as a bridge to recovery or as a means to delay progression to more advanced stages and, ultimately, transplantation. Efforts have also been made to further study the LV pacing site, single versus multisite pacing, and the use of periprocedural imaging for optimal lead placement. Advances in patient selection, LV pacing, and device programming should improve the efficacy of CRT, thereby slowing heart failure progression in select patients. Ongoing clinical trials will also assess whether VV optimization will aid in converting nonresponders to responders. A tremendous need exists in device therapy for risk stratification, identifying not only those who will benefit but also those who would not be expected to benefit and should be considered for alternative therapy. Device therapy with CRT and ICD offers the opportunity to reduce morbidity and increase survival in patients with drug refractory heart failure, and to retard, if not prevent, development of end-stage heart failure requiring cardiac transplantation, given the limited availability of this treatment option.

# REFERENCES

1. Ammar KA, Jacobsen SJ, Mahoney DW, et al. Prevalence and prognostic significance of heart failure stages: application of the American College of Cardiology/American Heart Association heart failure staging criteria in the community. Circulation 2007; 115:1563–70.

2. Taylor DO, Edwards LB, Aurora P, et al. Registry for the International Society of Heart and Lung Transplantation: twenty-fifth official adult heart transplantation report—2008. J Heart Lung Transplant 2008; 27:937–56.

3. Moss AJ, Hall WJ, Cannom DS, et al. Improved survival with an implantable defibrillator in patients with coronary disease at high risk for ventricular arrhythmia. Multicenter Automatic Defibrillator Implantation Trial Investigators. N Engl J Med 1996;335:1933–40.

4. Moss AJ, Fadl Y, Zarebl W, et al. Survival benefit with an implantable defibrillator in relation to mortality risk in chronic coronary heart disease. Am J Cardiol 2001;88:516–20.

5. Bardy GH, Lee KL, Mark DB, et al. Amiodarone or an implantable cardioverter-defibrillator for congestive heart failure (SCD-HeFT). N Engl J Med 2005;352: 225–37.

6. Abraham WT, Fisher WG, Smith AL, et al., for the Multisite Insync Randomized Clinical Evaluation (MIRACLE) Investigators and Coordinators. Double-blind, randomized controlled trial of cardiac resynchronization in chronic heart failure. N Engl J Med 2002;346:1845–53.

7. Linde C, Leclercq C, Rex S, et al., on behalf of the Multisite Stimulation in Cardiomyopathies (MUSTIC) Study Group. Long-term benefits of biventricular pacing in congestive heart failure: results from the Multisite Stimulation in Cardiomyopathy (MUSTIC) study. J Am Coll Cardiol 2002;40:111–8.

8. Bristow MR, Saxon LA, Boehmer J, et al. Cardiac-resynchronization therapy with or without an implantable defibrillator in advanced chronic heart failure (COMPANION). N Engl J Med 2004;350:2140–50.

9. Cleland JG, Daubert JC, Erdmann E, et al. The CARE-HF study (Cardiac Resynchronization in Heart Failure study): rationale, design, and end-points. Eur J Heart Fail 2001;3:481–9.

10. The Antiarrhythmics versus Implantable Defibrillators (AVID) Investigators. A comparison of antiarrhythmic-drug therapy with implantable defibrillators in patients resuscitated from near-fatal ventricular arrhythmias. N Engl J Med 1997;337:1576–84.

11. Connolly SJ, Gent M, Roberts RS, et al. Canadian Implantable Defibrillator Study (CIDS): a randomized trial of the implantable cardioverter-defibrillator against amiodarone. Circulation 2000;101:1297–302.

12. Kuck KH, Cappato R, Seibels J, et al. Randomized comparison of antiarrhythmic drug therapy with implantable defibrillators in patients resuscitated from cardiac arrest: the Cardiac Arrest Study Hamburg (CASH). Circulation 2000;102:748–54.

13. Moss AJ, Zareba W, Hall WJ, et al. Prophylactic implantation of a defibrillator in patients with myocardial infarction and reduced ejection fraction. N Engl J Med 2002;346:877–83.

14. Greenberg H, Case RB, Moss AJ, et al. Analysis of mortality events in the multicenter automatic defibrillator implantation trial (MADIT-II). J Am Coll Cardiol 2004;43:1459–65.

15. Strickberger SA, Hummel JD, Bartlett TG, et al. Amiodarone versus implantable cardioverter defibrillator: randomized trial in patients with nonischemic dilated cardiomyopathy and asymptomatic nonsustained ventricular tachycardia (AMIOVIRT). J Am Coll Cardiol 2003;41:1707–12.

16. Kadish A, Dyer A, Daubert JP, et al. Prophylactic defibrillator implantation in patients with nonischemic dilated cardiomyopathy. N Engl J Med 2004; 350:2151–8.

17. Sandner SE, Wieselthaler G, Zuckerman A, et al. Survival benefit of the implantable cardioverter defibrillator in patients on the waiting list for cardiac transplantation. Circulation 2001;104(Suppl I):I-171–6.

18. Ghosh N, Mangat I, O'Donnell SS, et al. Outcomes in heart failure patients referred for consideration of implantable cardioverter defibrillator for primary prophylaxis of sudden cardiac death: what are the risks of waiting? Can J Cardiol 2009;25(10):e342–6.

19. Packer DL, Prutkin JM, Hellkamp AS, et al. Impact of implantable cardioverter-defibrillator, amiodarone, and placebo on the mode of death in stable patients with heart failure: analysis from the Sudden Cardiac Death in Heart Failure Trial. Circulation 2009;120: 2170–6.

20. Wilkoff BL. The Dual Chamber and VVI Implantable Defibrillator (DAVID) trial: rationale, design, results, clinical implications and lessons for future trials. Card Electrophysiol Rev 2003;7(4):468–72.

21. Hohnloser SH, Kuhn KH, Dorian P, et al. Prophylactic use of an implantable cardioverter-defibrillator after acute myocardial infarction. N Engl J Med 2004; 351:2481–8.

22. Steinbeck G, Andresen D, Seidl K, et al. Defibrillator implantation early after myocardial infarction. N Engl J Med 2009;361(15):1427–36.

23. Bigger JT, Coronary Artery Bypass Graft (CABG) Patch Trial Investigators. Prophylactic use of implanted cardiac defibrillators in patients at high risk for ventricular arrhythmias after coronary artery bypass graft surgery. N Engl J Med 1996;335: 1933–40.

24. Epstein AE. Benefits of the implantable-cardioverter defibrillator. J Am Coll Cardiol 2008;52:1122–7.

25. Goldenberg I, Vyas AK, Hall WJ, et al. Risk stratification for primary implantation of a cardioverter-defibrillator in patients with left ventricular dysfunction. J Am Coll Cardiol 2008;51:288–96.

26. MERIT-HF Study Group. Effect of metoprolol CR/XL in chronic heart failure: Metoprolol CR/XL Randomised Intervention Trial in Congestive Heart Failure (MERIT-HF). Lancet 1999;353:2001–7.

27. Poole JE, Johnson GW, Hellkam AS, et al. Prognostic importance of defibrillator shocks in patients with heart failure. N Engl J Med 2008;359:1009–17.

28. Daubert JP, Zareba W, Cannon DS, et al. Inappropriate implantable cardioverter-defibrillator shocks in MADIT II: frequency, mechanisms, predictors, and survival impact. J Am Coll Cardiol 2008;51: 1357–65.

29. Kashani A, Barold SS. Significance of QRS complex duration in patients with heart failure. J Am Coll Cardiol 2005;46:2183–92.

30. Auricchio A, Stellbrink C, Block M, et al. Effect of pacing chamber and atrioventricular delay on acute systolic function of paced patients with congestive heart failure. Circulation 1999;99:2993–3001.

31. Bristow MR, Feldman AM, Saxon LA, for the COMPANION steering committee and COMPANION Clinical Investigators. Heart failure management using implantable devices for ventricular resynchronization: comparison of medical therapy, pacing, and defibrillation in chronic heart failure (COMPANION) trial. J Card Fail 2000;6:276–85.

32. Yu CM, Chau E, Sanderson JE, et al. Tissue Doppler echocardiographic evidence of reverse remodeling and improved synchronicity by simultaneously delaying regional contraction after biventricular pacing therapy in heart failure. Circulation 2002;105: 438–45.

33. Auricchio A, Stellbrink C, Sack S, et al, Pacing Therapies in Congestive Heart Failure (PATH-CHF) Study Group. Long-term clinical effect of hemodynamically optimized cardiac resynchronization therapy in patients with heart failure and ventricular conduction delay. J Am Coll Cardiol 2002;39:2026–33.

34. Auricchio A, Stellbrink C, Butter C, et al, Pacing Therapies in Congestive Heart Failure II Study Group, Guidant Heart Failure Research Group. Clinical efficacy of cardiac resynchronization therapy using left ventricular pacing in heart failure patients stratified by severity of ventricular conduction delay. J Am Coll Cardiol 2003;42:2109–16.

35. Cazeau S, Leclercq C, Lavergne T, et al, Multisite Stimulation in Cardiomyopathies (MUSTIC) Study Investigators. Effects of multisite biventricular pacing in patients with heart failure and intraventricular conduction delay. N Engl J Med 2001;344:873–80.

36. Abraham WT, on behalf of the Multisite InSync Randomized Clinical Evaluation (MIRACLE) Investigators and Coordinators. Rationale and design of a randomized clinical trial to assess the safety and efficacy of cardiac resynchronization therapy in patients with advanced heart failure: the Multicenter InSync Randomized Clinical Evaluation (MIRACLE). J Card Fail 2000;6:369–80.

37. Bader H, Garrigue S, Lafitte S, et al. Intra-left ventricular electromechanical asynchrony. A new independent predictor of severe cardiac events in heart failure patients. J Am Coll Cardiol 2004;43:248–56.

38. Cho GY, Song JK, Park WJ, et al. Mechanical dyssynchrony assessed by tissue Doppler imaging is a powerful predictor of mortality in congestive heart failure with normal QRS duration. J Am Coll Cardiol 2005;46:2237–43.

39. Beshai JF, Grimm RA. The resynchronization therapy in narrow QRS study (RethinQ study): methods and protocol design. J Interv Card Electrophysiol 2007; 19:149–55.

40. Beshai JF, Grimm RA, Nagueh SF, et al. Cardiac-resynchronization therapy in heart failure with narrow QRS complexes. N Engl J Med 2007;357:2461–71.

41. Bleeker GB, Schalij MJ, Holman ER, et al. Cardiac resynchronization therapy in patients with systolic left ventricular dysfunction and symptoms of mild heart failure secondary to ischemic or non-ischemic cardiomyopathy. Am J Cardiol 2006;98(2):230–5.

42. Kuhlkamp V, InSync 7272 ICD World Wide Investigators. Initial experience with an implantable cardioverter-defibrillator incorporating cardiac resynchronization therapy. J Am Coll Cardiol 2002;39: 790–7.

43. Landolina M, Lunati M, Gasparini M, et al. Comparison of the effects of cardiac resynchronization therapy in patients with class II versus class III and IV heart failure (from the InSync/InSync ICD Italian registry). Am J Cardiol 2007;100:1007–12.

44. Packer M. Proposal for a new clinical end point to evaluate the efficacy of drugs and devices in the treatment of chronic heart failure. J Card Fail 2001; 7:176–82.

45. Linde C, Abraham WT, Gold MR, et al. Randomized trial of cardiac resynchronization in mildly symptomatic heart failure patients and in asymptomatic patients with left ventricular dysfunction and previous heart failure symptoms. J Am Coll Cardiol 2008;52:1834–43.

46. Moss AJ, Hall WJ, Cannom DS, et al. Cardiac resynchronization therapy for the prevention of heart failure events. N Engl J Med 2009;361:1329–38.

47. McAlister FA, Ezekowitz JA, Wiebe N, et al. Systematic review: cardiac resynchronization in patients with symptomatic heart failure. Ann Intern Med 2004;141:381–90.

48. Freemantle N, Tharmanathan P, Calvert MJ, et al. Cardiac resynchronization for patients with heart failure due to left ventricular systolic dysfunction—a systematic review and meta-analysis. Eur J Heart Fail 2006;8:433–40.

49. Cattadori G, Francesco G, Berti M, et al. Assessment of cardiac resynchronization therapy response. Int J Cardiol 2009;136:240–2.

50. Hasan A. Optimizing cardiac resynchronization therapy. Curr Heart Fail Rep 2008;5:38–43.

51. Auricchio A, Salo RW. Acute hemodynamic improvements by pacing in patients with severe congestive heart failure. Pacing Clin Electrophysiol 1997;20: 313–24.

52. Jansen AH, Bracke FA, van Dantzig JM, et al. Correlation of echo-Doppler optimization of atrioventricular delay in cardiac resynchronization therapy with invasive hemodynamics in patients with heart failure secondary to ischemic or idiopathic dilated cardiomyopathy. Am J Cardiol 2006;97:552–7.

53. Sogaard P, Egeblad H, Pedersen AK, et al. Sequential versus simultaneous biventricular resynchronization for severe heart failure: evaluation by tissue Doppler imaging. Circulation 2002;106:2078–84.

54. Perego GB, Chianca R, Facchini M, et al. Sequential versus simultaneous biventricular pacing in heart failure: an acute hemodynamic study. Eur J Heart Fail 2003;5:305–13.

55. Boriani G, Muller CP, Seidl KH, et al, RHYTHM II Investigators. Randomized comparison of simultaneous biventricular stimulation versus optimized interventricular delay in cardiac resynchronization therapy. The Resynchronization for the Hemodynamic Treatment for Heart Failure Management II implantable cardioverter defibrillator (RHYTHM II ICD) study. Am Heart J 2006;151:1050–8.

56. Rao K, Kumar UN, Schafer J, et al. Reduced ventricular volumes and improved systolic function with cardiac resynchronization therapy; a randomized trial comparing simultaneous biventricular pacing, sequential biventricular pacing, and left ventricular pacing. Circulation 2007;115:2136–44.

57. Leon AR, Abraham WT, Brozena S, et al, InSync III Clinical Study Investigators. Cardiac resynchronization with sequential biventricular pacing for the treatment moderate-to-severe heart failure. J Am Coll Cardiol 2005;46:2298–304.

58. Cleland J, Freemantle N, Ghio S. Predicting the long-term effects of cardiac resynchronization therapy on mortality from baseline variables and the early response. J Am Coll Cardiol 2008;52: 438–45.

59. Cabrera-Bueno F, Molina-Mora MJ, Alzueta J. Persistence of secondary mitral regurgitation and response to resynchronization therapy. Eur J Echocardiogr 2010;11(2):131–7.

60. Adelstein EC, Saba S. Usefulness of baseline electrocardiographic QRS complex pattern to predict response to cardiac resynchronization. Am J Cardiol 2009;103:238–42.

61. Bleeker GB, Schalij MJ, Molhoek SG, et al. Relationship between QRS duration and left ventricular dyssynchrony in patients with end-stage heart failure. J Cardiovasc Electrophysiol 2004;15(5):544–9.

62. Yu CM, Lin H, Zhang Q, et al. High prevalence of left ventricular systolic and diastolic asynchrony in patients with congestive heart failure and normal QRS duration. Heart 2003;89(1):54–60.

63. Chung ES, Leon AR, Tavazzi A, et al. Results of the predictors of response to CRT (PROSPECT) trial. Circulation 2008;117:2608–16.

64. Anand IS, Fisher LD, Chiang YT, et al., Val-HeFT Investigators. Changes in brain natriuretic peptide and norepinephrine over time and mortality and morbidity in the Valsartan Heart Failure Trial (Val-HeFT). Circulation 2003;107:1278–83.

65. Erol-Yilmaz A, Verberne HJ, Schrama TA, et al. Cardiac resynchronization induces favorable neurohumoral changes. Pacing Clin Electrophysiol 2005; 28(4):304–10.

66. Sinha AM, Filzmaier K, Breithardt OA, et al. Usefulness of brain natriuretic peptide release as a surrogate marker of the efficacy of long-term cardiac resynchronization therapy in patients with heart failure. Am J Cardiol 2003;91(6):755–8.

67. Delgado RM, Palanichamy N, Radovancevic R, et al. Brain natriuretic peptide levels and response to cardiac resynchronization therapy in heart failure patients. Congest Heart Fail 2006;12(5):250–3.

68. Rose EA, Gelijns AC, Moskowitz AJ, et al. Longterm use of a left ventricular assist device for endstage heart failure. N Engl J Med 2001;345(20):1435–43.

69. INTERMACs Destination therapy registry, 2010.

70. Cantillon DJ, Tarakji KG, Kumbhani DJ, et al. Improved survival among ventricular assist device recipients with a concomitant implantable cardioverter-defibrillator. Heart Rhythm 2010;7(4):466–71.

71. Lietz K, Long JW, Kfoury AG, et al. Outcomes of left ventricular assist device implantation as destination therapy in the post-REMATCH era: implications for patient selection. Circulation 2007;116(5): 497–505.

72. John R, Kamdar F, Liao K, et al. Improved survival and decreasing incidence of adverse events with the HeartMate II left ventricular assist device as a bridge-to-transplant therapy. Ann Thorac Surg 2008;86(4):1227–34.

73. Delgado RM, Radovancevic B. Symptomatic relief: left ventricular assist devices versus resynchronization therapy. Heart Fail Clin 2007;3:259–65.

74. Tang AS, Wells GA, Arnold M, et al. Resynchronization/defibrillation for ambulatory heart failure trial: rationale and trial design. Curr Opin Cardiol 2009; 24(1):1–8.

75. Holzmeister J, Hürlimann D, Steffel J, et al. Cardiac resynchronization therapy in patients with a narrow QRS. Curr Heart Fail Rep 2009;6:49–56.

# Economic Implications and Cost-effectiveness of Implantable Cardioverter Defibrillator and Cardiac Resynchronization Therapy

Michael L. Bernard, MD, PhD, Michael R. Gold, MD, PhD*

## KEYWORDS

- Cost-effectiveness • ICD • CRT • Cost analysis
- ICER • Sudden cardiac death

Heart failure is a leading contributor to overall morbidity and mortality and, unlike coronary artery disease, has declining survival rates.[1] At the time of diagnosis, patients have a 1-year survival rate of 62%[2] and carry a 6- to 9-fold increase in the rate of sudden cardiac death (SCD).[3] SCD represents the leading cause of mortality with approximately 300,000 US deaths annually and is the first manifestation of cardiac disease in most patients who are affected.[3]

Implantable cardioverter defibrillators (ICDs) were developed as a method to combat SCD in survivors of sudden cardiac arrest and in those with increased risk, such as patients with depressed left ventricular function. For heart failure patients with prolonged QRS duration and left ventricular systolic dysfunction, cardiac resynchronization therapy (CRT) with biventricular pacing was developed to treat ventricular electric dyssynchrony and thereby, to improve hemodynamic parameters and clinical outcomes. Several landmark trials have demonstrated mortality benefits for select patient populations receiving ICDs and CRT for primary and secondary prevention of SCD.[4–8] CRT devices have also been shown to have a significant effect on patient quality of life as well as the rate of hospitalization, which is the largest contributor to overall health care costs in patients with heart failure.[7,9]

Despite the significant morbidity and mortality benefits of ICDs and CRTs, skepticism persists about the cost-effectiveness of providing an expensive therapy to a high-mortality population, such as those with advanced heart failure. To date, several ICD and CRT trials have been assessed from a cost-effectiveness perspective using both trial-based data and disease simulation models.[10–21] These analyses have been performed in several countries using separate health care economic systems.[22–29] The most influential factors in the incremental cost-effectiveness ratios (ICERs) were cost at implantation, time to device replacement, and time horizon of the study. Based on the available studies, the ICER of ICD and/or CRT device implantation is favorable for appropriately selected patients and is comparable to those of other common cardiovascular therapies.

Conflict of Interests: Dr Gold is a consultant to Boston Scientific and Medtronic; receives research grants from Boston Scientific, Medtronic, Sorin, and St Jude; and has received honoraria from Boston Scientific, Biotronik, Sorin, Medtronic, and St Jude. Dr Bernard has no conflict of interest.
Division of Cardiology, Medical University of South Carolina, ART 7031, MSC 592, Charleston, SC 29425, USA
* Corresponding author.
*E-mail address:* goldmr@musc.edu

Heart Failure Clin 7 (2011) 241–250
doi:10.1016/j.hfc.2010.12.007

## MEASURING COST-EFFECTIVENESS IN THE ICD/CRT-RECEIVING POPULATION

The economics of health care is a complex medical, social, and ethical issue. Whereas medical, technological, and pharmaceutical advances offer improvements in morbidity and mortality, they often come at an increased cost. Methods to assess the cost-effectiveness of new therapies were developed to assist health care providers and health care systems. When therapies are both less expensive and more effective they are considered economically dominant; however, most new interventions are more costly. These new therapies must provide adequate morbidity and mortality benefit to justify their widespread use as opposed to the available standard of care. One of the most commonly used financial evaluations for a new therapy is an estimate of the ICER.

The ICER compares the incremental cost of a new intervention, including increased costs as well as decreased costs of any subsequent care, to the overall medical benefit usually measured as quality-adjusted life-year (QALY).[30] The ICER is not a fixed formula because various health care systems around the world use distinct health care economic paradigms. In the United States, guidelines for cost-effectiveness studies recommend that incremental costs should include all costs of a new therapy including any follow-up care specific to the new therapy.[31] In addition, any decrease in health care costs, for example, shorter hospital stays or fewer hospitalizations, is deducted. More comprehensive studies include secondary costs such as travel, job productivity, and caregiver expenses. In contrast to cost-benefit studies, in which only absolute costs are evaluated, cost-effectiveness studies include nonmonetary benefits of a new therapy that are incorporated into the QALY figure. QALY is a value derived from the summation of time intervals weighted by a factor ranging from 0 (death) to 1 (perfect health) related to the patient's perceived sense of well-being. For each given time point, patients must rate their health usually through a standardized quality-of-life questionnaire. Although highly subjective, this type of analysis allows the inclusion of nonmortality benefits of a given therapy. Incremental costs are then divided by the QALYs to arrive at the ICER, with lower values representing more favorable trade-off between the cost and benefit. There is no current US standard for ICERs, although therapies generating less than $50,000 to $100,000 increased cost per QALY are generally considered favorable. However, these figures stem from an argument that interventions with values similar or equal to that of dialysis ($50,000 per QALY in 1982) should be provided to patients and are therefore subject to debate.[32] Published ICERs for common cardiovascular therapies are listed in **Fig. 1**. In countries with more nationalized health care systems, the ICER of a given therapy is compared with the national standards and thresholds before that therapy is approved for widespread use. For purposes of comparison,

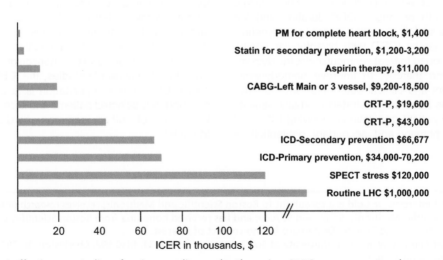

**Fig. 1.** Cost-effectiveness studies of various cardiovascular therapies. CABG, coronary artery bypass graft; CRT-P, CRT pacemaker, LHC, left heart catheterization, PM, pacemaker; SPECT, single-photon emission computed tomography. (*Data from* Refs.[36–38])

published non-US values are converted to US dollars based on the exchange rate on January 1, 2010 and placed in parentheses.

ICERs can be generated from trial-based studies, from disease simulation models based on trial data, or from a combination of both. The benefits of trial-based studies include interpretation of actual observed data from randomized studies, which minimizes the error generated by mathematical projections. The most limiting factor of trial-based studies is the finite period, or the time horizon, in which the study was performed. This factor can be particularly influential when a therapeutic benefit and/or cost is skewed toward the extremes of the given period. For example, as opposed to drug therapy, in which the costs are distributed over the duration of the study, ICD and CRT costs are weighted toward the start of the time horizon because of high costs of devices and implantation expenditures. In such instances, trials may not be of sufficient duration to derive accurately the true incremental cost to QALY ratio. As one method to address the shortcomings of trial-based studies, disease simulation models are commonly used. Using observed or predicted outcome data, a disease simulation model can generate estimated ICERs when trial data are not available or are limited. Furthermore, specific comparisons can be made that may not have been studied in a trial. Limitations of these studies stem from assumptions made in the models themselves. Hybrid studies, in which trial data are extrapolated to longer time points using models

based on the trial itself, combine the best of the trial- and model-based analyses. Such studies are particularly attractive in studying the cost-effectiveness of ICD and CRT.

## COST-EFFECTIVENESS OF ICDs
### Primary Prevention Studies

ICD implantation for primary prevention provides a substantial mortality benefit largely because of the reduction of SCD in patients with left ventricular systolic dysfunction. The largest primary prevention randomized trials, Multicenter Automatic Defibrillator Implantation Trial II (MADIT-II) and Sudden Cardiac Death in Heart Failure Trial (SCD-HeFT), demonstrated 31% and 23% reductions in all-cause mortality, respectively.[4,5] A meta-analysis of 9 randomized trials showed a 19% decrease in all-cause mortality.[10] To date, trial-based cost-effectiveness studies using both MADIT-II and SCD-HeFT data as well as several studies using disease simulation models in different health care systems have been published (**Table 1**).

Using a trial-based analysis of the MADIT-II population, Zwanziger and colleagues[11] reported an ICER of $235,000 per year of life saved at the end point of the trial, 3.5 years. When the survival curves were extrapolated to 12 years, the ICER ranged from $78,600 to $144,000 using different time-dependent hazard ratio models and assuming reimplantation at 5 and 10 years. Applying the MADIT-II criteria to the Duke Cardiovascular Database, incremental costs were

---

**Table 1**
**Cost-effectiveness studies of ICD implantation. Values in parentheses represent converted monetary values based on exchanges rates January 1, 2010**

| Author | Trial(s) | Nation(s) | Time | Cost-effectiveness |
|--------|----------|-----------|------|--------------------|
| Zwanziger[11] | MADIT II | USA | 3.5 y<br>12 y | $235,000<br>$78,000–$144,000 |
| Al Khatib[12] | MADIT II | USA | 3–15 y | $50,500 |
| Mark[13] | SCD-HeFT | USA | 5 y | $38,389 |
| Mushlin[14] | MADIT | USA | 4 y | $27,000 |
| Sanders[15] | Meta-analysis<br>Primary prevention | USA | Variable | $34,000–$70,200 |
| O'Brien[17] | CIDS | Canada | 6 y | $213,543 |
| Larsen[18] | AVID | USA | 3 y | $66,677 |
| Cowie[22] | Meta-analyais<br>Primary prevention | Europe | Variable | ($45,454) |
| Caro[23] | SCD-HeFT | UK & France | 5 y | 5:1 return |
| Deniz[25] | SCD-HeFT | Canada | 5 y | 20:1 retutn |

roughly $90,000 in the ICD group compared with the medical therapy group, with a gain of 1.8 discounted life-years resulting in an ICER of $50,500.[12] This study analyzed that cost-effectiveness at 3-year intervals had a maximum follow-up interval of 15 years. The Duke population, compared with the MADIT-II individuals, had similar 3-year survival rates. The largest influences on the ICER were the time horizon and the cost of implantation. The trial-based cost-effectiveness analysis of the SCD-HeFT ICD cohort generated an ICER of $38,389 relative to the medical therapy arm.[13] Extrapolating the trial-based survival curves, time horizon was found to be an important factor in the ICER. Subgroup analysis revealed a favorable $23,231 to $29,872 ICER in the New York Heart Association (NYHA) II population compared with no cost benefit for the NYHA III group. Analysis of the MADIT trial demonstrated an ICER of $27,000 per QALY.[14] Using a Markov model based on 6 randomized trials in which ICD implantation correlated with a mortality benefit, cost-effectiveness ranged between $34,000 and $70,200 per QALY.[15] The most important factors in the cost-effectiveness ratio included the cost of implantation and the duration of mortality benefit gained by ICD placement.[16] The investigators concluded that if the mortality benefit of ICD implantation lasted up to 7 years, the cost-effectiveness ratio would remain less than $100,000. One of the major limitations of these studies is the assumed survival rates of the ICD-recipient population. Most analyses assume a stable rate of survival that may not reflect the effect of comorbidities in patients with systolic dysfunction. Alternatively, technological advancements are most likely to reduce the costs and extend the longevity of implanted devices, which are 2 of the most influential factors determining the ICER. A meta-analysis of primary prevention trials estimated the ICERs as they varied with mortality rate, device longevity, and quality-of-life index (**Fig. 2**).[15] ICD implantation became less favorable when absolute mortality benefits were less than 20% and when device was implanted before 5 years. To summarize, in general, the ICER of an ICD for primary prevention purposes is favorable, given appropriate patient selection, and provides continued mortality benefit for several years after implantation.

### Secondary Prevention Studies

There are limited cost-effectiveness studies on ICD implantation for secondary prevention. Analysis of the Canadian Implantable Defibrillator Study (CIDS) revealed an ICER of $213,543 at an approximate 6-year interval.[17] Subgroup analysis demonstrated that patients with reduced left ventricular ejection fraction (<35%) had an ICER of approximately $100,000. When extrapolated to 12 years, the ICER was estimated between $100,000 to $150,000. The economic subgroup analysis of the Antiarrhythmic Versus Implantable Defibrillators (AVID) study demonstrated a base case cost-effectiveness ratio of $66,677 at the 3-year interval.[18] Cost-effective ratios obtained at 6 and 20 years were $68,378 and $80,358, respectively, assuming a constant survival rate. Using adjusted survival rates reflecting the high mortality of the AVID population, the cost-effectiveness ratio increased to more than $200,000 at the 6- and 20-year intervals. Subgroup analysis showed that patients with ventricular fibrillation had a more favorable cost-effectiveness ratio than those with ventricular tachycardia. Compared with results of primary prevention trials, the ICERs of secondary prevention trials were generally higher, which is counterintuitive because these patients seem at higher risk and more frequently experience appropriate shocks. This finding is most likely caused by lower mortality benefit and higher comorbidities in the AVID and CIDS populations. Moreover, these studies were older with lower overall survival and less frequent use of concomitant medical therapies, such as β-blockers, angiotensin-converting enzyme inhibitors, angiotensin receptor blockers, and statins.

### Cost-Effectiveness of ICD Therapy Worldwide

Analysis of ICD cost-effectiveness has been performed in several different countries and health care systems. Compared with the United States health care, worldwide health care organizations more commonly rely on cost-effectiveness ratios and ICERs to assist with use of particular therapies. Using a meta-analysis of 6 ICD primary prevention trials, Cowie and colleagues[22] demonstrated a cost-effectiveness ratio of €31,717 ($45,454), which was projected to be favorable for European health care systems. Using rates based on results from the SCD-HeFT trial, a 5-year projection of ICD implantation costs and benefits were obtained and analyzed under both United Kingdom and French health care paradigms.[23] Using cost-benefit rather that cost-effectiveness analysis, ICD implantation in the SCD-HeFT population was shown to have a 5:1 return on investment and therefore represent a worthwhile investment for appropriate patients. An Italian cost analysis study of patients receiving ICDs under MADIT-II criteria estimated a cost of €6.70 and €4.60 ($9.60 and $6.60) a day for

5-and 7-year intervals, respectively.[24] A simulation of 1000 patients in each arm of the SCD-HeFT trial yielded a favorable 20:1 return in investment at a 5-year interval, leading to the conclusion that ICDs are a worthwhile therapy for primary prevention of SCD in a Canadian population.[25] Based on available data, ICD implantation for primary prevention of SCD seems to be a cost-effective option for several different health care systems.

## COST-EFFECTIVENESS OF CRT

CRT combined with optimal medical therapy reduces all-cause mortality, mortality from heart failure, and mortality from SCD.[7–9] Furthermore, CRT pacing improves quality of life and reduces hospitalizations in the advanced heart failure population. The Cardiac Resynchronization-Heart Failure (CARE-HF) trial demonstrated a 40% reduction in mortality, 45% reduction in death from worsening heart failure, and a 46% reduction in SCD.[7] Hospitalizations due to worsening heart failure were reduced by 52% in the same study. The Myocardial Ischemia Reduction with Acute Cholesterol Lowering (MIRACLE) trial showed a 77% reduction in hospitalization days in patients receiving CRT when compared with those receiving optimal medical management.[9] Quality-of-life assessment in patients receiving CRT devices plus medical therapy was markedly improved as evidenced by the Comparison of Medical Therapy, Pacing, and Defibrillation in Heart Failure (COMPANION) trial.[8] The implications for cost-effectiveness when studying CRT versus ICD lies in the improvement of QALY and decrease in costs stemming from reduced hospitalizations.

### CRT-Pacemaker Studies

Few studies have assessed cost-effectiveness of CRT (**Table 2**). Nine randomized trials were used to generate a Markov model to assess the cost-effectiveness of providing CRT in symptomatic heart failure patients.[19] For patients receiving CRT, an ICER of $107,800 was derived from an additional cost of $30,000 that resulted in an additional 0.28 QALY relative to patients optimally treated medically. The limitations of the study included the diversity in selected patient populations in the different trials as well as the inability to standardize costs saved from reduced hospitalizations. Using the COMPANION trial data, the extrapolated 7-year ICER was $19,600, which was less than any value obtained from ICD trials.[20] Assessment of CRT in the CARE-HF trial in European enrollees resulted in an ICER of €19,319 ($27,686) when evaluated at a mean follow-up interval of 29.4 months.[26] A UK disease simulation

cost-effectiveness study using a 5-year interval based on the CARE-HF trial yielded an ICER of £15,247 ($25,645), with the largest factors including cost of implantation and time horizon.[27] A Scandinavian assessment of cost-effectiveness of CRT using the CARE-HF trial as a model resulted in favorable cost-effectiveness ratios in Denmark, Finland, and Sweden when survival data and costs were extended to 6 years.[28] Therefore, trial-based and disease simulation studies derived from the CARE-HF trial generated ICERs that were considered economically favorable in their respective health care systems. Similar to ICD trials, CRT cost-effectiveness was most affected by cost of implantation and time horizon.

### Cost-Effectiveness of CRT Defibrillator Compared with CRT-Pacemaker

Implantation of CRT defibrillator (D) compared with CRT pacemaker (P) devices is more expensive, and therefore CRT-D has potentially less-favorable ICER despite the decrease in mortality provided by the ICD component. Three studies have assessed the cost-effectiveness of CRT-D using available clinical trials. Compared with the ICER of $19,600 for CRT-P, the cost-effectiveness ratio for CRT-D implantation was $43,000 using a 7-year disease simulation model of the COMPANION trial.[20] Although a relative 0.17 QALY advantage was seen with CRT-D compared with CRT-P, it was offset by an increase in cost of $36,200 in the CRT-D group to $13,800 in the CRT-P group. A German disease simulation model using the COMPANION trial data resulted in an ICER of €88,143 ($126,320) for CRT-D implantation compared with optimal medical therapy at 2 years.[29] Extending the analysis to 7 years based on the average longevity of the device reduced the ICER to €24,650 ($35,327). The only assessment of CRT-D versus CRT-P cost-effectiveness used data from the CARE-HF and COMPANION trials to simulate 10,000 device implantations at 6 (CRT-P) and 7 (CRT-D) years.[21] The ICERs of CRT-P and CRT-D compared with that of optimal medical therapy were €7538 ($10,803) and €18,017 ($25,821), respectively, at the end point of the simulation. CRT-D compared with CRT-P generated an ICER of €47,909 ($68,960). There was minimal increase in ICER of CRT-P compared with medical therapy for different starting ages; however, increasing age resulted in significant increase in ICERs of CRT-D compared with CRT-P. Although CRT-D implantation results in increased cost compared with CRT-P implantation, it retains a favorable cost-effectiveness ratio when used in addition to medical therapy.

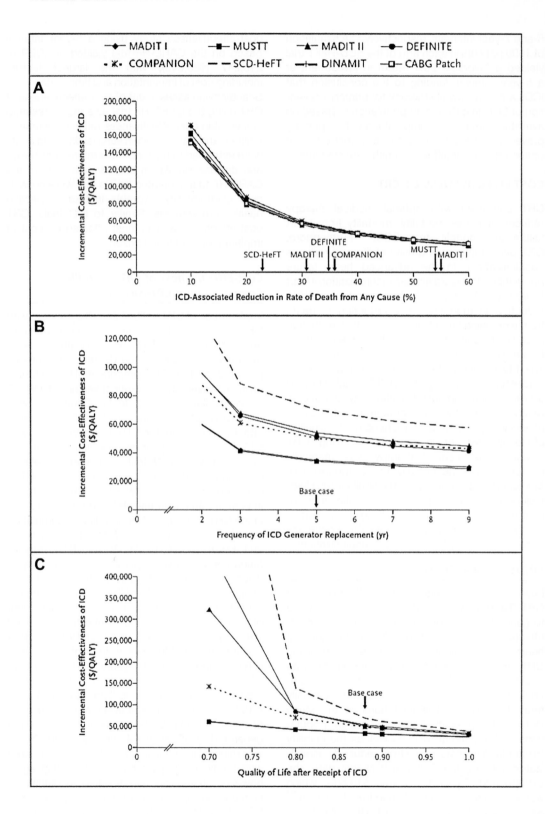

**Table 2**
Cost-effectiveness studies of CRT-P and CRT-D implantation. Values in parentheses represent converted monetary values based on exchanges rates January 1, 2010

| Author | Trial(s) | CRT mode | Nation(s) | Time | Cost-effectiveness |
|--------|----------|----------|-----------|------|--------------------|
| Nichol[19] | Meta-analysis | CRT-P | USA | Variable | $107,800 |
| Feldman[20] | COMPANION | CRT-P | USA | 7 y | $19,600 |
| | | CRT-D | | | $43,000 |
| Calvert[26] | CARE-HF | CRT-P | Europe | 29 m | ($27,686) |
| Caro[27] | CARE-HF | CRT-P | UK | 5 y | ($25,645) |
| Blomstrom[28] | CARE-HF | CRT-P | Scandanavia | 6 y | Favorable |
| Aidelsburger[29] | COMPANION | CRT-D | Germany | 2 y | ($126,320) |
| | | | | 7 y | ($35,327) |
| Yao[21] | CARE-HF | CRT-P | Europe | 6 y | ($10,803) |
| | COMPANION | CRT-D | | 7 y | ($25,821) |

## COST-EFFECTIVENESS OF ICDS IN SPECIAL POPULATIONS

Cost-effectiveness studies have also been performed among patient populations with risks of SCD not included in most primary and secondary prevention trials. Goldenberg and colleagues[33] estimated the cost-effectiveness of ICD implantation in congenital long QT syndrome (LQTS) and in hypertrophic cardiomyopathy (HCM) using simulation models of survival and incidences of SCD events. When stratifying patients into low risk (no known risk factors), high risk (risk factors but no previous events), and very high risk (survivors of SCD), the cost-effectiveness ratios were favorable for all groups except the low-risk group. The ICERs for low-risk patients with LQTS and HCM was $400,000 to $600,000, whereas the ICERs for high-risk patients ranged from $3328 to $7102 in LQTS and $17,526 to $17,892 in HCM populations. In very high–risk patients, the ICERs in patients with LQTS and HCM were $15,483 to $19,393 and $22,329 to $22,944, respectively. Based on these estimates, ICD implantation in high-risk and very high–risk patients with LQTS and HCM is more cost-effective than in the general primary and secondary prevention populations. These findings were similar to those of You and colleagues,[34] who analyzed the cost-effectiveness of ICD implantation, amiodarone therapy, and placebo in an HCM population model. Stratifying the patients by age and risk factors of SCD, the investigators estimated favorable ICERs for ICD implantation in younger patients with 1 risk factor and for middle-aged and older patients with 2 or more risk factors for SCD. Modeling of the cost-effectiveness of ICD implantation for high-risk patients with Brugada syndrome demonstrated an ICER of $9591, well within an acceptable range.[35] Although limited studies are available, ICDs seem to be cost-effective for patients with a high risk of SCD because of inherited channelopathies.

## DISCUSSION

ICD and/or CRT confers a demonstrated mortality benefit that is superior to medical therapy among several high-risk cohorts, primarily with left ventricular systolic dysfunction and heart failure. Since the advent of ICD and CRT technologies, concerns regarding the high initial costs of device

---

**Fig. 2.** Sensitivity analysis of the incremental cost-effectiveness of prophylactic implantation of an ICD when compared with control therapy with respect to the efficacy (A), the frequency of generator replacement (B), and the quality of life (C). Panel A reflects the efficacy of the ICD in reducing the risk of death from any cause. The arrows indicate the efficacy of the ICD in reducing the risk of death from any cause in the individual trials. The arrow in panel B indicates the base case estimate of replacing the generator every 5 years. The arrow in panel C indicates the base case estimate of the quality of life with an ICD of 0.88. For this analysis, the assumed quality of life with control therapy remains constant at 0.88. CABG Patch, Coronary Artery Bypass Graft Patch; COMPANION, Comparison of Medical Therapy, Pacing, and Defibrillation in Heart Failure; DEFINITE, Defibrillators in Non-Ischemic Cardiomyopathy Treatment Evaluation; DINAMIT, Defibrillator in Acute Myocardial Infarction; MUSTT, Multicenter Unsustained Tachycardia Trial. (*Reprinted from* Sanders GD, Hlatky MA, Owens DK. Cost-effectiveness of implantable cardioverter-defibrillators. N Engl J Med 2005;353(14):1477; with permission.)

implantation were a potential barrier to widespread use. Most of the major randomized clinical trials studying primary or secondary prevention of SCD, as well those investigating the benefit of CRT, were analyzed for cost-effectiveness. Despite the high initial costs of such devices, their use for primary or secondary prevention of SCD seems to be cost-effective when compared with the national standards. Moreover, ICDs were shown to be cost-effective by several different health care systems as well as in specialized populations such as high-risk patients with LQTS and HCM.

Despite these objective data, the perception that ICD and CRT are expensive persists for several reasons. First, many physicians or health care systems are influenced by the high initial device and implantation costs. Thus, it is common for primary care physicians to treat mild hyperlipidemia routinely with medical therapy in a young patient with no other risk factors and yet not refer patients for ICD implantation because of cost concerns, although the latter option is more cost-effective. Second, it is often hard to ascertain the benefit of device therapy (particularly ICD) among individual patients. If a patient does not receive a shock within the 5 to 7 years of initial battery life of the device, the perception is that this was an unnecessary device implantation. However, if an antihypertensive drug is given and the blood pressure decreases, it is considered effective, even if the patient experienced a myocardial infarction, stroke, or died. Thus, using cost-effectiveness analysis to make population decisions rather than extrapolating from individual responses to therapy is often difficult. Finally, device therapy is often not immediately life prolonging, such as some other expensive therapies including dialysis and heart transplantation. Accordingly, the perception of the appropriateness of these therapies from a societal perspective is often different.

CRT is also a highly cost-effective modality for advanced heart failure patients meeting requirements for implantation. Compared with ICDs, CRTs offer additional cost saving related to reduction in hospitalizations and improved quality-of-life measurements. These results are contingent on assumptions of patient mortality derived from trial-based data as well as for assumed device longevity of 5 to 7 years. The most influential criteria for cost-effectiveness for most cost-effectiveness studies were cost of device implantation, time horizon of the study, and the time to reimplant or upgrade. The Resynchronization Reverses Remodeling in Systolic Left Ventricular Dysfunction (REVERSE) and Multicenter Automatic Defibrillator Implantation CRT (MADIT-CRT) trials showed comparable benefits of CRT

in mild heart failure with regard to reductions of hospitalizations and quality of life, but had little effect on mortality. It will be interesting to compare the cost-effectiveness in these cohorts with ICD therapy that improves mortality but does not affect morbidity or quality-of-life measures.

As technology progresses, device cost and longevity will most likely change favorably, thereby reducing the ICERs of ICDs and CRTs. This change is particularly relevant for CRT devices, which have much higher complication rates and shorter device longevity because of the complexities and challenges of left ventricular lead implantation. Little progress has been made recently with the development of new classes of drugs to improve outcomes in heart failure or prevent sudden death. Consequently, most of the benefit for reducing pharmacologic costs in heart failure and SCD will be derived from reduced prices of medications due to generic forms of drugs as well as improved access and disease-based treatment programs. New technologies may also have a significant effect on the cost-effectiveness of device therapy, including subcutaneous defibrillators, leadless pacing, and better dissemination of automatic external defibrillators.

## REFERENCES

1. Swedberg K, Cleland J, Dargie H, et al. Task Force for the Diagnosis and Treatment of Chronic Heart Failure of the European Society of Cardiology. Guidelines for the diagnosis and treatment of Chronic Heart Failure: executive summary (update 2005). The Task Force for the Diagnosis and Treatment of CHF of the European Society of Cardiology. Eur Heart J 2005;26:1115–41.

2. Cowie MR, Wood DA, Coats AJ, et al. Incidence and aetiology of heart failure; a population based study. Eur Heart J 1999;20(6):421–8.

3. American Heart Association (AHA). 2000 Heart and stroke statistical update. Dallas (TX): American Heart Association; 2009. Update.

4. Moss AJ, Zareba W, Hall J, et al, Multicenter Automatic Defibrillator Implantation Trial II Investigators. Prophylactic implantation of a defibrillator in patients with myocardial infarction and reduced ejection fraction. N Engl J Med 2002;346(12):877–83.

5. Bardy GH, Lee KL, Mark DB, et al, Sudden Cardiac Death in Heart Failure Trial (SCD-HeFT) Investigators. Amiodarone or an implantable cardioverter-defibrillator for congestive heart failure. N Engl J Med 2005;352(3):225–37.

6. The Antiarrhythmics versus implantable defibrillators (AVID) investigators. A comparison of antiarrhythmic-drug therapy with implantable defibrillators in

patients resuscitated from near-fatal ventricular arrhythmias. N Engl J Med 1997;337(22):1576–83.

7. Cleland JGF, Daubert JC, Erdmann E, et al, Cardiac Resynchronization-Heart Failure (CARE-HF) Study Investigators. The effect of cardiac resynchronization on morbidity and mortality in heart failure. N Engl J Med 2005;352(15):1539–49.

8. Bristow MR, Saxon LA, Boehmer J, et al, Comparison of Medical Therapy, Pacing, and Defibrillation in Heart Failure (COMPANION) Investigators. Cardiac-resynchronization therapy with or without an implantable defibrillator in advanced chronic heart failure. N Engl J Med 2004;350(21):2140–50.

9. Abraham WT, Fischer WG, Smith AL, et al. Cardiac resynchronization in chronic heart failure. N Engl J Med 2002;346:1845–53.

10. Ezekowitz JA, Rowe BH, Dryden DM, et al. Systematic review: implantable cardioverter defibrillators for adults with left ventricular systolic dysfunction. Ann Intern Med 2007;147(4):251–62.

11. Zwanziger J, Hall WJ, Dick AW, et al. The cost effectiveness of implantable cardioverter-defibrillators: results from the Multicenter Automatic Defibrillator Implantation Trial (MADIT)-II. J Am Coll Cardiol 2006;47:2310–8.

12. Al Khatib SM, Anstrom KJ, Eisenstein EL, et al. Clinical and economic implications of the multicenter automatic defibrillator implantation trial II. Ann Intern Med 2005;142:593–600.

13. Mark DB, Nelson CL, Anstrom KJ, et al. Cost-effectiveness of defibrillator therapy or amiodarone in chronic stable heart failure. Results from the Sudden Cardiac Death in Heart Failure Trial (SCD-HeFT). Circulation 2006;114:135–42.

14. Mushlin AI, Hall WJ, Zwanziger, et al. The cost-effectiveness of automatic implantable cardiac defibrillators: results from MADIT, Multicenter Automatic Defibrillator Implantation Trial. Circulation 1998;97:2129–35.

15. Sanders GD, Hlatky MA, Owens DK. Cost-effectiveness of implantable cardioverter-defibrillators. N Engl J Med 2005;353(14):1471–80.

16. Goldman L. Cost-effectiveness in a flat world — can ICDs help the United States get rhythm? N Engl J Med 2005;353(14):1513–5.

17. O'Brien BJ, Connoly SJ, Goeree R, et al. Cost-effectiveness of the implantable cardioverter-defibrillator results from the Canadian Implantable Defibrillator Study (CIDS). Circulation 2001;103:1416–21.

18. Larsen G, Hallstrom A, McAnulty J, et al. Cost-effectiveness of the implantable cardioverter-defibrillator versus antiarrhythmic drugs in survivors of serious ventricular tachyarrhythmias: results from the Antiarrhythmics Versus Implantable Defibrillators (AVID) economic analysis substudy. Circulation 2002;105:2049–57.

19. Nichol G, Kaul P, Husztl E, et al. Cost-effectiveness of cardiac resynchronization therapy in patients with symptomatic heart failure. Ann Intern Med 2004;141:343–51.

20. Feldman AM, de Lissovoy G, Bristow MR, et al. Cost effectiveness of cardiac resynchronization therapy in the Comparison of Medical Therapy, Pacing, and Defibrillation in Heart Failure (COMPANION) trial. J Am Coll Cardiol 2005;46(12):2311–21.

21. Yao G, Freemantle N, Calvert MJ, et al. The long-term cost-effectiveness of cardiac resynchronization therapy with or without an implantable cardioverter-defibrillator. Eur Heart J 2007;28(1):42–51.

22. Cowie MR, Marshall D, Drummond M, et al. Lifetime cost-effectiveness of prophylactic implantation of a cardioverter defibrillator in patients with reduced left ventricular systolic function: results of Markov modeling in a European population. Europace 2009;11:716–26.

23. Caro JJ, Ward A, Deniz HB, et al. Cost-benefit analysis of preventing sudden cardiac deaths with an implantable cardioverter defibrillator versus amiodarone. Value Health 2007;10(1):13–22.

24. Boriani G, Biffi M, Russo M, et al. Primary prevention of sudden cardiac death: can we afford the cost of cardioverter-defibrillators? Data from the Search-MI Registry-Italian Sub-study. Pacing Clin Electrophysiol 2006;29:S29–34.

25. Deniz HB, Ward A, Caro JJ, et al. Cost-benefit analysis of primary prevention of sudden cardiac death with an implantable cardioverter defibrillator versus amiodarone in Canada. Curr Med Res Opin 2009;25(3):617–26.

26. Calvert MJ, Freemantle N, Yao G, et al. Cost-effectiveness of cardiac resynchronization therapy. Results from the Care-HF trial. Eur Heart J 2005;26(24):2681–8.

27. Caro JJ, Guo S, Ward A, et al. Modelling the economic and health consequences of cardiac resynchronization therapy in the UK. Curr Med Res Opin 2006;22(6):1171–9.

28. Blomstrom P, Ekman M, Lundqvist CB, et al. Cost-effectiveness of cardiac resynchronization therapy in the Nordic region: an analysis based on the Care-HF trial. Eur J Heart Fail 2008;10:869–77.

29. Aidelsburger P, Grabein K, Klauss V, et al. Cost effectiveness of cardiac resynchronization therapy in combination with an implantable cardioverter defibrillator (CRT-D) for the treatment of chronic heart failure from a German health care system perspective. Clin Res Cardiol 2007;9:89–97.

30. Cohen DJ, Reynolds MR. Interpreting the results of cost-effectiveness studies. J Am Coll Cardiol 2008;52(25):2119–26.

31. Gold MR, Siegel JE, Russell LB, et al. Cost-effectiveness in health and medicine. New York: Oxford University Press; 1996.

32. Ubel PA, Hirth RA, Chernew ME, et al. What is the price of life and why doesn't it increase at the rate of inflation? Arch Intern Med 2003;163:1637–41.

33. Goldenberg I, Moss AJ, Maron BJ, et al. Cost-effectiveness of implanted defibrillators in young people with inherited cardiac arrhythmias. Ann Noninvasive Electrocardiol 2005;10(Suppl 4):67–83.

34. You JJ, Woo A, Ko DT, et al. Life expectancy gains and cost-effectiveness of implantable cardioverter/defibrillators for the primary prevention of sudden cardiac death in patients with hypertrophic cardiomyopathy. Am Heart J 2007;154: 899–907.

35. Wang K, Yamauchi K, Li P, et al. Cost-effectiveness of implantable cardioverter-defibrillators in Brugada syndrome treatment. J Med Syst 2008;32(1):51–7.

36. Boriani G, Biffi M, Martignani C, et al. Expenditure and value for money: the challenge of implantable cardioverter defibrillators. QJM 2009;102(5):349–56.

37. Silver MT. Implantable defibrillators and beta-blockers in patients with left ventricular dysfunction: economic, ethical, and legal considerations. Am Heart J 2007;153:S59–64.

38. Tengs TO, Adams ME, Pliskin JS. Five-hundred life-saving interventions and their cost-effectiveness. Risk Anal 1995;15(3):369–90.

# Advances in Cardiopulmonary Resuscitation

Demetris Yannopoulos, MD[a],*, Kostantinos Kotsifas, MD[b],
Keith G. Lurie, MD[c]

## KEYWORDS

- CPR • Circulation • Cardiac arrest • Hypothermia
- Ventilation • Compression • Devices • Blood flow

Sudden cardiac death is one of the most common causes of death, accounting for approximately 1,000,000 deaths yearly in North America and Europe.[1,2] This clinical toll is enormous; more than 1000 adults die each day in the United States from an out-of-hospital cardiac arrest and a similar number die from in-hospital cardiac arrest. Survival from out-of-hospital and in-hospital cardiac arrest remains poor despite a significant improvement in many aspects of treatment of emergency clinical situations. Even in the most advanced emergency medical systems in Western societies[1] neurologically intact survival rates remain less than 20%. This article focuses on important advances in the science of cardiopulmonary resuscitation (CPR) in the last decade that have led to a significant improvement in understanding the complex physiology of cardiac arrest and critical interventions for the initial management of cardiac arrest and postresuscitation treatment. Special emphasis is given to the basic simple ways to improve circulation, vital organ perfusion pressures, and the grave prognosis of sudden cardiac death.

The complexity of cardiac arrest has led to a study theory that divides it into 3 phases. Although the existence of the 3 phases is not scientifically proven, they provide a useful construct for a more comprehensive understanding of the complexities of cardiac arrest.

Specific treatments targeting the pathophysiology of each phase increase the chances of a meaningful recovery.[3] The first phase after cardiac arrest is termed "the electrical phase." This lasts about 4 minutes after cardiac arrest; most patients present with ventricular fibrillation (VF) initially and often respond to immediate defibrillation. The second phase, called "the circulatory phase" begins at minute 4 and lasts to minute 10, depending on the surrounding temperature and conditions. High-quality CPR, with emphasis on improvement of the delivery of oxygenated blood to the brain and heart before defibrillation, is paramount, and techniques that increase circulation have been shown to improve outcomes. The third phase, or "metabolic phase," usually begins after 10 minutes. Current treatment strategies for patients in the metabolic phase are poor. These late efforts generally target the metabolic derangements associated with prolonged ischemia. Survival is inversely related to the time of untreated cardiac arrest. Most of the patients in cardiac arrest receive professional assistance during the second phase because of delays in arrival of paramedics or lack of bystander CPR. This is one of the reasons that extra emphasis has been placed on improving circulation and simplifying the delivery of compressions and ventilations in recent American Heart Association (AHA) Guidelines.

This article originally appeared in *Cardiac Electrophysiology Clinics*, volume 1, number 1.

[a] Department of Medicine, Interventional Cardiology, University of Minnesota, 420 Delaware Street, MMC 508, Minneapolis, MN 55455, USA
[b] Department of Pulmonary Medicine, Sotiria General Hospital, Goudi 10928, Athens, Greece
[c] Department of Emergency Medicine, Hennepin County Medical Center, Minneapolis Medical Research Foundation, University of Minnesota, 914 South 8th Street, 3rd Floor, Minneapolis, MN 55404, USA
* Corresponding author.
E-mail address: yanno001@umn.edu

## IMMEDIATE CPR

The earlier the intervention and targeted therapies are delivered after cardiac collapse, the higher the chances of survival. Because most patients in cardiac arrest are initially found by laypersons, a renewed emphasis has been placed on increasing bystander CPR. Studies have shown that when operators who receive 911 calls provide instruction by phone on how to provide CPR to lay rescuers who have not been previously trained in CPR, teaching only chest-compression CPR results in no worse outcomes compared with teaching mouth-to-mouth technique and chest compression.[4] This simplified approach to teaching CPR has only been shown to result in no harm in long-term outcomes. However, prolonged periods of chest-compression-only CPR have been shown to be dangerous in some animal studies, and high-quality studies are lacking in humans. Despite a lack of substantial improvement in outcomes with chest-compression-only CPR, fear of disease transmission from mouth-to-mouth ventilation and the challenges of trying to teach mouth-to-mouth by telephone have shifted the emphasis of phone instructions before arrival of the emergency medical services (EMS) to focus rescuers on chest compressions only. These efforts increase the chances of successful defibrillation because the "no-flow" state is reduced. Without bystander CPR the likelihood of neurologically intact survival is significantly reduced.

Early defibrillation is an essential therapy for the electrical phase of cardiac arrest. Direct current defibrillation can restore a perfusing rhythm in 80% of patients within 1 to 2 minutes. However, after 10 minutes the success rate falls to less than 5%. That is one of the reasons that broad deployment of public-access defibrillators in places where large numbers of people are likely to congregate has been encouraged. In one study that tested early defibrillation in casinos in the United States the survival of patients suffering VF was 50% overall. Patients who received defibrillation within 3 minutes of collapse had a 75% hospital discharge rate.[5] Based on a solid body of evidence, early defibrillation in a witnessed arrest is a class I recommendation based on the 2005 AHA CPR Guidelines.[6] Other studies have not shown so much promise for use of automated external defibrillators (AEDs).[7] The public-access defibrillation study funded by the US National Institutes of Health found a small but statistically significant difference in outcomes when thousands of AEDs were deployed and compared with defibrillation by first responders. In an equally important study from Seattle, Cobb and colleagues[8] showed

that survival rates decreased by 30% when AEDs were placed on all first-responder vehicles in Seattle. These investigators demonstrated that 90 seconds of CPR before delivery of a shock resulted in a significant increase in survival. These data stressed, for the first time, the importance of priming the pump to clear lactate and circulate blood through the heart before defibrillation.

Other issues related to defibrillation remain complicated. For example, Bardy and colleagues[9] showed that in survivors of anterior-wall myocardial infarction who were not candidates for implantation of a cardioverter-defibrillator, access to a home AED did not significantly improve overall survival, compared with reliance on conventional resuscitation methods, despite the higher theoretic probability for sudden cardiac death than controls. Similarly, although there are no clinical data demonstrating improved long-term survival rates between the monophasic and biphasic waveforms for treatment of VF during the electrical phase of cardiac arrest, a single high-energy (150–200 J) biphasic defibrillation shock is believed to be the treatment of choice of in- and out-of-hospital VF.

One of the biggest changes in cardiac arrest science in the past 15 years is that the frequency of VF as the initial cardiac arrest rhythm has decreased from about 50% to less than 30%.[10] The reasons for this change remain unknown but use of implantable defibrillators in high-risk patients and more aggressive preventative care with cholesterol-lowering agents, β-blockers and interventional cardiology procedures may contribute to this epidemiologic change. There are animal data to suggest that some drugs, including β-blockers and angiotensin-converting enzyme (ACE) inhibitors may decrease the duration of VF. Regardless of the cause, the change in the frequency of VF as the initial presenting rhythm to asystole (nearly 50%) and pulseless electrical activity focuses even more attention on finding better ways to improve circulation, as described in the next section.

## IMPROVING CIRCULATION

Most prehospital cardiac arrests cannot be treated within 4 minutes from the time of arrest. Initiation of therapy for cardiac arrest after 4 to 5 minutes of a nonperfusing rhythm calls for immediate compressions to generate blood flow and partially replete the membrane energy required for generation of an organized rhythm. When the time between the 911 call and paramedic arrival is longer than 4 to 5 minutes, CPR before shock significantly improves survival and hospital discharge rates up to 5-fold (from 4% to 22%). If the time to defibrillation is less than 5 minutes, there are no differences in survival.[11]

The focus of modern CPR is on improved circulation during CPR; this means more effective compressions, fewer interruptions, and less frequent ventilations. For basic life support (BLS) the compression/ventilation ratio is 30:2, to provide fewer interruptions of compressions for ventilation. During CPR, even in the best of circumstances, the generated cardiac output is less than 20% of normal. Respiratory exchange is adequate with less-than-normal minute ventilation, in part because gas exchange is limited by the severely reduced pulmonary flow. For advanced life support (ALS), continuous chest compressions without interruption for ventilations are strongly recommended to improve circulation and enhance vital-organ perfusion and oxygenation. Equally important is starting chest compressions immediately, as soon as they are indicated.

This recommendation is based on a consensus of experts in CPR. However, it has been shown in pigs that with the shift from a 15:2 to a 30:2 compression/ventilation ratio the common carotid blood flow doubles and there is a 25% increase in cardiac output without any compromise in oxygenation and acid-base balance (**Fig. 1**).[12] Further efforts to reduce the ventilation frequency are harmful in animals, as described later.[13,14]

During ALS uninterrupted compressions with a rate of 100/min are recommended. The rescuers that are responsible for the ventilation should deliver 8 to 10 breaths/min with special care not to hyperventilate. Continuous delivery of high-quality chest compressions with attention to full chest-wall recoil is tiring and rescuers should rotate frequently (every 2–3 minutes) to avoid excessive fatigue, which diminishes the quality of CPR.[15]

## VENTILATIONS

Periodic positive-pressure ventilation during CPR is fundamental to providing oxygen to the blood and tissues.[16] Recent studies have shown that each positive-pressure ventilation is associated with an increase in intrathoracic pressure, which

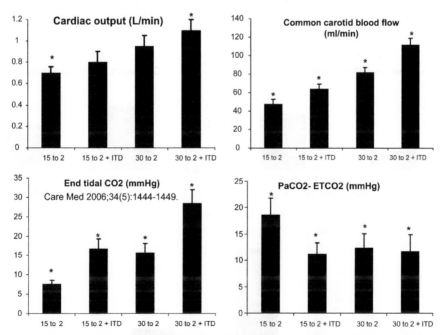

**Fig. 1.** After 6 minutes of untreated VF 6 minutes of either 15:2 or 30:2 compression/ventilation ratio CPR was performed. At the end the inspiratory ITD was added for another 4 minutes. There was a significant increase of cardiac output, common carotid artery flow, end tidal $CO_2$ in the animals that received 30:2 C/V ratio. There was a further increase with the addition of an ITD although it was applied late. $Paco_2$-$Etco_2$ is a marker of pulmonary ventilation/perfusion matching. * means statistically significant difference when compared with the ratio of 15:2 with a $P<.05$. (*From* Yannopoulos D, Aufderheide TP, Gabrielli A, et al. Clinical and hemodynamic comparison of 15:2 and 30:2 compression-to-ventilation ratios for cardiopulmonary resuscitation. Crit Care Med 2006;34:1444; with permission.)

increases intracranial pressure and decreases cardiac filling; the hemodynamic consequences reduce cerebral and coronary perfusion. Too frequent or too few ventilations can be harmful, if not deadly.[17,18] The frequency of ventilation during CPR should be reduced to 8 to 10 breaths/min once the airway has been secured, and each 500-mL tidal-volume breath should be delivered rapidly (in <1 second) to minimize the duration of positive airway pressures. These subtle but fundamental changes in ventilation technique ensure optimal circulation during conventional, manual, closed-chest CPR.[19] The benefits of positive-pressure ventilation must be weighed against the harm associated with too much ventilation. In addition, the unwillingness of the layperson to provide CPR because of the fear of communicating diseases and the inherent aversion to mouth-to-mouth ventilation should be taken into consideration.

Excessive ventilation rates and volumes increase intrathoracic pressure and intracranial pressures and concomitantly decrease coronary perfusion pressure, mean arterial pressure, and survival rates in animals (**Fig. 2**).[18] Intracranial pressures are regulated, in part, by intrathoracic pressures: each time ventilation is delivered there is an increase in the pressure inside the thorax

and the brain, which reduces cardiac and cerebral perfusion pressures.[19]

Maintaining an open and secure airway is paramount during CPR. However, stopping chest compressions and taking time to intubate stops all circulation. Techniques and devices that allow rescuer personnel to provide ventilation without having to interrupt chest compressions, including use of a 2-handed face-mask technique and some of the supraglottic airway devices, are simple but significant advances. Thus, although endotracheal intubation is still recommended, many advanced EMS systems perform CPR with a face-mask technique or supraglottic airway initially and then intubate 10 minutes later or after a return of spontaneous circulations. Thus, use of a Combitube or other supraglottic airway device (eg, KING LTS-D, King Systems, Noblesville, IN, USA), which are placed in the oropharyngeal cavity and allow for nonselective airway isolation for the purpose of ventilation, and the laryngeal mask airway, is recommended. These devices have not been shown to alter outcomes after cardiac arrest but they do maintain airway patency.

When using a face-mask for ventilation, a 2-person technique is recommended. One person maintains the correct head position, the

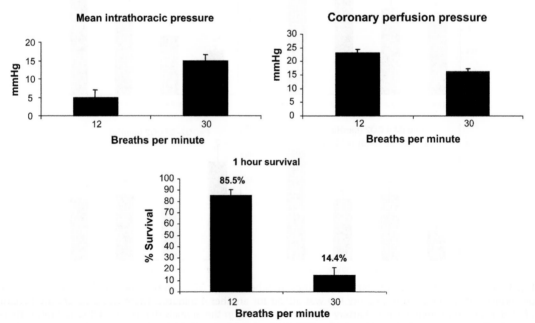

**Fig. 2.** Hyperventilation and survival. When after 6 minutes of untreated VF pigs received CPR with either 12 or 30 breaths/min (as observed frequently in a clinical trial), the mean intrathoracic pressure was inversely related to coronary perfusion pressure and 1-hour survival rates; P<.05. (*From* Aufderheide TP, Sigurdsson G, Pirrallo RG, et al. Hyperventilation-induced hypotension during cardiopulmonary resuscitation. Circulation 2004;109:1960; with permission.)

complete seal, and a jaw thrust to maintain airway patency, and the second person squeezes the resuscitator bag. This approach can be used for a more prolonged period when adequate personnel are available as it enables rescuers to perform high-quality CPR without stopping compressions and interrupting circulation to place an advanced airway device. This approach works well when using an impedance threshold device (ITD), as described later in this article, and is inexpensive. Delaying intubation by providing good face-mask ventilation technique is an important way to maximize chest compression time.

## COMPRESSIONS

Chest compressions or "external cardiac massage" was first introduced into the modern medical literature by Kouwenhoven and colleagues in 1960.[20] Generation of blood flow during compressions results from an increase in intrathoracic pressure (thoracic pump theory), the mechanical effect of compressing the heart between the sternum and spine (cardiac pump theory), and the cardiac valvular system, which allows mainly unidirectional flow. The recommendation for pushing "hard and fast" results from the understanding of the importance of compressions during CPR. However, pushing too hard and too fast can be harmful; like the ventilation frequency, understanding the subtleties of the chest-compression technique is essential for good outcomes. A depth of 3 to 5 cm is considered adequate compression depth (**Fig. 3**).[21] The rate should be 100 compressions/min because lower rates decrease forward blood flow.[22] Interruptions should be minimized, because every time compressions are stopped, it takes a significant amount of time to reestablish adequate aortic pressure and coronary perfusion pressure.[23] For example, pulse checks should not last more than 10 seconds. CPR should be delivered continuously for 2 minutes before pulse or rhythm checks. In observational studies the average time without compressions during resuscitation varies from 25% to 50% (**Fig. 4**).[24] This variation can be extremely detrimental as no compressions means no perfusion.

One of the recommendations by the AHA is that uninterrupted chest compressions should be delivered before the delivery of a shock, and chest compressions should be resumed immediately thereafter for 2 minutes. Although performing chest compression immediately after direct current shock was based on consensus opinion, the overall thrust of the recommendation is the importance of circulation before defibrillation (**Fig. 5**). Chest compressions for 90 seconds to 3 minutes before defibrillation help to "prime" the pump, making successful return of spontaneous circulation most likely after defibrillation. Chest compressions for 60 seconds to 2 minutes immediately after defibrillation are believed to help prevent the hypotension and asystole that is often observed when a defibrillation shock is delivered. As a result, rather than check for a pulse after a defibrillation shock in a patient who has been in VF for more than 4 minutes, the rescuers should immediately resume CPR to maintain circulation, even if the heart is spontaneously beating. Although a theoretic risk of reinducing fibrillation with chest compression exists, there are no human data to support a significant risk or benefit in performing 2 minutes of CPR immediately after defibrillation and before checking for rhythm and pulses.

## COMPRESSION-ONLY (HANDS-ONLY) CPR

Because uninterrupted chest compressions are easier to perform and possibly a more attractive and simpler method to teach bystander CPR (as

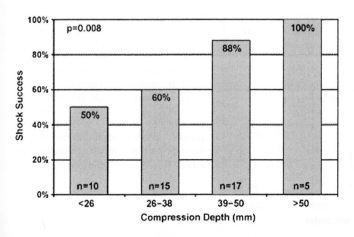

**Fig. 3.** Association between chest compression depth and shock success. Cases are grouped by 30-second average compression depth in approximately 11-mm (0.5-in) intervals. Chest compression depth of 38 to 50 mm (1.5–2 in) represents current CPR guidelines recommendations. Deeper chest compressions are significantly associated with increased probability of shock success. (*From* Edelson DP, Abella BS, Kramer-Johansen J, et al. Effects of compression depth and pre-shock pauses predict debrillation failure during cardiac arrest. Resuscitation 2006;71(2):141; with permission.)

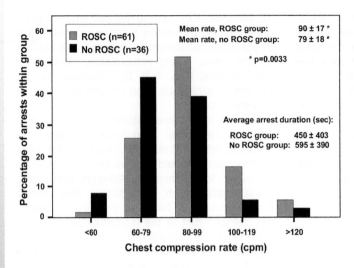

**Fig. 4.** Chest compression rates correlation with initial resuscitation outcome. Subgroup of patients attaining ROSC is shown in gray; subgroup that did not, in black. Note 2 overlapping but distinct distributions, with mean rates for each group shown. Note mean durations of resuscitation for 2 groups, demonstrating that the group that expired received longer resuscitation efforts on average, arguing against a "slow-code" bias. Asterisk denotes statistical significance from a 2-tailed *t*-test as shown. (*From* Abella BS, Sandbo N, Vassilatos P, et al. Chest compression rates during cardiopulmonary resuscitation are suboptimal: a prospective study during in-hospital cardiac arrest. Circulation 2005;111:428; with permission.)

shown by the Survey of Survivors of Out-of-Hospital Cardiac Arrest in the Kanto Region of Japan [SOS-KANTO] study)[25] the Emergency Cardiovascular Care Committee of the AHA has released a science advisory recommending an alternative strategy of compression-only or "hands-only" CPR for layperson bystanders witnessing an adult cardiac arrest.[4]

The recommendations summarized include the following 3 possibilities: (1) If an adult suddenly collapses, trained or untrained bystanders should (at a minimum) activate their community emergency medical response system (call 911) and provide high-quality chest compressions by pushing hard and fast in the center of the chest, minimizing interruptions according to the published guidelines (class I). (2) If a bystander has not received training in CPR, then hands-only CPR is strongly encouraged (class IIa). The

rescuer should continue hands-only CPR until an AED arrives and is ready for use or EMS providers take over care of the victim. (3) When the bystander has received training in CPR, he or she can provide conventional CPR using a 30:2 compression/ventilation ratio (class IIa) or hands-only CPR (class IIa). CPR with either of the 2 techniques should be continued until defibrillation is possible or EMS providers take over. When the bystander, regardless of training status, is not confident in his or her ability to provide conventional CPR, including high-quality chest compressions with rescue breaths (compressions of adequate rate and depth with minimal interruptions), then hands-only CPR is recommended (class IIa).

There is no evidence to support the adoption of this approach by trained EMS paramedics. There is, on the contrary, a significant body of evidence

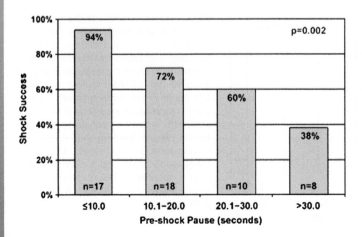

**Fig. 5.** Association between preshock pause and shock success. Cases are grouped by preshock pause in 10-second intervals. Note that longer preshock pauses are significantly associated with a smaller probability of shock success. (*From* Edelson DP, Abella BS, Kramer-Johansen J, et al. Effects of compression depth and pre-shock pauses predict debrillation failure during cardiac arrest. Resuscitation 2006;71(2):141; with permission.)

that disputes the notion that prolonged CPR can be performed without the presence of ventilation. It has recently been shown that when delivered ventilations decrease from 10 beats/min to 2 beats/min, a significant decrease in brain tissue oxygen tension and carotid blood flow occurs.[13] In addition, in a 24-hour neurologic and survival evaluation study, animals with no assisted ventilation had significantly worse neurologic outcomes with evidence of significant respiratory and metabolic acidosis and profound hypoxemia within the first of 4 minutes of chest-compression-only CPR despite open airways compared with standard CPR (**Fig. 6**).[14] This new investigation is in concordance with 2 previously published studies that showed worsening rates of return of spontaneous circulation (ROSC) and evidence of severe respiratory acidosis and hypoxemia when prolonged CPR is performed without ventilations.[16,26] There are data in support of a chest-compression-only strategy for lay rescuers, but there are no prospective randomized trials that demonstrate a benefit to this approach by professional first responders. By contrast, EMS systems in Europe and the United States that follow the AHA Guidelines on compressions show the highest survival rates in the history of CPR (Rae, King County, WA, USA; White, Rochester, MN, USA; Sunde, Oslo, Norway).

## CHEST-WALL DECOMPRESSION

With each chest-wall decompression, the negative intrathoracic pressure naturally generated by the elastic recoil properties of the chest wall promotes venous return to the heart, thereby increasing preload for the next compression cycle. The decompression-induced vacuum within the chest is transmitted to the brain and as a result intracranial pressure is transiently reduced, thereby reducing resistance to forward brain flow. Incomplete decompression, like hyperventilation, is a common mistake and is harmful. Incomplete chest-wall recoil decreases blood flow to the heart and brain during CPR. Fatigue and ineffective technique, inappropriate hand positioning, or poorly designed mechanical CPR adjuncts can result in incomplete chest-wall recoil. Data from recent trials

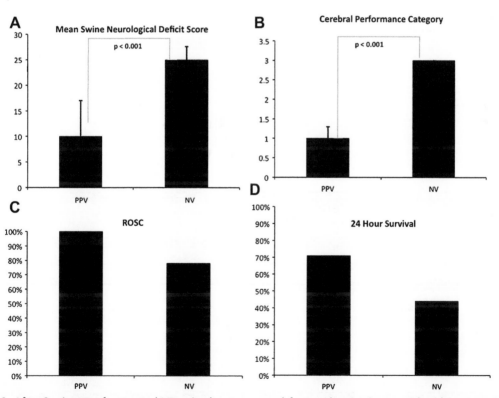

**Fig. 6.** After 8 minutes of untreated VF, animals were treated for another 8 minutes with either 10 positive-pressure ventilation (PPV)/min or with no assisted ventilation (NAV) before defibrillation. Survivors were followed for 24 hours. *A*, Mean neurologic score; *B*, CPC score; *C*, rate of return to spontaneous circulation; *D*, 24-hour survival rate in percentage. The number of animals that survived of the total number of animals in the group is shown in parentheses.

demonstrated that many rescuers fail to decompress completely,[27,28] which results in a sustained end diastolic increase of intrathoracic pressure. This phenomenon, when examined in a porcine model of cardiac arrest, revealed 2 fundamental effects. First, incomplete chest-wall recoil caused a significant decrease of mean arterial pressure, an increase in right atrial pressure, and thus decreased coronary perfusion pressures. Second, incomplete chest-wall recoil led to a significant increase in intracranial pressure and a decrease in cerebral and systemic perfusion pressures (**Fig. 7**).[19] When incomplete decompression and positive-pressure ventilation occurred simultaneously, cerebral perfusion ceased; the cerebral perfusion gradient was essentially zero for at least 3 to 4 compression-decompression cycles (**Fig. 8**).

### Devices

Mechanical devices have been developed with the intent to improve circulation and promote air exchange and ventilation. Those devices are discussed in detail in this section.

### *Harnessing negative intrathoracic pressure to increase venous return and increase vital organ perfusion during CPR*

**Inspiratory ITD** The dynamic energy of the expanding chest wall during the decompression phase can be harnessed to increase venous return, increase aortic pressure, lower intracranial pressure, and increase circulation to the heart and brain. The inspiratory ITD regulates the entry of air through the airways into the chest during the decompression phase of CPR. It causes a decrease in intrathoracic pressure of −2 to 10 mmHg, depending on the method used to perform chest compressions. The intrathoracic vacuum that develops with the ITD helps to draw blood back to the heart and lower intracranial pressure during the recoil phase of CPR.[29] Although this device is attached to an airway, it is used during CPR to enhance circulation (**Fig. 9**).

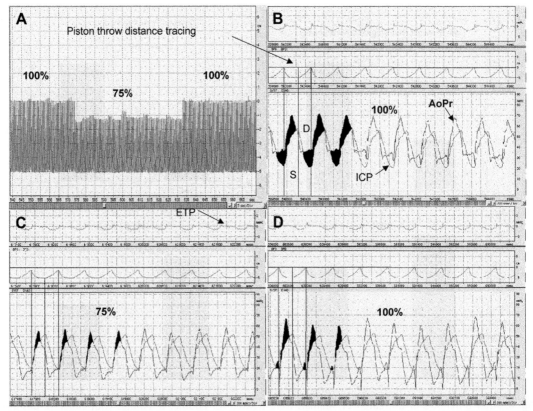

**Fig. 7.** The effect of incomplete chest-wall recoil on cerebral perfusion pressure (*A–D*). (*From* Yannopoulos D, McKnite S, Aufderheide TP, et al. Effects of incomplete chest wall decompression during cardiopulmonary resuscitation on coronary and cerebral perfusion pressures in a porcine model of cardiac arrest. Resuscitation 2005;64:363; with permission.)

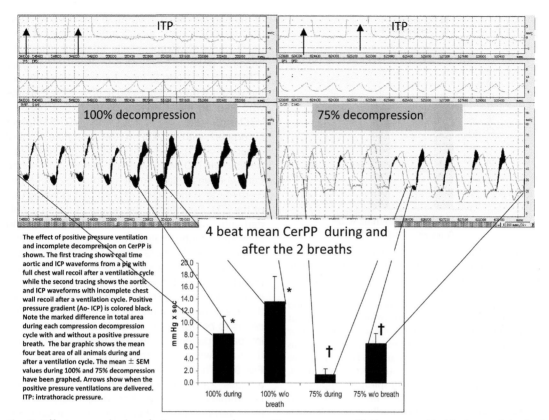

ITP

ITP

100% decompression

75% decompression

The effect of positive pressure ventilation and incomplete decompression on CerPP is shown. The first tracing shows real time aortic and ICP waveforms from a pig with full chest wall recoil after a ventilation cycle while the second tracing shows the aortic and ICP waveforms with incomplete chest wall recoil after a ventilation cycle. Positive pressure gradient (Ao- ICP) is colored black. Note the marked difference in total area during each compression decompression cycle with and without a positive pressure breath. The bar graphic shows the mean four beat area of all animals during and after a ventilation cycle. The mean ± SEM values during 100% and 75% decompression have been graphed. Arrows show when the positive pressure ventilations are delivered. ITP: intrathoracic pressure.

**4 beat mean CerPP during and after the 2 breaths**

(y-axis: mmHg x sec; values 0.0, 2.0, 4.0, 6.0, 8.0, 10.0, 12.0, 14.0, 16.0, 18.0, 20.0)

(x-axis categories: 100% during, 100% w/o breath, 75% during, 75% w/o breath)

**Fig. 8.** Effect on cerebral perfusion pressure when positive-pressure ventilations are added to incomplete chest decompressions. (*From* Yannopoulos D, McKnite S, Aufderheide TP, et al. Effects of incomplete chest wall decompression during cardiopulmonary resuscitation on coronary and cerebral perfusion pressures in a porcine model of cardiac arrest. Resuscitation 2005;64:363; with permission.)

Demonstration of ITD benefit in animal and clinical studies form the basis for the level IIa recommendation for the ITD in the 2005 AHA Guidelines. One of the first animal studies performed with the ITD demonstrated that use of the active ITD increased 24-h survival and preserved neurologic function after induced cardiac arrest in pigs.[30] There was a statistically significant increase in these key outcome parameters, as shown in **Fig. 10**. There was improved neurologic function in the overall study group, and in the subset of pigs that were resuscitated with defibrillation shock therapy and epinephrine. Blood gas data demonstrated that relative tissue

- <u>Concept</u>: Lower intrathoracic pressure in the chest during the decompression phase of CPR enhances venous return to the thorax.

- <u>Design</u>: Each time the chest wall recoils following a compression, the ITD transiently blocks air/oxygen from entering the lungs, creating a small vacuum in the chest, resulting in improved preload.

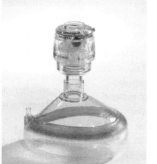

**Fig. 9.** The concept and design of the inspiratory ITD. The ITD can be placed on an endotracheal tube or on a specially designed face-mask for bag- mask ventilation provided that a good air seal is applied. Timing lights flash at a rate of 10/min to guide ventilations and compressions (10 compressions between 2 flashes).

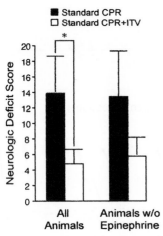

**Fig. 10.** Pittsburgh neurologic deficit score for all animals receiving standard CPR with either sham (n = 11 of 20 survivors 24 hours after resuscitation) or active (n = 17 of 20 survivors 24 hours after resuscitation) valve (ITV is the old term for the ITD) and subgroup of animals that were resuscitated without (w/o) epinephrine. All values are mean ± stander error of the mean; *P<.03. Twenty-four-hour survival was 55% in the sham valve group and 85% in the active valve group (P<.05). (*From* Lurie KG, Zielinski T, McKnite S, et al. Use of an inspiratory impedance valve improves neurologically intact survival in a porcine model of ventricular fibrillation. Circulation 2002;105:124; with permission.)

oxygenation was considered adequate in both groups and no differences were observed between groups on autopsy. The intrathoracic pressures were significantly lower in the ITD group. Subsequent studies have demonstrated that use of the ITD lowers intracranial pressures more rapidly than in pigs treated with standard CPR alone. It is hypothesized that this observation helps to explain the markedly improved neurologic outcomes in this porcine survival study.

After the animal studies, Pirrallo and colleagues[31] demonstrated with a double-blind, randomized, control trial that systolic blood pressures were twice as high with an active ITD when compared with a sham device. A concurrent study demonstrated that 24-hour survival rates were twice as high in patients presenting with pulseless electrical activity with the active device.[32] More recently, Aufderheide and colleagues[33] reported beneficial outcomes from the use of the ITD in 5 US EMS systems and Davis and colleagues[34] showed a nearly 2-fold survival improvement when the ITD was used on patients with an in-hospital cardiac arrest. Aufderheide and colleagues[33] showed that the changes in CPR practice resulted in a significant increase of hospital discharge rates for all patients, regardless

of presenting heart rhythm, from 10% to 13% (P = .007) and significantly improved the percentage of neurologically intact or minimally impaired patients (cerebral performance category [CPC] scores 1 and 2) who were discharged from the hospital from 33% to 60% (P = .03). Patients who had an initial rhythm of VF had a hospital discharge rate of 31.1% with ITD treatment compared with 20.4% in the historical control group (P = .01). These more recent studies incorporated the ITD into a systems-based approach to care wherein multiple small but important changes were made in the quality of CPR that included use of the ITD. Specifically the recent studies by Aufderheide and colleagues and Davis and colleagues incorporated improvements including: (1) emphasis on more compressions and fewer ventilations; (2) allowing complete chest-wall recoil; (3) uninterrupted chest compressions during advanced airway management; and (4) the use of an ITD during BLS and ALS.[33] The ITD needs to be applied early and it can be used with intubated patients connected to the endotracheal tube and with a face-mask and a good seal (see **Fig. 9**).[35] The ITD is the only CPR device to receive a class 2a recommendation by the AHA; this recommendation was based in part on the observed doubling of blood pressure observed in a randomized double-blind, out-of-hospital, cardiac arrest trial with the ITD.[15,31] It is important to emphasize that no device, including the ITD, is a panacea; this and other new technologies need to be used in a systems-based approach to improve survival rates significantly.

**Intrathoracic pressure regulator** The second generation of intrathoracic pressure regulation devices to improve cardiorespiratory interactions during CPR is the intrathoracic pressure regulator (ITPR). This device is not dependent on the elastic properties of the expanding chest wall to generate negative intrathoracic pressure. The device provides continues negative airway pressure in intubated animals and allows for positive-pressure ventilation delivery. This device improves all basic hemodynamic parameters during CPR and the rates of return to spontaneous circulation. In addition. it has shown significant improvement in hemodynamic parameters during hypovolemic cardiac arrest (hemorrhage).[36] This device is cleared for sale by the US Food and Drug Administration and clinical trials are under way to determine its potential benefit.

### Compression devices
The load-distributing band (LDB) device (Autopulse, Zoll Circulation, Sunnyvale, CA, USA), an

automated band-compression device, has been shown to increase perfusion pressures in animals and humans.[37,38] It is based on the physiologic principal that circumferential thoracic compression increases intrathoracic pressure without significant cardiac compression and can effectively produce forward flow. Increasing intrathoracic pressure results in forward blood flow. There is some controversy, however, as use of this device has been reported to be associated with positive and adverse outcomes. For example, a recent large randomized trial (ASPIRE) was prematurely stopped because of safety concerns. Rates of survival to discharge from hospital were found to be lower in the LDB-CPR group (5.8% vs 9.9% [P = .04]; adjusted for covariates and clustering, P = .06). In addition, survival with a CPC score of 1 or 2 was recorded in 7.5% (28 of 371) of patients in the manual CPR group compared with 3.1% (12 of 391) in the LDB-CPR group (P = .006).[39] In contrast, a second non-randomized historical control-based study on the LDB-CPR, published in the same issue of *JAMA*, showed that when the LBD-CPR device was used in a systems-based approach to care that included CPR before shock and therapeutic hypothermia, survival rates increased. The second study compared resuscitation outcomes before and after an urban EMS system switched from manual CPR to LDB-CPR. A total of 499 patients were included in the manual CPR phase (2001–2003) and 284 patients in the LDB-CPR phase (2003–2005); of these latter patients, the LDB device was applied in 210 patients. Patients in the manual CPR and LDB-CPR phases were comparable except for more EMS-witnessed arrests (18.7% vs 12.6%) with LDB. Rates of survival to discharge from hospital were poor in the historical phase (2.9%) and increased to 9.7% (P<.01) with the new system. In a secondary analysis of the 210 patients in whom the LDB device was applied, 38 patients (18.1%) survived to hospital admission, and only 12 patients (5.7%) survived to hospital discharge. Among patients in the manual CPR and LDB-CPR groups who survived to discharge from hospital, there was no significant difference between groups in CPC or overall performance category. Thus, in a nonrandomized study a new resuscitation strategy that included using LDB-CPR on EMS ambulances was associated with improved survival to discharge from hospital in adults with out-of-hospital nontraumatic cardiac arrest, but the study design was controversial.[40] Based on the fundamental physiologic relationships described earlier in this article related to the importance of incomplete chest-wall recoil and potential harm associated with increasing the intrathoracic pressure too much, the authors speculate that better regulation of changes in intrathoracic pressure with LBD-CPR types of devices would result in more consistent results (**Fig. 11**).

### Active compression decompression device

The active compression decompression (ACD) CPR device turns the thorax into an active bellows, drawing respiratory gases into the lungs with each decompression, along with a small amount of blood back to the heart. With each compression air and blood are propelled out of the thorax.[41] Multiple out-of-hospital and in-hospital hemodynamic and survival studies have been performed with ACD CPR. Some have shown significant improvements in up to 1-year survival, whereas others have shown no significant benefit with the device.[42] The combination of an ACD device with the inspiratory ITD offers significant hemodynamic improvement during CPR.[43] The ITD activates ACD CPR by harnessing the bellowslike action of the thorax. The device combination results in a significant augmentation in coronary and cerebral circulation. The device combination was shown to improve short-term survival outcomes: 24-hour survival rates were increased by 50% in 2 separate randomized controlled trials.[42,44] At present the manual ACD CPR device is not approved by the US Food and Drug Administration (FDA) for sale in the United States.

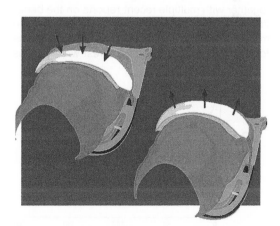

**Fig. 11.** Autopulse configuration. During compression (*left*) the band is tightened by the motor, and compression force is directed inward. During relaxation (*right*), the band is released, and the chest expands. (*From* Halperin HR, Paradis N, Ornato JP, et al. Cardiopulmonary resuscitation with a novel chest compression device in a porcine model of cardiac arrest: improved hemodynamics and mechanisms. J Am Coll Cardiol 2004;44:2214; with permission.)

Another ACD device, which is automated rather than manual, is the Lund University Compression Assist Device or LUCAS device. There are no randomized controlled trials with this device. However, this device provides an alternative to manual CPR and allows for complete chest-wall recoil with some degree of active decompression. FDA regulations currently limit the decompression phase forces to 3 pounds (1.3 kg).

## THERAPEUTIC HYPOTHERMIA

Although the benefits of therapeutic hypothermia were first described 50 years ago for patients after cardiac arrest, only recently have clinicians adopted this postresuscitation technique to help preserve brain function.[45] Animal and humans studies have shown that the rapid lowering of core temperature to 33°C for 24 hours improves neurologically intact survival rates for patients with an initial rhythm of VF. Two randomized human trials published in the *New England Journal of Medicine* in 2002 demonstrated that mild to moderate hypothermia (32–34°C), post resuscitation, resulted in an improvement (16%–23% absolute risk reduction) for poor neurologic outcomes in patients who had a witnessed VF arrest. There was a significant improvement in 6-month survival rates in the hypothermic groups (**Fig. 12** and **Table 1**).[46,47] Current AHA Guidelines support this approach, with a level 2a recommendation for patients who present with a witnessed arrest and VF as the presenting rhythm. These data, together with multiple recent reports on the benefits of therapeutic hypothermia, have resulted in more widespread use of therapeutic hypothermia for any patient after a cardiac arrest who remains comatose. The authors strongly support this more liberalized approach to this significant clinical advance.

Recent studies have shown that it is possible to cool during CPR before reperfusion is achieved to further minimize tissue damage before it occurs. Cooling during CPR in animals with venovenous access systems or with cold intravenous saline and use of ACD CPR plus the ITD may eventually offer a means to rapidly decrease cerebral temperatures during CPR and improve neurologic outcomes.[48,49] Based on data in support of therapeutic hypothermia, the guidelines recommend cooling of comatose patients after successful resuscitation when possible, as long as there is a protocol in place to assure careful monitoring of core temperatures and hemodynamics, prevention of shivering, and maintenance of adequate perfusion pressures during the recommended 24-hour period of cooling. Further study is needed to evaluate the therapeutic potential of early cooling and to investigate the best way of achieving cerebral hypothermia in a timely and practical manner.

## PHARMACOLOGIC MANAGEMENT

There have been few advances in the pharmacologic management of patients in cardiac arrest.

### Vasoactive Medications

Evidence for the broad use of vasoactive medication during CPR comes primarily from animal studies. There are no placebo-controlled trials to demonstrate long-term benefit of epinephrine or vasopressin. The 2005 AHA Guidelines recommend the use of either of these agents with a class IIb level of recommendation.

Epinephrine is the most commonly used vasopressor during CPR. The beneficial hemodynamic effects of epinephrine during CPR are caused by its potent α-adrenergic effects. The significant increase in central aortic pressures results in significant increase in coronary and cerebral perfusion pressures and possibly rates of successful resuscitation.[50]

However, based on multiple clinical trials, use of high-dose epinephrine is contraindicated and harmful in patients in cardiac arrest (class III recommendation). The guidelines continue to recommend 1 mg of epinephrine every 3 to 5 minutes (recommendation class IIb) for adults in cardiac arrest. If no venous access has been obtained, endotracheal or intraosseous administration can be effective.

Vasopressin is recommended as an alternative vasopressor during CPR. It too has potent

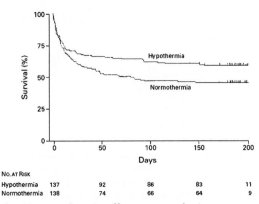

No. at Risk

| | | | | | |
|---|---|---|---|---|---|
| Hypothermia | 137 | 92 | 86 | 83 | 11 |
| Normothermia | 138 | 74 | 66 | 64 | 9 |

**Fig. 12.** Hypothermia effect on neurologic outcomes and survival. Censored data are indicated by tick marks. (*From* Hypothermia after Cardiac Arrest Study Group. Mild therapeutic hypothermia to improve the neurologic outcome after cardiac arrest. N Engl J Med 2002;346:549; with permission.)

**Table 1**
**Neurologic outcome and mortality at 6 months**

| Outcome | Normothermia | Hypothermia | Risk Ratio (95% CI)[a] | P Value[b] |
|---|---|---|---|---|
| | Number/Total Number (%) | | | |
| Favorable neurologic outcome[c] | 54/137 (39) | 75/136 (55) | 1.40 (1.08–1.81) | .009 |
| Death | 76/138 (55) | 56/137 (41) | 0.74 (0.58–0.95) | .02 |

[a] The risk ratio was calculated as the rate of a favorable neurologic outcome or the rate of death in the hypothermia group divided by the rate in the normothermia group. CI denotes confidence interval.
[b] Two-sided P values are based on Pearson's $\chi^2$ tests.
[c] A favorable neurologic outcome was defined as a cerebral-performance category of 1 (good recovery) or 2 (moderate disability). One patient in the normothermia group and 1 in the hypothermia group were lost to neurologic follow-up.
   *From* Hypothermia after Cardiac Arrest Study Group. Mild therapeutic hypothermia to improve the neurologic outcome after cardiac arrest. N Engl J Med 2002;346:549; with permission.

vasoconstricting properties. No study has shown that vasopressin use increases hospital discharge rates when used in patients in cardiac arrest. A recent study showed the combination of epinephrine plus vasopressin resulted in higher rates of ROSC, and no increase in long-term survival rates, but a strong trend toward worsening of neurologic outcomes, except in those with an initial rhythm of asystole arrest.[51] However, the quality of CPR was an important uncontrolled variable in that study. Another more recent randomized clinical trial showed no significant benefit with the combination of epinephrine plus vasopressin compared with epinephrine alone.[52] The authors of this article recommend that 1 to 2 doses of epinephrine are used before using vasopressin, given the lack of definitive data and levels of recommendation in the new guidelines to epinephrine and vasopressin.

There is no good treatment of asystole. Atropine, a vagolytic medication, has no known negative effects in patients with asystole, and can be given for severe bradycardiac and asystole with doses of 1 mg intravenously every minute to a total dose of 3 mg. There is no randomized animal or human study to support the administration of atropine for improvement of outcomes.

## Antiarrhythmic Agents

As with the other intravenous medications, there are insufficient levels of data or consensus among the experts regarding the use of antiarrhythmic agents during CPR. Amiodarone is considered the drug of choice and as an intravenous bolus of 150 to 300 mg for VF or pulseless ventricular tachycardiac that are unresponsive to the initial sequences of CPR-shock-CPR-vasoconstrictors. The recommendation is based on limited clinical trials,[53,54] showing improvement in hospital admission but no definitive increase in hospital discharge rates, when compared with placebo or lidocaine. Given the lack of definitive data, lidocaine (initial dose of 1–1.5 mg/kg intravenously) can also be used in patients in cardiac arrest.

## REPERFUSION THERAPY

Because of the high incidence of obstructive coronary artery disease (70% of autopsy patients document active thrombus in the coronary tree and from patients undergoing cardiac catheterization another 70% show evidence of severe coronary artery stenosis) in the cardiac-arrest population and the inability to make the diagnosis of ST elevation myocardial infarction based on the postresuscitation ECG, elective angiogram and primary angioplasty should be considered in all survivors without any other clear cause for the cardiac arrest.[55] Long-term prognosis after primary percutaneous coronary intervention (PCI) in survivors of cardiac arrest is good, with 2-year survival rates reported up to 70%.[56] A body of evidence that primary PCI should be considered in survivors of cardiac arrest is currently being evaluated and will be addressed in the next AHA/ECC Guidelines in 2010. In a recent study, reperfusion therapy (PCI or coronary artery bypass graft) had the most profound effect on outcome (adjusted odds ratio = 4.47) when compared with no reperfusion therapy. Patients were transported directly from the emergency department to the PCI suite when clinically stable.[57]

## SYSTEMS-BASED APPROACH TO RESUSCITATION

Perhaps one of the biggest advances in CPR is the systems-based approach. The notion that one single intervention can significantly improve

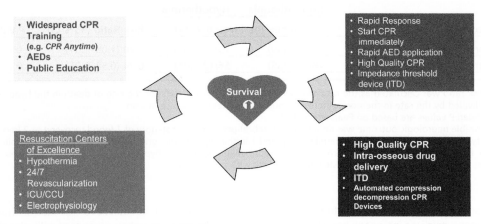

**Fig. 13.** A systems-based approach to resuscitation.

outcomes in cardiac arrest has been fading because of the complexity and severity of multiorgan dysfunction that develops from the systemic hypoperfusion and hypoxemia. Data from Seattle demonstrating that the introduction of AEDs in all of the first-responder vehicles resulted in a decrease in survival rates for nearly a decade was a warning of the importance of circulation during resuscitation. When CPR was performed for 90 seconds before defibrillation, survival rates were shown to improve with AED implementation. Different efforts to address the issue have shown promise, with significant improvement in mortality and hospital discharge. Application of

**Table 2**
**The effect of various sudden cardiac arrest interventions: a combination of all of the interventions could theoretically result in a 24% to 37% increase in survival**

| Intervention | Effect | Expected Absolute Survival Rate ↑ Compared with Baseline (%) |
|---|---|---|
| Bystander CPR<br>CPR anytime in schools, homes, and public meeting places | ☐ Rapid EMS notification<br>☐ Start circulation | 2–5[58–61] |
| AED use<br>Widespread strategic AED deployment | ☐ Reduce time to first shock in VF patients | 4–6[6,62–66] |
| Improved CPR quality and drug delivery<br>Prevent hyperventilation, continuous chest compressions, CPR pre/post shock, intraosseous drug delivery, automated compression-decompression devices | ☐ Increase circulation to heart and brain<br>☐ Increase oxygen and drug delivery | 6–10[17,27,67,68] |
| ITD eg, ResQPOD (Advanced Circulatory Systems, Eden Prairie, MN, USA)<br>BLS and ALS deployment | ☐ Increase circulation to heart and brain<br>☐ Increase oxygen and drug delivery | 5[31,32,44,69] |
| Resuscitation centers<br>Standard hypothermia protocols, cardiac angiography, intensive care/electrophysiology evaluation, device placement | ☐ Revascularization<br>☐ Organ preservation<br>☐ Prevent sudden cardiac death | 5–10[46,47,70–73] |
| | | Total: 22–36 |

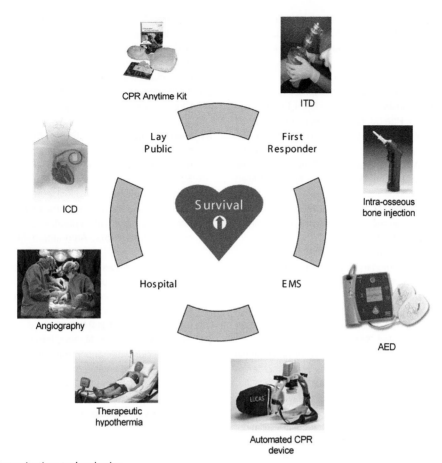

Fig. 14. Resuscitation technologies.

good-quality CPR, limitation of compression interruptions and ventilations, addition of an inspiratory ITD, and early postresuscitation hypothermia and reperfusion therapies have shown promise when implemented as a system rather than unique interventions.[57]

One program that focuses on this systems-based approach is called Take Heart America. The approach is shown in **Fig. 13**. This technology-based approach implements all of the most highly recommended changes in the 2005 AHA Guidelines. **Table 2** describes the key interventions and their anticipated benefits. This approach includes using new techniques and devices to train lay and professional rescuers in a faster and more reliable way on how to perform CPR, increase circulation during CPR, and focus on skilled postresuscitation care (see **Fig. 14**). Some of these technologies, which have been available only within the past 5 years, are shown in **Fig. 14**.

When these technologies have been deployed, survival rates have increased from 9% to 17% in sites that have implemented this approach (see

http://www.takeheartamerica.org/). This kind of approach, akin to treating other complex diseases like cancer or human immunodeficiency virus syndromes, focuses on the criticality of integrating multiple time-sensitive interventions with state-of-the art technology for the care of patients in cardiac arrest. The authors believe that the synergy associated with this approach underlies the foundation for the future of CPR and will result in a fundamental shift in the treatment of all patients in cardiac arrest.

## REFERENCES

1. Cobb LA, Fahrenbruch CE, Olsufka M, et al. Changing incidence of out-of-hospital ventricular fibrillation, 1980–2000. JAMA 2002;288:3008–13.
2. Zheng ZJ, Croft JB, Giles WH, et al. Sudden cardiac death in the United States, 1989 to 1998. Circulation 2001;104:2158–63.
3. Weisfeldt ML, Becker LB. Resuscitation after cardiac arrest: a 3-phase time-sensitive model. JAMA 2002; 288:3035–8.

4. Sayre MR, Berg RA, Cave DM, et al. Hands-only (compression-only) cardiopulmonary resuscitation: a call to action for bystander response to adults who experience out-of-hospital sudden cardiac arrest: a science advisory for the public from the American Heart Association Emergency Cardiovascular Care Committee. Circulation 2008;117:2162–7.

5. Valenzuela TD, Roe DJ, Nichol G, et al. Outcomes of rapid defibrillation by security officers after cardiac arrest in casinos. N Engl J Med 2000;343:1206–9.

6. Caffrey SL, Willoughby PJ, Pepe PE, et al. Public use of automated external defibrillators. N Engl J Med 2002;347:1242–7.

7. Marijon E, Combes N, Boveda S. Home automated defibrillators after myocardial infarction. N Engl J Med 2008;359:533–4.

8. Cobb LA, Fahrenbruch CE, Walsh TR, et al. Influence of cardiopulmonary resuscitation prior to defibrillation in patients with out-of-hospital ventricular fibrillation. JAMA 1999;281:1182–8.

9. Bardy GH, Lee KL, Mark DB, et al. Home use of automated external defibrillators for sudden cardiac arrest. N Engl J Med 2008;358:1793–804.

10. Nichol G, Thomas E, Callaway CW, et al. Regional variation in out-of-hospital cardiac arrest incidence and outcome. JAMA 2008;300:1423–31.

11. Wik L, Hansen TB, Fylling F, et al. Delaying defibrillation to give basic cardiopulmonary resuscitation to patients with out-of-hospital ventricular fibrillation: a randomized trial. JAMA 2003;289:1389–95.

12. Yannopoulos D, Aufderheide TP, Gabrielli A, et al. Clinical and hemodynamic comparison of 15:2 and 30:2 compression-to-ventilation ratios for cardiopulmonary resuscitation. Crit Care Med 2006;34:1444–9.

13. Lurie KG, Yannopoulos D, McKnite SH, et al. Comparison of a 10-breaths-per-minute versus a 2-breaths-per-minute strategy during cardiopulmonary resuscitation in a porcine model of cardiac arrest. Respir Care 2008;53:862–70.

14. Yannopoulos D, Matsuura T, McKnite S, et al. No assisted ventilation CPR and 24-hour neurological outcomes in a porcine model of cardiac arrest. Crit Care Med 2009. [Epub ahead of print].

15. 2005 AHA guidelines of CPR and emergency cardiovascular care. Circulation 2005;112.

16. Idris AH, Becker LB, Fuerst RS, et al. Effect of ventilation on resuscitation in an animal model of cardiac arrest. Circulation 1994;90:3063–9.

17. Aufderheide TP, Lurie KG. Death by hyperventilation: a common and life-threatening problem during cardiopulmonary resuscitation. Crit Care Med 2004;32:S345–51.

18. Aufderheide TP, Sigurdsson G, Pirrallo RG, et al. Hyperventilation-induced hypotension during cardiopulmonary resuscitation. Circulation 2004;109:1960–5.

19. Yannopoulos D, McKnite S, Aufderheide TP, et al. Effects of incomplete chest wall decompression during cardiopulmonary resuscitation on coronary and cerebral perfusion pressures in a porcine model of cardiac arrest. Resuscitation 2005;64:363–72.

20. Kouwenhoven WB, Jude JR, Knickerbocker GG. Closed-chest cardiac massage. JAMA 1960;173:1064–7.

21. Halperin HR, Tsitlik JE, Guerci AD, et al. Determinants of blood flow to vital organs during cardiopulmonary resuscitation in dogs. Circulation 1986;73:539–50.

22. Kern KB, Sanders AB, Raife J, et al. A study of chest compression rates during cardiopulmonary resuscitation in humans. The importance of rate-directed chest compressions. Arch Intern Med 1992;152:145–9.

23. Berg RA, Sanders AB, Kern KB, et al. Adverse hemodynamic effects of interrupting chest compressions for rescue breathing during cardiopulmonary resuscitation for ventricular fibrillation cardiac arrest. Circulation 2001;104:2465–70.

24. Abella BS, Sandbo N, Vassilatos P, et al. Chest compression rates during cardiopulmonary resuscitation are suboptimal: a prospective study during in-hospital cardiac arrest. Circulation 2005;111:428–34.

25. SOS-KANTO study group. Cardiopulmonary resuscitation by bystanders with chest compression only (SOS-KANTO): an observational study. Lancet 2007;369:920–6.

26. Idris AH, Banner MJ, Wenzel V, et al. Ventilation caused by external chest compression is unable to sustain effective gas exchange during CPR: a comparison with mechanical ventilation. Resuscitation 1994;28:143–50.

27. Aufderheide TP, Pirrallo RG, Yannopoulos D, et al. Incomplete chest wall decompression: a clinical evaluation of CPR performance by EMS personnel and assessment of alternative manual chest compression-decompression techniques. Resuscitation 2005;64:353–62.

28. Aufderheide TP, Pirrallo RG, Yannopoulos D, et al. Incomplete chest wall decompression: a clinical evaluation of CPR performance by trained laypersons and an assessment of alternative manual chest compression-decompression techniques. Resuscitation 2006;71:341–51.

29. Aufderheide TP, Alexander C, Lick C, et al. From laboratory science to six emergency medical services systems: New understanding of the physiology of cardiopulmonary resuscitation increases survival rates after cardiac arrest. Crit Care Med 2008;36:S397.

30. Lurie KG, Zielinski T, McKnite S, et al. Use of an inspiratory impedance valve improves neurologically intact survival in a porcine model of ventricular fibrillation. Circulation 2002;105:124–9.

31. Pirrallo RG, Aufderheide TP, Provo TA, et al. Effect of an inspiratory impedance threshold device on hemodynamics during conventional manual cardiopulmonary resuscitation. Resuscitation 2005;66:13–20.

32. Aufderheide TP, Pirrallo RG, Provo TA, et al. Clinical evaluation of an inspiratory impedance threshold device during standard cardiopulmonary resuscitation in patients with out-of-hospital cardiac arrest. Crit Care Med 2005;33:734–40.

33. Aufderheide TP, Birnbaum M, Lick C, et al. A tale of seven EMS systems: an impedance threshold device and improved CPR techniques double survival rates after out-of-hospital cardiac arrest. Circulation 2007;116(Suppl II):II936–7.

34. Davis S, Thigpen K, Basol R, et al. Implementation of the 2005 American Heart Association Guidelines together with the Impedance Threshold Device improves hospital discharge rates after in-hospital cardiac arrest. Circulation 2008;118:S765.

35. Plaisance P, Soleil C, Lurie KG, et al. Use of an inspiratory impedance threshold device on a facemask and endotracheal tube to reduce intrathoracic pressures during the decompression phase of active compression-decompression cardiopulmonary resuscitation. Crit Care Med 2005;33:990–4.

36. Yannopoulos D, Nadkarni VM, McKnite SH, et al. Intrathoracic pressure regulator during continuous-chest-compression advanced cardiac resuscitation improves vital organ perfusion pressures in a porcine model of cardiac arrest. Circulation 2005;112:803–11.

37. Halperin HR, Paradis N, Ornato JP, et al. Cardiopulmonary resuscitation with a novel chest compression device in a porcine model of cardiac arrest: improved hemodynamics and mechanisms. J Am Coll Cardiol 2004;44:2214–20.

38. Halperin HR, Tsitlik JE, Gelfand M, et al. A preliminary study of cardiopulmonary resuscitation by circumferential compression of the chest with use of a pneumatic vest. N Engl J Med 1993; 329:762–8.

39. Hallstrom A, Rea TD, Sayre MR, et al. Manual chest compression vs use of an automated chest compression device during resuscitation following out-of-hospital cardiac arrest: a randomized trial. JAMA 2006;295:2620–8.

40. Ong ME, Ornato JP, Edwards DP, et al. Use of an automated, load-distributing band chest compression device for out-of-hospital cardiac arrest resuscitation. JAMA 2006;295:2629–37.

41. Shultz JJ, Coffeen P, Sweeney M, et al. Evaluation of standard and active compression-decompression CPR in an acute human model of ventricular fibrillation. Circulation 1994;89:684–93.

42. Plaisance P, Lurie KG, Vicaut E, et al. A comparison of standard cardiopulmonary resuscitation and active compression-decompression resuscitation for out-of-hospital cardiac arrest. French Active Compression-Decompression Cardiopulmonary Resuscitation Study Group. N Engl J Med 1999;341: 569–75.

43. Lurie KG, Coffeen P, Shultz J, et al. Improving active compression-decompression cardiopulmonary resuscitation with an inspiratory impedance valve. Circulation 1995;91:1629–32.

44. Wolcke BB, Mauer DK, Schoefmann MF, et al. Comparison of standard cardiopulmonary resuscitation versus the combination of active compression-decompression cardiopulmonary resuscitation and an inspiratory impedance threshold device for out-of-hospital cardiac arrest. Circulation 2003;108: 2201–5.

45. Benson DW, Williams GR Jr, Spencer FC, et al. The use of hypothermia after cardiac arrest. Anesth Analg 1959;38:423–8.

46. Hypothermia after Cardiac Arrest Study Group. Mild therapeutic hypothermia to improve the neurologic outcome after cardiac arrest. N Engl J Med 2002; 346:549–56.

47. Bernard SA, Gray TW, Buist MD, et al. Treatment of comatose survivors of out-of-hospital cardiac arrest with induced hypothermia. N Engl J Med 2002; 346:557–63.

48. Nozari A, Safar P, Stezoski SW, et al. Critical time window for intra-arrest cooling with cold saline flush in a dog model of cardiopulmonary resuscitation. Circulation 2006;113:2690–6.

49. Srinivasan V, Nadkarni VM, Yannopoulos D, et al. Rapid induction of cerebral hypothermia is enhanced with active compression-decompression plus inspiratory impedance threshold device cardiopulmonary resusitation in a porcine model of cardiac arrest. J Am Coll Cardiol 2006;47:835–41.

50. Michael JR, Guerci AD, Koehler RC, et al. Mechanisms by which epinephrine augments cerebral and myocardial perfusion during cardiopulmonary resuscitation in dogs. Circulation 1984;69:822–35.

51. Wenzel V, Krismer AC, Arntz HR, et al. A comparison of vasopressin and epinephrine for out-of-hospital cardiopulmonary resuscitation. N Engl J Med 2004; 350:105–13.

52. Gueugniaud PY, David JS, Chanzy E, et al. Vasopressin and epinephrine vs. epinephrine alone in cardiopulmonary resuscitation. N Engl J Med 2008; 359:21–30.

53. Dorian P, Cass D, Schwartz B, et al. Amiodarone as compared with lidocaine for shock-resistant ventricular fibrillation. N Engl J Med 2002;346:884–90.

54. Kudenchuk PJ, Cobb LA, Copass MK, et al. Amiodarone for resuscitation after out-of-hospital cardiac arrest due to ventricular fibrillation. N Engl J Med 1999;341:871–8.

55. Spaulding CM, Joly LM, Rosenberg A, et al. Immediate coronary angiography in survivors of

out-of-hospital cardiac arrest. N Engl J Med 1997; 336:1629–33.

56. Bendz B, Eritsland J, Nakstad AR, et al. Long-term prognosis after out-of-hospital cardiac arrest and primary percutaneous coronary intervention. Resuscitation 2004;63:49–53.

57. Sunde K, Pytte M, Jacobsen D, et al. Implementation of a standardised treatment protocol for post resuscitation care after out-of-hospital cardiac arrest. Resuscitation 2007;73:29–39.

58. Holmberg M, Holmberg S, Herlitz J. Factors modifying the effect of bystander cardiopulmonary resuscitation on survival in out-of-hospital cardiac arrest patients in Sweden. Eur Heart J 2001;22:511–9.

59. Holmberg M, Holmberg S, Herlitz J, et al. Survival after cardiac arrest outside hospital in Sweden. Swedish Cardiac Arrest Registry. Resuscitation 1998;36:29–36.

60. Larsen MP, Eisenberg MS, Cummins RO, et al. Predicting survival from out-of-hospital cardiac arrest: a graphic model. Ann Emerg Med 1993;22:1652–8.

61. Valenzuela TD, Roe DJ, Cretin S, et al. Estimating effectiveness of cardiac arrest interventions: a logistic regression survival model. Circulation 1997;96:3308–13.

62. Auble TE, Menegazzi JJ, Paris PM. Effect of out-of-hospital defibrillation by basic life support providers on cardiac arrest mortality: a metaanalysis. Ann Emerg Med 1995;25:642–8.

63. Stiell IG, Wells GA, DeMaio VJ, et al. Modifiable factors associated with improved cardiac arrest survival in a multicenter basic life support/defibrillation system: OPALS Study Phase I results. Ontario Prehospital Advanced Life Support. Ann Emerg Med 1999;33:44–50.

64. Stiell IG, Wells GA, Field BJ, et al. Improved out-of-hospital cardiac arrest survival through the

inexpensive optimization of an existing defibrillation program: OPALS study phase II. Ontario Prehospital Advanced Life Support. JAMA 1999;281:1175–81.

65. Weaver WD, Hill D, Fahrenbruch CE, et al. Use of the automatic external defibrillator in the management of out-of-hospital cardiac arrest. N Engl J Med 1988; 319:661–6.

66. White RD, Bunch TJ, Hankins DG. Evolution of a community-wide early defibrillation programme experience more than 13 years using police/fire personnel and paramedics as responders. Resuscitation 2005;65:279–83.

67. Abella BS, Alvarado JP, Myklebust H, et al. Quality of cardiopulmonary resuscitation during in-hospital cardiac arrest. JAMA 2005;293:305–10.

68. Wik L, Kramer-Johansen J, Myklebust H, et al. Quality of cardiopulmonary resuscitation during out-of-hospital cardiac arrest. JAMA 2005;293:299–304.

69. Plaisance P, Lurie KG, Vicaut E, et al. Evaluation of an impedance threshold device in patients receiving active compression-decompression cardiopulmonary resuscitation for out of hospital cardiac arrest. Resuscitation 2004;61:265–71.

70. Bernard S, Buist M, Monteiro O, et al. Induced hypothermia using large volume, ice-cold intravenous fluid in comatose survivors of out-of-hospital cardiac arrest: a preliminary report. Resuscitation 2003;56: 9–13.

71. Lurie KG, Idris A, Holcomb JB. Level 1 cardiac arrest centers: learning from the trauma surgeons. Acad Emerg Med 2005;12:79–80.

72. Merchant RM, Abella BS, Khan M, et al. Cardiac catheterization is underutilized after in-hospital cardiac arrest. Resuscitation 2008;79:398–403.

73. Yannopoulos D, Aufderheide T. Acute management of sudden cardiac death in adults based upon the new CPR guidelines. Europace 2007;9:2–9.

# Public Access Defibrillation

Robert W. Rho, MD[a,b,*], Richard L. Page, MD[a,c]

**KEYWORDS**
- Ventricular fibrillation • Defibrillation • Cardiac arrest
- Resuscitation • Automated external defibrillator

In the United States, 50 to 60 people suffer a cardiac arrest each hour, amounting to approximately 250,000 deaths every year. In the first 5 minutes of a cardiac arrest, ventricular tachycardia and ventricular fibrillation (VF) are the most frequent cardiac arrhythmias encountered. Despite emergency medical response systems, the long-term survival from out-of-hospital cardiac arrest remains poor in most United States cities. Paramount to achieving successful resuscitation of a cardiac arrest victim is providing early defibrillation. The likelihood of survival decreases by 7% to 10% for every 1-minute delay in defibrillation. If defibrillation is delayed more than 10 minutes, the likelihood of survival is very poor. Modern living with vertical high-rise buildings, heavy traffic, and sprawling suburbs pose significant obstacles to emergency medical services (EMS) within cities. In 1995, in response to the abysmal survival of out-of-hospital cardiac arrest, the American Heart Association challenged the medical industry to develop a defibrillator that could be placed in public settings, used safely by lay responders, and provide earlier defibrillation to cardiac-arrest victims. Over the last decade, there have been significant technological advancements in automated external defibrillators (AEDs) and clinical studies have demonstrated their benefits and limitations in public locations. This article discusses the modern AED and the data to support public access defibrillation (PAD).

## THE MODERN AUTOMATED EXTERNAL DEFIBRILLATOR

The AED is designed to accurately analyze electrocardiograms obtained via defibrillation pads placed by lay responders on an arrest victim's chest. The device was first clinically introduced in 1979 by Diack and colleagues.[1] This "automatic cardiac resuscitator" was field tested in 21 cardiac-arrest victims in VF and resulted in 35 successful defibrillations to sinus rhythm.

Since this original "proof of concept" report, significant important advancements in AEDs have occurred. Today, the AED is a lightweight, small, portable device designed to be safe, reliable, and easy to use. The device is equipped with a highly accurate algorithm that accurately detects ventricular tachycardia and VF and is able to distinguish it from supraventricular arrhythmias and artifact with nearly 100% sensitivity and specificity. The device provides visual instructions and voice prompts to the lay responder as to whether a shock is advised. When a shock is advised, the responder pushes a button on the unit to deliver the shock. Many modern devices are programmed to comply with the most recent International Liaison Committee on Resuscitation–American College of Cardiology–American Heart Association (ILCOR/ACC/AHA) guidelines for cardiac resuscitation and can coach the responder through cardiopulmonary resuscitation (CPR), sensing and adapting to the

This article originally appeared in *Cardiac Electrophysiology Clinics*, volume 1, number 1.
a Department of Medicine, University of Washington, Seattle, WA 98195-6422, USA
b Division of Cardiology, University of Washington Medical Center, 1959 NE Pacific Street, HSB, Room AA121C, Box 356422, Seattle, WA 98195-6422, USA
c Division of Cardiology, University of Washington Medical Center, 1959 NE Pacific Street, HSB, Room AA510A, Box 356422, Seattle, WA 98195-6422, USA
* Corresponding author. Division of Cardiology, University of Washington Med Center, 1959 NE Pacific Street, Room AA121C, Box 356422, Seattle, WA 98195-6422.
*E-mail address:* rrho@u.washington.edu

Heart Failure Clin 7 (2011) 269–276
doi:10.1016/j.hfc.2011.01.006

responder's actions.[2] Modern devices also have automatic self-tests ensuring that the battery and all other components of the AED are operational when it is needed.

## THE USE OF AUTOMATED EXTERNAL DEFIBRILLATORS BY LAY RESPONDERS

To achieve shorter call-to-defibrillation times, many communities have equipped nontraditional first responders (eg, police officers, firefighters) with AEDs. These nontraditional first responders are able to arrive at the scene of a cardiac-arrest victim before paramedics and, therefore, provide earlier defibrillation. Additionally, these nontraditional first responders may be the first to arrive at other situations where a cardiac arrest may have occurred, such as at the scene of an accident, and can administer early defibrillation. Investigators have reported significant improvements in survival when earlier defibrillation was achieved by nontraditional emergency-response personnel equipped with an AED. Weaver and colleagues[3] demonstrated that among 276 cardiac-arrest victims treated initially by firefighters, 84 (30%) survived to hospital discharge. This is compared to the survival of 44 of 228 (19%) victims when firefighters performed CPR only and defibrillation was performed only after arrival of paramedics (odds ratio, 1.8; 95% CI, 1.1–2.9). The average call-to-defibrillation time was 3.6 minutes with firefighters compared to 5.1 minutes with paramedics. This study and others[4,5] demonstrated that non–emergency medical team rescuers were able to safely and effectively provide earlier defibrillation with an AED and improve survival significantly.

Further insights on the use of AEDs by lay responders have been gained from experience of AED use in aircrafts and casinos, locations where traffic is heavy and stressful situations are common. The recognition and resuscitation of patients aboard an aircraft pose significant challenges. Until recently, victims of cardiac arrest aboard aircraft suffered from significant delays in defibrillation and therefore rarely survived. Quantas Airlines had a limited program that provided AEDs on some international flights. Results were promising.[6] American Airlines was the first carrier to equip all aircraft with AEDs and train all flight attendants in their use. Over a 2-year period, the AED was used in 200 instances, 191 events in aircraft and 9 events in the airport terminal. Electrocardiographic data was available in 185 patients. The AED advised a shock in 14 of 14 patients who had VF diagnosed as their initial arrhythmia. No shock was advised in the remaining patients. The sensitivity and

specificity of identifying VF was 100%. The first shock successfully defibrillated 13 of 14 patients and defibrillation was withheld in 1 patient at the request of the family. The rate of survival to hospital discharge after defibrillation was 40%.[7]

These studies demonstrate the feasibility, efficacy, and safety of the AED and its use by lay persons on aircraft and in airport terminals (**Fig. 1**). Subsequently, in April 2001, the US Federal Aviation Administration made AEDs

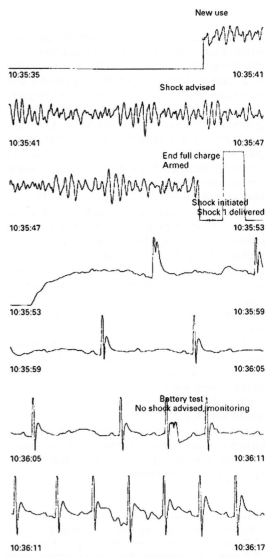

**Fig. 1.** An actual recording from an AED used on a passenger found to be in VF. A shock is advised, delivered, and followed by a pause, then sinus rhythm with 2:1 conduction, and eventual sinus rhythm with 1:1 conduction. The patient survived to hospital discharge. (*From* Page RL, Joglar JA, Kowal RC, et al. Use of automated external defibrillators by a U.S. airline. N Engl J Med 2000;343:1212; with permission.)

mandatory on all United States domestic and international flights.

Another important study assessed the feasibility, safety, and efficacy of AEDs used by trained security officers in casinos. AEDs were placed in locations where a rescuer could retrieve the AED and apply it to a victim within 3 minutes of an arrest. Because all casinos are equipped with surveillance cameras, investigators were able to report accurate times from collapse to defibrillation. One hundred and forty-eight patients had a cardiac arrest. VF was the initial rhythm in 105 patients and shock was advised in all cases. Four patients (4%) were pronounced dead at the scene, 35 patients (33%) died in the emergency department, and 56 patients (53%) survived to hospital discharge. The mean time from collapse to attachment of the AED was $3.5 \pm 2.9$ minutes; the mean time from collapse to first defibrillation shock was $4.4 \pm 2.9$ minutes; and the mean time from collapse to arrival of paramedics was $9.8 \pm 4.3$ minutes. Among patients with witnessed cardiac arrest and defibrillation no later than 3 minutes after collapse, the survival rate to hospital discharge was 74%.[8]

These studies illustrate the feasibility, safety, and efficacy of the use of the AED in specific environments characterized by heavy traffic of people under stressful situations and the presence of trained lay-rescuers.

The effectiveness of AEDs placed in more general public locations as part of an integrated PAD system has also been studied. Capucci and colleagues[9] reported the experience of the Piacenza Progetto Vita (PPV), a PAD system in which 12 AEDs were placed in high-risk locations, 12 were placed in lay-staffed ambulances, and 15 were placed in police cars serving the Piacenza region of Italy. In this study, 1287 lay volunteers were trained in the use of AEDs and responded to all cases of suspected cardiac arrest. The time from emergency call to arrival on the scene was $4.8 \pm 1.2$ minutes for the PPV responders versus $6.2 \pm 2.3$ minutes for EMS ($P = .05$). Survival to hospital discharge was 10.5% for the PPV group versus 3.3% for the EMS-treated group ($P = .006$). A "shockable" rhythm (ventricular tachycardia or VF) was present in 23.8% of the PPV group versus 15.6% for the EMS group ($P = .05$), probably because the PPV responder was able to arrive sooner than the EMS. This study demonstrated that a PAD system manned by lay-responders could triple overall survival above and beyond a well-developed EMS system by providing defibrillation approximately 1.5 minutes earlier than the EMS system.

In Austria, a national PAD program was initiated in 2002. During the study period, 1865 devices were deployed and, over a 2-year period, the use of an AED was documented in 73 cases. Eleven cases were excluded from the analysis because the devices were activated by EMS dispatchers and considered part of the local EMS system. Survival to hospital discharge was 17 of 62 (27%) among patients who required use of the AED. Evaluation of a historical control prior to the PAD system demonstrated a survival to hospital discharge rate of 4.3%.[10] In the United Kingdom, the government decided in 1999 that PAD should become a part of a core service provision under the National Health Service. Results of the initial phase of the implementation, which placed AEDs in fixed sites at airports and railway stations, have been reported. Out of 172 patients in whom the AED was used, a shockable rhythm was detected in 135 (78%). Thirty-eight of 172 (28%) persons who suffered a cardiac arrest in these locations survived to hospital discharge.[11]

The first randomized study of AEDs was the PAD (Public Access Defibrillation) trial, a National Institutes of Health–sponsored, prospective, multicenter trial of AEDs placed in prespecified public places. Community units were assigned to a structured emergency-response system involving lay volunteers trained in CPR, with half the community units being provided with AEDs. The primary outcome was survival to hospital discharge. This study included 19,000 volunteer responders in 993 community units in 24 North American regions. A total of 30 of 128 arrests (23%) survived to hospital discharge in the CPR + AED arm of the study compared to 15 of 107 (14%) in the CPR-only arm ($P = .03$; relative risk, 2.0; 95% CI, 1.07–3.77). Although large, multiunit, residential complexes represented 16% of the study locations, 28% of all cardiac arrests occurred at these locations. This finding is important because survival from cardiac arrest in residential locations was very poor in this study (0.6%).[12]

An important observation relevant to the overall impact of AEDs in public places is that over 75% of out-of-hospital cardiac arrests occur in the home.[13,14] Given the high frequency of arrest in the home, and the poor survival in residential units in the PAD trial, the Home AED Trial (HAT) was undertaken. HAT enrolled 7001 patients who had suffered an anterior myocardial infarction but were not candidates for an implantable cardiac defibrillator. In each case, someone in the home was instructed in CPR and activation of EMS, but half were randomized to receive a home AED. During a median follow-up of 37.3 months, 450 patients died (6.5% in the control group and 6.4% in the AED group; $P = .77$). The average mortality in this study was 2.1% in the control group and 2.0% in the AED group, which were lower than the historical data employed to calculate the power of the study. This reduced overall mortality is attributed to better medical management and high rate of revascularization following the index myocardial infarction. Among patients with death from tachyarrhythmias, less than one half of arrests that occurred at home were witnessed (58 of 160). Among all patients who died, only 41% died at home in this study. The AED was used in 32 patients in the study. A shock was advised for 13 patients and delivered in 12 patients. Five patients survived to hospital discharge but 1 died several days later. Overall, 4 of 14 (28.6%) patients who had VF and were shocked by the AED survived long term. Interestingly, the AED was used in 7 neighbors who had suffered a cardiac arrest but were not enrolled in the study. A shock was advised in 4 of 7 patients and 2 of 4 survived to hospital discharge. There were no documented inappropriate shocks in this study. Although the HAT study demonstrated no significant difference in mortality with home AEDs, it is important to re-emphasize that the study population had an event rate that was considerably lower than expected. Whether the home AED would be more effective in a higher-risk population remains unknown. The HAT study also demonstrated (1) that cardiac arrests occur less often in the home (41%) than what has been reported previously, (2) that the usefulness of home AEDs is limited because many arrests in the home are not witnessed despite the best-case scenario of a spouse educated in sudden death and the use of an AED, and (3) that, when the AED was used, it was accurate and effective and resulted in a long-term survival of 33%. Furthermore, neighbors of homes with AEDs also benefited with 2 of 4 patients in whom a shock was advised surviving to hospital discharge.[15]

Based on the HAT data, patients who wish to have an AED at home should not be discouraged, but general policy decisions or third-party coverage about home AEDs cannot be supported by the available data on home AEDs. On the other hand, in households that include a higher-risk patient (eg, patients with myocardial infarction with severely depressed ejection fraction refusing a defibrillator, patients with long-QT syndrome, patients with arrhythmogenic right ventricular cardiomyopathy, and patients with hypertrophic cardiomyopathy) along with a motivated and educated companion, a home AED may be reasonable. In addition, homeowners who frequently entertain large numbers of older guests may consider providing the added security of an AED.

## PUBLIC ACCESS DEFIBRILLATION PROGRAMS: WHERE DO WE BEGIN?

Several variables influence the potential impact that an AED will have in a given location. These include (1) the likelihood that a cardiac arrest would be witnessed and a potential rescuer would be present in that location, (2) the EMS response time to that location, and (3) the demographics and number of patients in that location. Simply having an AED present does not save lives if a cardiac arrest is not likely to be witnessed, even if that locale has very heavy traffic (such as public restrooms or residential complexes). At a population level, to make any significant impact on the total number of cardiac arrests due to ventricular arrhythmias, it would seem reasonable to conclude that an AED should be disseminated widely throughout the community. However, the issues discussed above, along with cost constraints, suggest that initial efforts in any community should focus first on locations where AEDs are most likely to be used. The American Heart Association suggests that such a place should be defined as a location where at least one cardiac arrest is likely to occur every 2 years. In a study by Becker and colleagues[12] conducted in King County, Washington, from 1990 to 1994, public sites where cardiac arrests may occur were divided into 23 location categories. Ten sites were found to have a "high" incidence of cardiac arrests, although only the international airport, county jail, and a large shopping mall reached the American Heart Association threshold. The placement of 276 AEDs in the 172 high-incidence sites was estimated to provide treatment for 134 cardiac-arrest patients in a 5-year period. Because 80 of 134 (60%) of patients were found to be in VF, assuming a survival rate of between 10% and 40%, the investigators estimated that between 8 and 32 lives might have been saved over a period of 5 years. However, to cover the remaining 347 arrests that occurred in public, AEDs would have to have been placed in more than 70,000 sites. In the PAD study, AEDs were placed only in locations thought to be generally suitable for AEDs. Among these prespecified sites, cardiac arrest occurred most frequently in fitness centers (5.1 per 1000 persons) and golf courses (4.8 per 1000 persons) and least frequently in office complexes (0.7 per 1000 persons) and hotels (0.7 per 1000 persons). Survival in PAD sites from treatable cardiac arrest was highest in recreational complexes, public transportation sites, and fitness centers. Survival was poor in residential facilities, reflecting the low likelihood that a bystander rescuer will be available at these sites.[12]

Based on the data available, communities establishing a PAD program should focus initial efforts on placing AEDs at locations where cardiac arrests are most likely to occur, especially where emergency medical team response times of less than 5 minutes cannot be reliably achieved. This may include large transportation terminals, exercise facilities, sports complexes, golf courses, and shopping centers. Ideally, the work of planning and maintaining the PAD program and the job of training individuals in the program should be supervised and coordinated by the local EMS and supervised by a physician. The PAD program should be integrated and coordinated through the local EMS system and each AED should be registered and "on-line" so that the local EMS system is aware of any instance that the AED is in use as well as its precise location. The precise location within each venue for each AED should be carefully selected to allow for the most efficient use of the AED for that location (ie, reached within 3 minutes) and the location of the AED should be clearly marked.

The cost for such a system does not need to be assumed entirely by local government but can be shared by local businesses who may benefit from the worthy charitable donation and "good will" advertisement that the AED may provide. As an example of some innovations in widespread dissemination of AEDs, Japan has placed AEDs in vending machines situated in locations where people congregate. The AED is installed behind an unlocked, transparent door and clearly marked. The cost of the AED is shared by the manufacturer of the drinks, the provider of the vending machine, the distributor of the AED, and the proprietor of the vending machine. Another innovative way to help pay for AEDs is through paid advertising above boxes in which AEDs are stored.[16]

An area of significant attention has been the placement of AEDs at elementary and high schools. Despite parental expectation that teachers and staff be trained in CPR, most surveys of elementary and high schools demonstrate that up to one third of teachers have no training in CPR.[17] In a cross-sectional survey of high schools in Washington state, the principal at each high school in the Washington Interscholastic Activities Association (n = 407) was asked to complete a Web-based questionnaire. One hundred and eighteen (29%) completed the survey. Sixty-four (54%) schools reported having at least one AED on school grounds (mean 1.6, range 1–4 AEDs). As for funding for the AEDs, 60% came from donations, 27% came from the school district, and 11% came from individual schools or athletic departments. AED training was completed by 78% of coaches, 72% of administrators, 70% of school nurses, and 48% of teachers. Only 25% of schools coordinated the implementation of AEDs with an outside medical agency and only 6% of schools coordinated the AED with the local EMS system. One school used the AED on a basketball official, who survived after a single shock. This study illustrates that significant improvements need to made to the structuring and coordination of emergency response plans in public high schools.[18] The placement of AEDs at National Collegiate Athletic Association Division I universities may also benefit spectators, coaches, and referees in that up to 77% of sudden cardiac arrests in college sporting venues occur in older non-students.[19]

Data on the efficacy of AEDs on young athletes are limited but raise some concern regarding the low survival rate. In a study by Drezner and Rogers,[20] the timing and detail of nine athletes who had a sudden cardiac arrest was analyzed. All nine athletes had a witnessed cardiac arrest and seven athletes received immediate defibrillation with an average time to defibrillation of 3.1 minutes. Despite early defibrillation, only one of the nine athletes survived. The lower-than-expected survival rates may be due to structural heart disease (hypertrophic cardiomyopathy and arrhythmogenic right ventricular cardiomyopathy), which is common among young athletes who present with a sudden cardiac arrest. These findings should not discourage the implementation of PAD programs in school athletic venues but should stimulate increased work in improving on existing emergency action plans at athletic events.

Teachers, physical education instructors, and administrators should all be trained and certified in basic life support. Emergency response systems for cardiac-arrest scenarios on campus should be carefully planned, and those plans should be carefully reviewed and integrated with the local EMS system. Goals of these response plans should strive for a collapse-to-EMS-call time of less than 1 minute and a collapse-to-first-shock time of less than 3 minutes. Because the sudden death of a child is an especially tragic event for a family and community, the carefully planned distribution of AEDs on school campuses and athletic venues may be justified even though cardiac arrests are rare. Many states have legislation supporting the placement of AEDs in schools and at school sporting events.[21]

## PUBLIC AWARENESS AND EDUCATION

A critical factor in the success of a PAD program is public awareness and widespread training in basic life support and in the basic operation of an AED.

Strong evidence shows that lay responders are capable of safely and effectively administering treatment with an AED. Even naïve sixth graders have been demonstrated to perform well in mock simulations of the use of the AED and, in some cases, performed better than trained professionals.[22] The importance of broad public awareness and training cannot be overemphasized because of the high likelihood that a non–medically trained bystander will be responsible for the initial treatment of cardiac-arrest victims.

## AUTOMATED EXTERNAL DEFIBRILLATORS AND CIVIL LIABILITY

A potential barrier to the effectiveness of a PAD program is the fear of lawsuits that may arise because of complications during the resuscitation attempt. To protect layperson responders involved in the resuscitation attempts of a cardiac-arrest victim, state and federal legislators have been actively involved in providing "good Samaritan" liability protection to organizations and individuals. The Aviation Medical Assistance Act (Public Law 105–170) was signed by President Clinton on April 24, 1998, and provided liability protection to airlines and individuals attempting to obtain or provide medical assistance on airplanes. On November 13, 2000, President Clinton signed the Cardiac Arrest Survival Act, now Public Law 106–505, which requires the placement of AEDs in federal buildings and provides civil immunity to users of the AED. The Cardiac Arrest Survival Act has played a pivotal role in setting the standards for immunity protection for rescuers using AEDs and for those who acquire an AED. As of 2001, all 50 states passed laws providing limited immunity protection for lay rescuers using AEDs to resuscitate a cardiac-arrest victim. A complete list of state legislation and regulations regarding AED and PAD programs can be obtained on the Internet.[21,23]

## ADVANCED DIRECTIVES

With the implementation of an aggressive resuscitation system within communities, it is important for patients with chronic or terminal illnesses and for our extremely elderly patients to carefully consider advanced directives. Physicians should remind such patients to carefully consider whether they wish to be resuscitated in the event of a cardiac arrest. Aggressive resuscitation of a patient who has little chance at long-term survival may lead to unnecessary morbidity, unnecessary physical and psychological distress to the patient and family, and unnecessary healthcare expenditures. Patients who do not wish to be resuscitated should have this clearly marked on a necklace or bracelet.

## COST-EFFECTIVENESS

PAD programs will be more cost-effective in regions where the likelihood is high that an AED will be used and where survival from the standard EMS system is very poor (<5%). Cram and colleagues[24] estimated that in locations where an AED would be used at a rate of once every 5 years as recommended by the American Heart Association, each AED in a public place would cost $30,000 per each quality-adjusted life-year (QALY) gained compared to EMS response alone. The AED would be much more cost-effective in some locations, such as international airports, public sports venues, golf courses, jails, health clubs, and large shopping malls. The AED would be less cost-effective in community centers, primary care centers, and hotels, where the cost is estimated to be more than $200,000 per QALY gained. However, the analysis of the cost-effectiveness of AEDs in PAD programs has significant limitations. The cost of these programs will vary from community to community. Every location has unique characteristics influencing the cost-effectiveness of an AED at that location, such as frequency of events (number of times the AED is likely to be used related to the demographics and number of people frequenting this location), likelihood of an available rescuer at the location, local EMS response times to that location, and the impact the AED would have on survival at that location. Even the likelihood of vandalism requiring replacement of the AED at the location should be taken into consideration. Determining which entities (private or public) may contribute to the cost of implementing such a program further complicates assessment of the cost of a PAD program.

## KEEPING PACE WITH THE SCIENCE OF RESUSCITATION

In November 2005, the International Liaison Committee on Cardiac Resuscitation and the American Heart Association (ILCOR/AHA) published new guidelines for CPR and emergency cardiac care. These updated guidelines were based on the evaluation of 22,000 peer-reviewed publications conducted by 281 physicians and scientists from the international resuscitation community.[2]

After an updated review of the literature and science of resuscitation, the guidelines committee recommended the following:

An emphasis on good quality CPR and minimizing interruptions

In the case of a witnessed cardiac arrest, a one-shock protocol followed by five cycles of CPR (one cycle equals 30 compressions to two breaths) before checking for a pulse

In the case of an unwitnessed cardiac arrest, five cycles of CPR preceding defibrillation.

Since publication of these guidelines in 2005, all AEDs manufactured currently are in compliance. Changes to the programming of AEDs have included a one-shock protocol and the addition of voice prompts to continue CPR immediately after the first shock.

## SUMMARY

The AED is a safe and effective tool that can significantly improve survival of cardiac-arrest victims. However, the effectiveness of this device depends on it being available at the site of arrest. Based on solid clinical evidence of the safety, accuracy, and effectiveness of AED use by lay responders, many communities are adopting PAD programs. These efforts have been supported in the United States with legislation at the state and federal level mandating the placement of AEDs in selected locations, providing funding for the development of local PAD programs, and providing liability protection to organizations and individuals who become involved in the execution of PAD. Further research into the relative effectiveness of AEDs in specific locations, financial support from private sources, improvements in public awareness and education on the use of AEDs will guide the development of community PAD programs and save lives that may otherwise be lost prematurely.

## REFERENCES

1. Diack AW, Welborn WS, Rullman RG, et al. An automatic cardiac resuscitator for emergency treatment of cardiac arrest. Med Instrum 1979;13:78–83.
2. 2005 American Heart Association guidelines for cardiopulmonary resuscitation and emergency cardiovascular care. Circulation 2005;112(24 Suppl):IV1–203.
3. Weaver WD, Hill D, Fahrenbuch CE, et al. Use of automated external defibrillators in the management of out-of-hospital cardiac arrest. N Engl J Med 1988; 319:661–6.
4. White RD, Vukov LF, Bugliosi TF. Early defibrillation by police: initial experience with measurement of critical time intervals and patient outcome. Ann Emerg Med 1994;23:1009–13.
5. Mossesso VN Jr, Davis EA, Auble TE, et al. Use of automated external defibrillators by police officers for treatment of out-of-hospital cardiac arrest. Ann Emerg Med 1998;32:200–7.
6. O'Rourke MF, Donaldson E, Geddes JS. An airline cardiac arrest program. Circulation 1997;96: 2849–53.
7. Page RL, Joglar JA, Kowal RC, et al. Use of automated external defibrillators by a U.S. airline. N Engl J Med 2000;343:1210–6.
8. Valenzuela TD, Roe DJ, Nichol G, et al. Outcomes of rapid defibrillation by security officers after cardiac arrest in casinos. N Engl J Med 2000;343:1206–9.
9. Capucci A, Aschieri D, Piepoli MF, et al. Tripling survival from sudden cardiac arrest via early defibrillation without traditional education in cardiopulmonary resuscitation. Circulation 2002;106: 1065–70.
10. Fleischhackl R, Roessler B, Domanovits H, et al. Results from Austria's nationwide public access defibrillation (ANPAD) programme collected over 2 years. Resuscitation 2008;77:195–200.
11. Davies CS, Colquhoun MC, Boyle R, et al. A national programme for on-site defibrillation by lay persons in selected high risk areas: initial results. Heart 2005; 91:1299–302.
12. Hallstrom A, Ornato JP, Weisfeldt M, et al. Public-access defibrillation and survival after out-of-hospital cardiac arrest. N Engl J Med 2004;351: 637–46.
13. Becker LB, Eisenberg M, Fahrenbruch C, et al. Public locations of cardiac arrest: implications for public access defibrillation. Circulation 1998;97: 2106–9.
14. Pell JP, Sirel JM, Marsden AK, et al. Potential impact of public access defibrillators on survival after out of hospital cardiopulmonary arrest: retrospective cohort study. Br Med J 2002;325:515.
15. Bardy GH, Lee KL, Mark DB, et al. Home use of automated external defibrillators for sudden cardiac arrest. N Engl J Med 2008;358:1793–804.
16. Mitamura H. Public access defibrillation: advances from Japan. Nat Clin Pract Cardiovasc Med 2008; 5(11):690–2.
17. Gagliardi M, Neighbors M, Spears C, et al. Emergencies in the school setting: Are public school teachers adequately trained to respond? Prehosp Disaster Med 1994;9:222–5.
18. Rothmier JD, Drezner JA, Harmon KG. Automated external defibrillators in Washington State high schools. Br J Sports Med 2007;41:301–5.
19. Drezner JA, Rogers KJ, Zimmer RR, et al. Use of automated external defibrillators at NCAA Division I universities. Med Sci Sports Exerc 2005;37:1487–92 State Legislation.
20. Drezner JA, Rogers KJ. Sudden cardiac arrest in intercollegiate athletes: detailed analysis and outcomes of resuscitation in nine cases. Heart Rhythm 2006;3:755–9.

21. National Conferences of State Legislatures Web site. Health care program state laws on heart attacks: cardiac arrest and defibrillators. Available at: http://www.ncsl.org/programs/health/aed.htm. Accessed March 31, 2009.

22. Gundry JW, Comess KA, DeRook FA, et al. Comparison of naïve sixth grade children with trained professionals in the use of an automated external defibrillator. Circulation 1999;100:1703–7.

23. Department of Health and Human Services Program Support Center Web site. Guidelines for public access defibrillation programs in federal facilities. Available at: http://www.foh.dhhs.gov/public/whatwedo/AED/HHSAED.asp. Accessed May 31, 2009.

24. Cram P, Vijan S, Fendrick AM. Cost effectiveness of automated external defibrillator deployment in selected public locations. J Gen Intern Med 2003; 18:745–54.

# Optimizing Community Resources to Address Sudden Cardiac Death

Younghoon Kwon, MD[a], Tom P. Aufderheide, MD[b],*

**KEYWORDS**

- Sudden cardiac death • Cardiac arrest
- Community resources
- Cardiopulmonary resuscitation (CPR) • Bystander CPR
- Public access defibrillation

Sudden cardiac arrest occurring outside the hospital is one of the leading causes of death in the developed world and claims 350,000 to 450,000 lives per year in the United States.[1] Despite recent advancements in resuscitative care and continuing efforts to improve public awareness of sudden cardiac arrest in the community, overall survival still remains low.[2]

The well-established "chain of survival" (early access, early cardiopulmonary resuscitation [CPR], early defibrillation, and early advanced care) incorporates scientifically proven interventions necessary for successful resuscitation and survival for patients with cardiac arrest (**Fig. 1**).[3,4] It is becoming increasingly evident, however, that low survival rates from cardiac arrest are not due to lack of understanding of effective interventions, but instead are due to weak links in the chain of survival and the inability of communities to ensure these links function in an efficient, timely, and coordinated fashion.

This article identifies for each link in the chain of survival aspects that define the link's quality, explains how communities can strengthen each link, and describes how communities can optimize local leadership and community stakeholder collaboration to forge a strong relationship between each link so that the sequence of interventions provided to patients with cardiac arrest are consistently efficient, timely, and well coordinated.

## EARLY ACCESS—BYSTANDER CARDIOPULMONARY RESUSCITATION

Studies have demonstrated convincingly that the odds of surviving out-of-hospital cardiac arrest (OHCA) increase two to four times when bystander CPR occurs before the arrival of emergency medical services (EMS).[5–7] Both the quality of bystander CPR and the interval from collapse to initiation of CPR have been associated with survival and good quality of life in survivors.[8,9] Therefore, the frequency of early initiation of bystander CPR significantly influences a community's overall performance in achieving successful outcome from cardiac arrest.

Despite these proven and marked benefits, rates of bystander CPR in communities are low.[10] The bystander CPR rate in most communities is less than 20%—in some it is only a few percent—and the variation between communities is large. Proposed theories to explain the low rate of bystander CPR include unpreparedness and lack of knowledge of the bystander to implement appropriate actions,[11,12] fear during the emergency, fear of causing harm, unfounded fear of legal consequences,[13] and unfounded fear of contracting a communicable disease by providing mouth-to-mouth breathing.[14–16] Although actual barriers may be a combination of these factors, all of them derive from the lack of public

This article originally appeared in *Cardiac Electrophysiology Clinics*, volume 1, number 1.
[a] Division of Cardiology, Department of Medicine, Healthcare East System, University of Minnesota, 45 West 10th Street, St Joseph Hospital, St Paul, MN 55102, USA
[b] Department of Emergency Medicine, Medical College of Wisconsin, 9200 West Wisconsin Avenue, FH/Pavilion 1P, Milwaukee, WI 53226, USA
* Corresponding author.
*E-mail address:* taufderh@mcw.edu

Heart Failure Clin 7 (2011) 277–286
doi:10.1016/j.hfc.2011.01.004

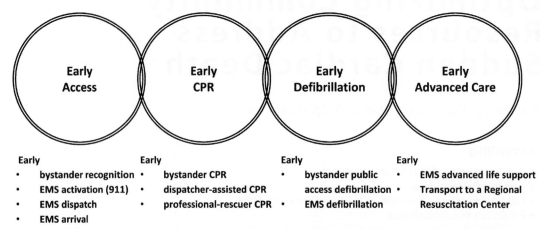

**Fig. 1.** The chain of survival. The chain of survival defines the proven interventions necessary for successful resuscitation and survival for patients with cardiac arrest. (*Adapted from* Cummins RO, Ornato JP, Thies WH, et al. Improving survival from sudden cardiac arrest: the "chain of survival" concept. A statement for health professionals from the Advanced Cardiac Life Support Subcommittee and the Emergency Cardiac Care Committee, American Heart Association. Circulation 1991;83:1833; with permission.)

awareness of sudden cardiac arrest and lack of training in CPR. Although American Heart Association CPR courses train more than 8 million Americans each year in CPR, this represents only between 2% to 3% of the American public. Clearly, more efficient and effective methods to train the public are required to comprehensively train a community and national population in bystander CPR.

## Bystander Cardiopulmonary Resuscitation Training

It is now recognized that it is impossible to train large populations using classroom-based CPR training methods.[17] The time demands of most American lifestyles preclude taking a 4-hour CPR course for all but those with an employment obligation for formal CPR training and certification. Recognizing these barriers, alternative training formats and materials have been developed and proposed to make training shorter, more accessible, and cost-effective.

Video self-instruction (VSI) is a successful alternative to traditional CPR courses for laypersons. This approach includes compact training materials combined in an inexpensive "CPR kit" (including an inflatable CPR manikin and training CD or video) that allows the participant to train in the privacy of his or her home at any time and that teaches high-quality CPR skills in approximately 20 minutes. Studies comparing CPR training with VSI versus a traditional 4-hour CPR course demonstrated VSI training resulted in similar, if not superior, CPR performance and skills retention initially and at 2 and 6 months.[18,19] The educational materials also provide permanent access

to intermittent refresher training, when desired. Furthermore, VSI participants provide the training materials to two to three additional family members or friends, significantly multiplying the educational impact of this approach.[18,19]

Thus, for the first time, VSI provides a proven, effective CPR training approach that enables communities to train a significantly larger portion of the layperson population in these basic life-saving skills and increases the community's incidence of bystander CPR.

## Cardiopulmonary Resuscitation in the Schools

Mandating CPR training in the schools holds the potential to train a generation of Americans in CPR. With time, the entire United States population could be trained in CPR (and in the use of automated external defibrillators [AEDs]).[20] Video-mediated instruction, no longer than a total of 30 minutes, now makes training possible in a single classroom period. This short time of training has removed a previous barrier (a 4-hour course) to widespread implementation of CPR in the schools.

Communities with receptive school boards that have adopted this approach (such as the Take Heart America [THA] project) have significantly increased the portion of the community trained in CPR.[21] Use of video-mediated instruction "CPR kits" further expands the impact of this approach as junior and senior high school students can take the materials home and train additional family and friends.

Although low, the cost of training materials (CPR kits) continues to be a potential barrier to budget-challenged school boards. The lack of a federal mandate for CPR in the schools currently precludes universal national implementation. Nonetheless, this concept, rigorously supported by the American Heart Association, is becoming increasingly popular in schools that are early adopters and that have recognized its importance. Such schools have enjoyed the success of this approach. CPR in the schools, then, is another potentially effective tool for communities to increase citizen CPR training.

### Simplified Cardiopulmonary Resuscitation Technique

Simplifying the CPR technique used by laypersons has the potential to increase the frequency of citizen action in an emergency and pave the way for innovative and new methods for mass CPR training. Animal studies have demonstrated that continuous chest compressions without rescue breathing are effective for a witnessed arrest during the first several minutes of CPR.[22,23] Clinical studies subsequently have confirmed that outcomes are acceptable after 'hands-only" bystander CPR (compared with bystander CPR with rescue breathing in untrained and trained laypersons).[24,25] This new concept removes the potential barriers to layperson action during an emergency, including fear of contracting a communicable disease by providing mouth-to-mouth breathing and concern by laypersons for the complexity of administering CPR. The American Heart Association recently published a recommendation that bystanders who witness a sudden collapse in an adult should perform chest-compression-only CPR if the rescuer is a bystander without CPR training or is previously trained but not confident in his or her ability to provide conventional CPR, including high-quality chest compressions with rescue breathing.[26]

### Mass Cardiopulmonary Resuscitation Training

The demonstrated success of VSI[18,19] and simplification of layperson CPR technique[26] has opened a window of opportunity for effective and simple mass training in CPR. Training the public to recognize cardiac arrest, call 911, and perform chest-compression-only CPR is now possible in 30-second public service announcements on television or shown at innovative locations, such as doctors' offices and emergency department waiting rooms. These short video clips, which also can be downloaded to cell phones and other electronic devices used by most Americans, have the potential to vastly increase public awareness as well as the rate of bystander CPR in the community. Such approaches are being studied in selected communities and hold promise to train entire populations in this life-saving technique. Communities should consider this as a potential option to improve the rate of bystander CPR locally.

## EARLY DEFIBRILLATION—PUBLIC ACCESS DEFIBRILLATION

Early defibrillation is a critical link in the chain of survival that can significantly improve outcome from OHCA.[27] For ventricular fibrillation cardiac arrest, the likelihood of survival substantially decreases for every minute of delay to defibrillation from the onset of cardiac arrest.[3,28] The concept of public access defibrillation (PAD) has emerged with advances in technology that have made AEDs reliable and simple to operate, enabling trained lay rescuers to perform early defibrillation (if they have access to an AED at the site of the cardiac arrest).[29]

PAD programs, which place AEDs in public locations throughout the community and train lay rescuers in CPR and use of the AEDs, incorporate an effective internal emergency response plan linked with the local EMS system. PAD programs are a crucial adjunct to a community's EMS-based efforts to achieve earlier defibrillation. They have been demonstrated to be safe, to consistently provide effective defibrillation minutes earlier than the EMS system, and to double survival rate from ventricular fibrillation OHCA.[30–33]

The American Heart Association recommends the following critical elements to achieve high-quality PAD programs[34]:

- The community should focus on strengthening each link in the chain of survival.
- Ideally, the PAD program should be under the supervision of a qualified health care provider with expertise in emergency cardiac care. The PAD director can optimize and coordinate training, site evaluation, AED placement, communication with the EMS system, lay-rescuer retraining, and quality-improvement monitoring.
- All lay rescuers should be trained in both CPR and AED use. Members of the PAD program should practice their internal emergency response several times each year, with unannounced drills.
- A written response plan should be implemented at each site, targeting a collapse-to-first-shock time of 4 to 5 minutes or less.
- The AED should be placed in a central, highly visible, and accessible location near a telephone. Residents or employees at

the site should be aware of the location. AEDs should ideally be placed no farther than a 1- to 1.5-minute walk from any location in the PAD site. AEDs should not be placed in locked offices or cabinets.

- The PAD program should be integrated with the local EMS system.
- The program should include a method to ensure data retrieval and quality assurance review of any AED use.
- The AED should be maintained according to manufacturer's recommendations.

Priority of PAD implementation should be given to public locations in the community expected to have the highest frequency of cardiac arrest. Locations where large crowds gather, such as public transportation terminals (eg, airports and train stations), sports arenas, shopping malls, recreational complexes, large industrial complexes, and federal buildings, should be considered strongly for PAD programs. Other public locations expected to have a relatively higher frequency of cardiac arrest due to physical activity or higher-risk populations include golf courses, health clubs, medical offices, and non–patient care areas of hospitals.[35,36]

## Automated External Defibrillators in the School

Most pediatric cardiac arrests occur among adolescents with previously undiagnosed congenital heart abnormalities in the setting of rigorous sports activity.[37–39] Although the incidence of pediatric cardiac arrest is low, the consequences are devastating.[40] When prompt and effective resuscitation is given, pediatric cardiac arrest survivors have the highest number of life-years salvaged. Furthermore, many at-risk adults are located at schools, including faculty, parents, and members of the community attending extramural activities.[20] As with CPR, the school is an ideal place to implement training programs in AED use, since students are more willing to learn and have the potential to spread the knowledge they have acquired.[41]

One example of successful PAD program implementation in the schools is Project ADAM (Automated Defibrillators in Adam's Memory), which began after a series of sudden deaths among high school athletes in Wisconsin.[42] This project has facilitated PAD program implementation in schools nationally by providing comprehensive resources that schools need to plan, fund, and implement a PAD program.

## Automated External Defibrillators in the Home

The most common location of OHCA is the home.[43] While the PAD Trial doubled ventricular fibrillation survival rate by placing AEDs in public locations, it also demonstrated a markedly low survival rate in residential facilities.[33] The subsequent Home AED Trial (HAT) failed to demonstrate a survival benefit by placing AEDs in the home compared with reliance on conventional resuscitation methods.[44] Given these results, placement of AEDs in the home is considered an ineffective strategy and should not be pursued by communities at this time.

## Communities and Public Access Defibrillation Programs

Despite these proven and marked benefits, PAD programs in communities remain underutilized. PAD programs are typically implemented by early-adopting companies and organizations. The programs (although highly effective) are independent, sporadically implemented, and variably maintained. Communities lack local leadership to champion strategic development of PAD programs, optimize locations of highest incidence of cardiac arrest in the community, and provide comprehensive coverage to the community. Moreover, communities lack public awareness of the importance of these programs, initiatives to generate funding to support these programs, and the administrative and political will to support a comprehensive community initiative. Thus, this proven and effective intervention, which doubles survival rate from cardiac arrest, remains grossly underutilized and prohibited from realizing its survival potential.

## EARLY ADVANCED CARE—EMERGENCY MEDICAL SERVICES
### The Coordinating Role of Emergency Medical Services in the Community

The EMS system represents a pivotal and coordinating component in the care of cardiac arrest for the community. As such, it is critically important to the community's cardiac arrest survival performance. EMS implements and coordinates crucial, time-sensitive interventions, including facilitating early access through 911, deploying rapid EMS, providing dispatcher-assisted bystander CPR, integrating with local PAD programs, delivering high-quality professional resuscitation, and selecting optimal hospital transport destinations for resuscitated cardiac arrest patients. Accordingly, the local EMS cardiac arrest survival rate is an accurate reflection of community performance and should be evaluated continuously as a community's quality assurance measure.[45]

## Dispatcher-assisted Telephone Cardiopulmonary Resuscitation

Communities should implement every strategy to encourage laypersons to perform CPR until EMS arrives. One of the most effective ways to immediately increase the incidence of bystander CPR in the community is to provide verbal instruction by the EMS dispatcher over the telephone. Dispatcher-assisted CPR dramatically increases the rate and quality of bystander-delivered CPR.[46] More importantly, dispatcher-assisted bystander CPR has been shown to improve survival in OHCA compared with no bystander CPR.[7] Since most bystanders are untrained in CPR and must provide this intervention during the initial few minutes before EMS arrival, simple instructions are necessary. Under these circumstances, chest-compression-only CPR has been shown to be just as effective (if not more so) for untrained laypersons.[26]

Communities should implement aggressive dispatcher-assisted bystander CPR programs. Success of the program requires training, retraining, and continuous quality improvement.

## Professional Cardiopulmonary Resuscitation

The quality of CPR delivered by trained medical professionals directly correlates with successful resuscitation.[47] However, the quality of CPR delivered varies. When electronically recorded and then evaluated, well-established, excellent EMS systems have been shown to provide chest compressions that are too shallow, long interruptions in chest compressions, incomplete chest-wall recoil, and excessive ventilation rates.[48–50] Because the quality of CPR provided correlates with successful resuscitation, it is a critical component of the community's cardiac arrest survival performance.

Accordingly, every EMS director should comprehensively educate and train first- and second- responding EMS personnel to provide high-quality CPR. Equally important, the quality of CPR needs to be electronically measured to provide real-time feedback to rescuers (while resuscitative efforts are being performed) and to provide continuous quality improvement for the EMS system. EMS directors can use readily available equipment now capable of electronically monitoring CPR performance during resuscitation.[51]

A suggested list of the important components of high-quality CPR (many of which have been demonstrated to be correlated with improved hemodynamics during CPR) include[52]:

- Chest compression depth: 1.5 to 2 in
- Chest compression rate: 100/min
- Ventilation rate: 6 to 10 breaths/min; ventilation duration: no more than 1 s/breath; tidal volume: 500 to 600 mL/breath
- Complete chest recoil following each compression
- Maximize hands-on time; minimize interruptions to CPR; no pauses in chest compressions more than 10 seconds
- CPR immediately before and immediately after defibrillation
- Use of Impedance Threshold Device (ITD; Advanced Circulatory Systems, Inc, Eden Prairie, Minnesota)
- Minimization of rescuer fatigue.

## OPTIMIZING POSTARREST CARE—REGIONALIZATION OF RESUSCITATION CENTERS

### Postarrest Cardiac Care

Optimizing hospital-based care for patients resuscitated from cardiac arrest has been shown to increase survival rate greater than any single intervention the community can make. One-year neurologically intact survival was more than doubled (from 26% to 56%) after implementing optimal postresuscitation care.[53]

There is wide variation in hospital-based survival rates following treatment of patients resuscitated from OHCA.[54–59] In-hospital factors found to be associated with improved survival include increased size of the hospital, availability of a cardiac catheterization laboratory, increased volume of patients treated for cardiac arrest, and available staffing (ratio of beds to nurses).[57–59] Furthermore, optimal postarrest cardiac care is complex and requires sophisticated hospital-based capabilities as well as protocol-driven, comprehensive care delivered by a coordinated, multidisciplinary team. The demands of such optimal care are often beyond the capabilities of most paramedic-receiving hospitals.

Optimized postarrest hospital-based care should include (1) therapeutic hypothermia, (2) hemodynamic support, (3) services of a cardiac catheterization laboratory, (4) optimal intensive care unit care, (5) option of using implantable cardioverter-defibrillators, and (6) social services.

### Therapeutic hypothermia

The most significant advance in postarrest cardiac care is implementation of therapeutic hypothermia (rapidly reducing core body temperature to 32°C to 34°C for 12 to 48 hours followed by controlled rewarming). This novel therapy significantly reduces mortality and improves neurologic outcome in comatose survivors of OHCA.[60,61] Therapeutic hypothermia should be an integral part of a standardized treatment strategy. Numerous techniques are available to induce and maintain hypothermia. These techniques include topical application of ice, use of cutaneous cooling devices, and intravascular cooling. Implementation of therapeutic hypothermia requires planning, education, and integration of emergency medicine, cardiology, and intensive care unit services within an institution.

### Hemodynamic support
Post–cardiac arrest myocardial dysfunction, which is common and usually transient in patients resuscitated from cardiac arrest, requires appropriate (and sometimes aggressive) hemodynamic support. Treatment often requires use of inotropes and vasopressors to maintain hemodynamic stability. Mechanical hemodynamic support, including an intra-aortic balloon pump, should be available and implemented if pharmacologic measures fail. Other measures include percutaneous cardiopulmonary bypass, extracorporeal membrane oxygenation, and the use of transthoracic ventricular assist devices.[62,63]

### Services of cardiac catheterization laboratory
Because the majority of OHCA patients have coronary artery disease that often precipitates cardiac arrest, prompt coronary arteriography followed by percutaneous intervention is life-saving in appropriate patients. Immediate access to interventional cardiology and availability of a cardiac catheterization laboratory at the treating hospital are essential.[64,65]

### Optimal intensive care unit care
Post–cardiac arrest patients are at risk of developing multiorgan dysfunction. Accordingly, they require optimal intensive care, including advanced hemodynamic monitoring, neurologic assessment, hemodynamic optimization, and the highest standards of critical care.

### Expert neurologic prognostication
Early determination of outcome after OHCA is a complicated issue requiring expert neurologic care. Accurate neurologic outcome prediction requires neurologists experienced in treating patients resuscitated from cardiac arrest and additionally may require electrophysiological examinations and neuroimaging tests. Comatose survivors of cardiac arrest often take longer than other patient populations to regain consciousness and achieve return to neurologic baseline (especially with therapeutic hypothermia treatment). Decisions to withdraw life support are critically important and need to be based on extensive experience with these newer treatments in the cardiac arrest patient population.[66,67]

### Implantable cardioverter-defibrillators
Insertion of implantable cardioverter-defibrillators is indicated in many patients who survive cardiac arrest. Such therapy is lifesaving, potentially increases quality of life, and should be implemented in all appropriate cardiac arrest survivors.[68]

### Social services
The complex nature of postarrest cardiac care demands appropriate psychosocial support for patients and their families throughout their hospitalization. Social service care should be integrated into optimal hospital-based care of cardiac arrest patients.

### Regionalization of Postarrest Hospital-based Care
Given the profound variability in hospital-based survival rates and the need for sophisticated hospital-based capabilities to optimize outcome for patients resuscitated from OHCA, communities should establish selected resuscitation centers regionally and transport resuscitated OHCA patients directly and exclusively to those resuscitation centers. Using the successful concept of the trauma center, local regionalization of resuscitation centers will provide resuscitated victims of OHCA with the highest quality hospital-based care and the community with a doubling of survival rates.[53,69,70] Establishing regional resuscitation centers requires a community-wide plan and collaboration among EMS directors, hospital administrators, emergency departments, cardiologists, and intensive care specialists throughout the community.

## A COMMUNITY-WIDE APPROACH TO CARDIAC ARREST
A very successful model of a community-wide approach to cardiac arrest is the THA Project.[21] THA is a demonstration project designed to show how cardiac arrest survival rates in America's cities can be significantly increased through a comprehensive, community-wide approach. THA has deployed state-of-the art resuscitation science strategies and outreach programs in four demonstration communities: St Cloud, Minnesota;

Anoka County, Minnesota; Columbus, Ohio; and Austin, Texas.

Key aspects of the THA approach are centered on strengthening and coordinating each link in the chain of survival throughout an entire community by increasing community awareness of cardiac arrest; implementing innovative CPR training programs in schools and media to increase the rate of bystander CPR; comprehensively implementing PAD programs in high-risk public locations; improving the quality of resuscitation skills of professional rescuers; and establishing resuscitation centers to optimize care of patients resuscitated from OHCA.

Combining the efforts of doctors, nurses, paramedics, health educators, and community leaders, THA already has demonstrated the validity of this general concept by increasing community-wide survival rates from OHCA more than two-fold.

## COORDINATION AND ADMINISTRATION OF COMMUNITY RESOURCES
### What a Community Needs to Succeed

### Cardiac arrest registry
Without an established cardiac arrest registry (capturing outcome of all cardiac arrests in the community), it is impossible to identify the current performance of the community and barriers to potential improvement. The CARES (Cardiac Arrest Registry to Enhance Survival) project is an excellent example of an immediately available cardiac arrest database that can be adopted by any community interested in improving outcome from cardiac arrest. It captures all essential data elements for OHCA events using an Internet-based network. The program is rapidly being adopted in many communities.[71]

### Cardiac arrest champion
To implement and coordinate a sustained and effective program to significantly improve the local survival rate from cardiac arrest, a community needs a cardiac arrest champion. This individual should have knowledge and expertise in the field of cardiac arrest as well as passion for improving cardiac arrest outcome. An effective community program needs this leadership to succeed.

### Medical leadership and collaboration
A community also needs an EMS medical director who has the will and capacity to provide medical leadership, oversight, and coordination to ensure the highest quality care for cardiac arrest patients. This person should take responsibility for training EMS rescuers in high-quality CPR, acquiring EMS equipment to electronically monitor the performance of CPR, and implementing a CPR

continuous quality-assurance program. The EMS medical director is pivotal in optimizing rapid access through 911, implementing dispatcher-assisted CPR, minimizing EMS response time, integrating EMS response with PAD programs, and establishing EMS transport policy to resuscitation centers. The EMS medical director also plays a collaborative role in working with community hospitals that receive EMS patients (heightening awareness of the medical community to optimal standards of practice).

Collaboration among hospitals and medical specialties can be challenging. Lack of collaboration and competing interests frequently represent barriers to a coordinated community plan. Common ground should be established in a genuine interest in improving outcome from cardiac arrest and a community-wide multidisciplinary committee instituted to meet on a regular basis. The formation of such a committee is a necessity for community progress. Continued communication and established common interests eventually achieve consensus on an action plan for improved cardiac arrest care in the community.

### Political leadership
Efforts to improve care of OHCA cannot be maximized unless there is support from local government, including the mayor's office and city council. In general, governmental departments recognize the public health impact of cardiac arrest and the potential benefit to local citizens of improved care. Communities should contact the appropriate local governmental agencies once a community plan has been defined.[72]

### Community support
Promoting CPR training in the schools, video-mediated CPR instruction, and innovative media techniques heightens awareness of cardiac arrest in the community. Every member of the community should be encouraged to actively participate in the chain of survival.

The community should establish a cardiac arrest survivors' network. Cardiac arrest survivors can promote a community initiative better than any other spokespeople. Fund-raising campaigns can be responsibly linked to public cardiac arrest survivor events to generate income for PAD programs and other critical initiatives.

### Administrative assistance
A dedicated administrative assistant is a necessity for scheduling, for organizational planning, and for maintaining continuous progress on multiple initiatives. Communities must find creative ways to

initially fund and maintain this critically important support.

### Communication and collaboration

For communities to forge a strong relationship between each link so that efficient, timely, and coordinated sequences of interventions can be provided to patients with cardiac arrest, community stakeholders must establish an infrastructure for scheduled meetings on an ongoing basis. Stakeholders at these regularly scheduled meetings should include (but not necessarily be limited to) EMS directors, hospital administrators, EMS personnel, emergency physicians, and community leaders. Collectively, this consortium of stakeholders should identify weaknesses in the community's links in the chain of survival and implement appropriate short-term and long-range action plans. Coordination among the sequences of cardiac arrest interventions should be continually addressed. A community-wide continuous quality-assurance program should be implemented to continuously evaluate the community's performance. Although other interests will compete, commitment and collaboration among stakeholders will result in transformation of the community's survival rate from cardiac arrest.

### Additional resources

Such organizations as the Citizen CPR Foundation (http://www.citizencpr.org), whose mission is to save lives from sudden death by stimulating citizen and community action, represent a valuable and comprehensive resource to communities and community leaders interested in improving outcome from cardiac arrest.

### SUMMARY

The chain of survival (early access, early CPR, early defibrillation, and early advanced care [see **Fig. 1**]) defines the proven interventions necessary for successful resuscitation and survival of patients with cardiac arrest. Low survival rates from cardiac arrest are not due to lack of understanding of effective interventions but are instead due to weak links in the chain of survival and the inability of communities to make certain these links function in an efficient, timely, and coordinated fashion. This article has reviewed how quality is defined for each link, how communities can strengthen each link, and how communities can forge a strong relationship between each link. By optimizing local leadership and stakeholder collaboration, communities have the potential to vastly improve outcomes from this devastating disease.

### ACKNOWLEDGMENTS

We gratefully acknowledge Ms Dawn Kawa for her valuable and gracious assistance in preparation of this manuscript.

### REFERENCES

1. Callans DJ. Out-of-hospital cardiac arrest—the solution is shocking. N Engl J Med 2004;351:632–4.
2. Rea TD, Eisenberg MS, Becker LJ, et al. Temporal trends in sudden cardiac arrest: a 25-year emergency medical services perspective. Circulation 2003;107:2780–5.
3. Cummins RO, Ornato JP, Thies WH, et al. Improving survival from sudden cardiac arrest: the "chain of survival" concept. Circulation 1991;83:1832–47.
4. ECC Committe, Subcommittees and Task Forces of the American Heart Association. 2005 American Heart Association guidelines for cardiopulmonary resuscitation and emergency cardiovascular care. Circulation 2005;112(24 Suppl):IV1–203.
5. Gallagher EJ, Lombardi G, Gennis P. Effectiveness of bystander cardiopulmonary resuscitation and survival following out-of-hospital cardiac arrest. JAMA 1995;274:1922–5.
6. Cummins RO, Eisenberg MS, Hallstrom AP, et al. Survival of OHCA with early initiation of cardiopulmonary resuscitation. Am J Emerg Med 1985;3:114–9.
7. Rea TD, Eisenberg MS, Culley LL, et al. Dispatcher-assisted cardiopulmonary resuscitation and survival in cardiac arrest. Circulation 2001;104(21):2513–6.
8. Stiell IG, Wells GA, De Maio VJ, et al. Modifiable factors associated with improved cardiac arrest survival in a multicenter basic life support/defibrillation system: OPALS study phase I results. Ann Emerg Med 1999;33:44–50.
9. Stiell IG, Nichol G, Wells G, et al. Health-related quality of life is better for cardiac arrest survivors who received citizen cardiopulmonary resuscitation. Circulation 2003;08:1939–44.
10. De Maio VJ, Stiell IG, Spaite DW, et al. OPALS study group. CPR-only survivors of OHCA: implications for out-of-hospital care and cardiac arrest research methodology. Ann Emerg Med 2001;37:602–8.
11. Swor R, Khan I, Domeier R, et al. CPR training and CPR performance: do CPR-trained bystanders perform CPR? Acad Emerg Med 2006;13:596–601.
12. Coon SJ, Guy MC. Performing bystander CPR for sudden cardiac arrest: behavioral intentions among the general adult population in Arizona. Resuscitation 2009;80(3):334–40.
13. Nolan RP, Wilson E, Shuster M, et al. Readiness to perform cardiopulmonary resuscitation: an emerging strategy against sudden cardiac death. Psychosom Med 1999;61:546–51.

14. Locke CJ, Berg RA, Sanders AB, et al. Bystander cardiopulmonary resuscitation—concerns about mouth-to-mouth contact. Arch Intern Med 1995; 155:938–43.

15. Shibata K, Taniguchi T, Yoshida M, et al. Obstacles to bystander cardiopulmonary resuscitation in Japan. Resuscitation 2000;44:187–93.

16. Johnston TC, Clark MJ, Dingle FA, et al. Factors influencing Queenslanders' willingness to perform bystander cardiopulmonary resuscitation. Resuscitation 2003;56:67–75.

17. Flint LS, Billi JE, Kelly K, et al. Education in adult basic life support training programs. Ann Emerg Med 1993;22:468–74.

18. Lynch B, Einspruch EL, Nichol G, et al. Effectiveness of a 30-minute CPR self-instruction program for lay responders: a controlled randomized study. Resuscitation 2005;67(1):31–43.

19. Einspruch EL, Lynch B, Aufderheide TP, et al. Retention of CPR skills learned in a traditional Heartsaver course versus 30-minute video self-training: a controlled randomized study. Resuscitation 2007; 74(3):476–86.

20. Lotfi K, White L, Rea T, et al. Cardiac arrest in schools. Circulation 2007;116:1374–9.

21. Take Heart America. Available at: http://takeheart america.org. Accessed September 15, 2009.

22. Berg RA, Kern KB, Hilwig RW, et al. Assisted ventilation does not improve outcome in a porcine model of single-rescuer bystander cardiopulmonary resuscitation. Circulation 1997;95(6):1635–41.

23. Chandra NC, Gruben KG, Tsitlik JE, et al. Observations of ventilation during resuscitation in a canine model. Circulation 1994;90(6):3070–5.

24. SOS-KANTO Study Group. Cardiopulmonary resuscitation by bystanders with chest compression only (SOS-KANTO): an observational study. Lancet 2007;369(9565):920–6.

25. Hallstrom A, Cobb L, Johnson E, et al. Cardiopulmonary resuscitation by chest compression alone or with mouth-to-mouth ventilation. N Engl J Med 2000;342(21):1546–53.

26. Sayre MR, Berg RA, Cave DM, et al. Hands-only (compression-only) cardiopulmonary resuscitation: a call to action for bystander response to adults who experience out-of-hospital cardiac arrest. A science advisory for the public from the Emergency Cardiovascular Care Committee, American Heart Association. Circulation 2008; 117(16):2162–7.

27. Eisenberg MS. Improving survival from out-of-hospital cardiac arrest: back to the basics. Ann Emerg Med 2007;49(3):314–6.

28. Marenco JP, Wang PJ, Link MS, et al. Improving survival from sudden cardiac arrest: the role of the automated external defibrillator. JAMA 2001;285: 1193–200.

29. Cummins RO, Eisenberg M, Bergner L, et al. Sensitivity, accuracy, and safety of an automatic external defibrillator. Lancet 1984;2:318–20.

30. Valenzuela TD, Roe DJ, Nichol G, et al. Outcomes of rapid defibrillation by security officers after cardiac arrest in casinos. N Engl J Med 2000;343:1206–9.

31. Page RL, Joglar JA, Kowal RC, et al. Use of automated external defibrillators by a U.S. airline. N Engl J Med 2000;343:1210–6.

32. van Alem AP, Vrenken RH, de Vos R, et al. Use of automated external defibrillator by first responders in out-of-hospital cardiac arrest: prospective controlled trial. BMJ 2003;327(7427):1312.

33. The public access defibrillation trial investigators. Public access defibrillation and survival after out-of-hospital cardiac arrest. N Engl J Med 2004;351: 637–46.

34. Guidelines 2000 for CPR and Emergency Cardiovascular Care. Part 4: the AED: key link in the chain of survival. The American Heart Association in collaboration with the International Liaison Committee on Resuscitation. Circulation 2000; 102(Suppl 8):60–76.

35. Becker L, Eisenberg M, Fahrenbruch C, et al. Public locations of cardiac arrest: implications for public access defibrillation. Circulation 1998;97(21): 2106–9.

36. Gratton M, Lindholm DJ, Campbell JP. Public access defibrillation: Where do we place the AEDs? Prehosp Emerg Care 1999;3(4):303–5.

37. Myerburg RJ, Mitrani R, Interian A Jr, et al. Identification of risk of cardiac arrest and sudden death in athletes. In: Estes NA 3rd, Salem DN, Wang PJ, editors. Sudden cardiac death in the athlete. Armonk (NY): Futura Publishing Co; 1997. p. 25–56.

38. Maron BJ, Gohman TE, Aeppli D. Prevalence of sudden cardiac death during competitive sports activities in Minnesota high school athletes. J Am Coll Cardiol 1998;32(7):1881–4.

39. Liberthson RR. Sudden death from cardiac causes in children and young adults. N Engl J Med 1996; 334(16):1039–44.

40. Topjian AA, Nadkarni VM, Berg RA. Cardiopulmonary resuscitation in children. Curr Opin Crit Care 2009;15(3):203–8.

41. Garza M. An AED in every school: the next step for public access defibrillation. J Exp Med Sci 2003;28: 22–3.

42. Project ADAM. Available at: http://www.chw.org/ display/PPF/DocID/26050/router.asp. Accessed September 15, 2009.

43. Litwin PE, Eisenberg MS, Hallstrom AP, et al. The location of collapse and its effect on survival from cardiac arrest. Ann Emerg Med 1987;16(7):787–91.

44. HAT investigators. Home use of automated external defibrillators for sudden cardiac arrest. N Engl J Med 2008;358:1793–804.

45. Cayten CG. Evaluation. In: Kuehl AE, editor. Prehospital systems and medical oversight. 2nd edition. St. Louis: Mosby Lifeline; 1994. p. 159–67.

46. Culley LL, Clark JJ, Eisenberg MS, et al. Dispatcher-assisted telephone CPR: common delays and time standards for delivery. Ann Emerg Med 1991;20(4): 362–6.

47. Abella BS, Sandbo N, Vassilatos P, et al. Chest compression rates during cardiopulmonary resuscitation are suboptimal: a prospective study during in-hospital cardiac arrest. Circulation 2005;111(4):428–34.

48. Wik L, Kramer-Johansen J, Myklebust H, et al. Quality of cardiopulmonary resuscitation during OHCA. JAMA 2005;293:299–304.

49. Aufderheide TP, Lurie KG. Death by hyperventilation: a common and life-threatening problem during cardiopulmonary resuscitation. Crit Care Med 2004; 32(Suppl 9):S345–51.

50. Aufderheide TP, Pirrallo RG, Yannopoulos D, et al. Incomplete chest wall decompression: a clinical evaluation of CPR performance by EMS personnel and assessment of alternative manual chest compression-decompression techniques. Resuscitation 2005;64(3):353–62.

51. Abella BS, Edelson DP, Kim S, et al. CPR quality improvement during in-hospital cardiac arrest using a real-time audiovisual feedback system. Resuscitation 2007;73(1):54–61.

52. Bobrow BJ, Aufderheide TP, Brady WJ. Maximizing survival from out-of-hospital cardiac arrest. Emerg Med Rep 2008;29(11):121–32.

53. Sunde K, Pytte M, Jacobsen D, et al. Implementation of a standardized treatment protocol for post-resuscitation care after out-of-hospital cardiac arrest. Resuscitation 2007;73:29–39.

54. Langhelle A, Tyvold SS, Lexow K, et al. In-hospital factors associated with improved outcome after out-of hospital cardiac arrest. A comparison between four regions in Norway. Resuscitation 2003;56:247–63.

55. Herlitz J, Engdal J, Svensson L, et al. Major differences in 1-month survival between hospitals in Sweden among initial survivors of out-of-hospital cardiac arrest. Resuscitation 2006;70:404–9.

56. Engdahl J, Abrahamsson P, Bang A, et al. Is hospital care of major importance for outcome after out-of-hospital cardiac arrest? Experience acquired from patients with out-of-hospital cardiac arrest resuscitated by the same emergency medical service and admitted to one of two hospitals over a 16-year period in the municipality of Goteborg. Resuscitation 2000;43:201–11.

57. Liu JM, Yang Q, Pirrallo RG, et al. Hospital variability of out-of-hospital cardiac arrest survival. Prehosp Emerg Care 2008;12(3):339–46.

58. Carr BG, Goyal M, Band RA, et al. A national analysis of the relationship between hospital factors and post-cardiac arrest mortality. Intensive Care Med 2009;35(3):505–11.

59. Carr B, Kahn J, Merchant RM, et al. Inter-hospital variability in post–cardiac arrest mortality. Resuscitation 2009;80:30–4.

60. Hypothermia after Cardiac Arrest Study Group. Mild therapeutic hypothermia to improve the neurologic outcome after cardiac arrest. N Engl J Med 2002; 346(8):549–56.

61. Bernard SA, Gray TW, Buist MD, et al. Treatment of comatose survivors of out-of-hospital cardiac arrest with induced hypothermia. N Engl J Med 2002; 346(8):557–63.

62. Hovdenes J, Laake JH, Aaberge L, et al. Therapeutic hypothermia after out-of-hospital cardiac arrest: experiences with patients treated with percutaneous coronary intervention and cardiogenic shock. Acta Anaesthesiol Scand 2007;51(2):137–42.

63. Nichol G, Karby-Jones R, Salerno C, et al. Systematic review of percutaneous cardiopulmonary bypass for cardiac arrest or cardiogenic shock states. Resuscitation 2006;70:381–94.

64. Spaulding CM, Joly LM, Rosenberg A, et al. Immediate coronary angiography in survivors of out-of-hospital cardiac arrest. N Engl J Med 1997;336: 1629–33.

65. Knafelj R, Radsel P, Ploj T, et al. Primary percutaneous coronary intervention and mild induced hypothermia in comatose survivors of ventricular fibrillation with ST-elevation acute myocardial infarction. Resuscitation 2007;74:227–34.

66. Geocadin RG, Buitrago MM, Torbey MT, et al. Neurologic prognosis and withdrawal of life support after resuscitation from cardiac arrest. Neurology 2006; 67:203–10.

67. Yannopoulos D, Kotsifas K, Aufderheide TP, et al. Cardiac arrest, mild therapeutic hypothermia, and unanticipated cerebral recovery. Neurologist 2007; 13(6):369–75.

68. The AVID investigators. A comparison of antiarrhythmic-drug therapy with implantable defibrillators in patients resuscitated from near-fatal ventricular arrhythmias. N Engl J Med 1997;337:1576–83.

69. Lurie KG, Idris A, Holcomb JB. Level 1 cardiac arrest centers: learning from the trauma surgeons. Acad Emerg Med 2005;12:79–80.

70. Kahn JM, Branas C, Schwab W, et al. Regionalization of medical critical care: what can we learn from the trauma experience? Crit Care Med 2008; 36:3085–9.

71. McNally B, Stokes A, Crouch A, et al. CARES: cardiac arrest registry to enhance survival. Ann Emerg Med 2009. [Epub ahead of print].

72. Eisenberg MS. A plan of action, . Resuscitate!: how your community can improve survival from sudden cardiac arrest. Seattle (WA): University of Washington Press; 2009. p. 179–206.

# Subcutaneous Implantable Cardioverter-Defibrillator Technology

Anurag Gupta, MD, Amin Al-Ahmad, MD*,
Paul J. Wang, MD

**KEYWORDS**

- Subcutaneous ICD • Implantable cardioverter-defibrillator
- Defibrillation • Sudden death • Tachyarrhythmias

The first human implant of the implantable cardioverter-defibrillator (ICD) in 1980 ushered in an era of improved recognition and therapy for sudden cardiac death (SCD).[1] Initial epicardial ICD lead systems required a thoracotomy for placement of epicardial defibrillation patches and epicardial rate-sensing leads. Advances in ICD technology over the last 3 decades have led to decreased device size and the design of effective transvenous defibrillation leads. In addition, there have been significant improvements in ICD detection and discrimination algorithms and improved shock waveforms. This had led to the current paradigm of endocardial ICD lead systems in which endocardial leads (including pace-sense components and shocking coils) are placed transvenously, thus obviating the need for thoracotomy.

Indications for ICD therapy have also changed over the years based upon the results of well-conducted large-scale clinical trials. Whereas, initially, the ICD was only indicated after aborted SCD, current ICD indications have expanded to include prophylactic implantation in individuals who have a high risk of SCD, greatly increasing the pool of potentially eligible candidates.[2–5]

Despite these advancements, there continues to be significant barriers in offering this therapy to appropriately indicated patients. ICD delivery can be technically challenging and expensive. Furthermore, current ICD systems have associated risk, including but not limited to procedural risks, inappropriate device therapy, and long-term device-related complications that prominently include lead failure.

Recently, subcutaneous or so-called leadless ICD systems have been developed that offer a potential new paradigm for facilitating ICD implantation. Though heterogeneous in design, these systems typically share a common theme of using electrodes that are placed subcutaneously without requirement for leads in or on the heart. Although not clinically approved, this article will examine studies investigating the subcutaneous ICD and discuss its possible advantages and disadvantages as compared with current transvenous ICD systems.

## EXPERIMENTAL EVIDENCE FOR THE SUBCUTANEOUS ICD
### Initial Studies

Defibrillation with implantable devices using noncardiac electrodes is not a new concept. In 1970, Schuder and colleagues[6] demonstrated the efficacy of a completely automatic implantable defibrillator that weighed approximately 1037 g and that used extrathoracic electrodes in three canines. Energy delivery across the chest wall ranged between approximately 23 to 37 J, and the time between induction of ventricular

This article originally appeared in *Cardiac Electrophysiology Clinics*, volume 1, number 1.
Division of Cardiovascular Medicine, Department of Internal Medicine, Cardiac Arrhythmia Service, Stanford University School of Medicine, 300 Pasteur Drive, Room H2146, Stanford, CA 94305-5233, USA
* Corresponding author.
*E-mail address:* aalahmad@cvmed.stanford.edu

Heart Failure Clin 7 (2011) 287–294
doi:10.1016/j.hfc.2011.01.005
1551-7136/11/$ – see front matter © 2011 Elsevier Inc. All rights reserved.

fibrillation to shock delivery ranged between 14 seconds to 40 seconds with later inductions. The first shock was successful in terminating ventricular fibrillation in 67 of 73 induced episodes, and no animal required external defibrillation.

### Subcutaneous Defibrillation in Children

Subcutaneous defibrillation has only been more recently reported in humans. Clinicians wishing to avoid or unable to place fully transvenous or epicardial ICD systems in pediatric patients with complex cardiac disease have reported cases of effective defibrillation using a subcutaneous array as the high-voltage lead.[7–12] For example, Gradaus and colleagues[7] reported successful subcutaneous defibrillation in two patients aged 12- and 14-years-old with a single-chamber ICD with a transvenous and epicardial bipolar pace-sense lead, respectively. Using an active abdominal can and a single subcutaneous array placed dorsolaterally in the left thorax, they reported successful conversion of ventricular fibrillation with defibrillation threshold (DFT) less than or equal to 20 J. Likewise, Berul and colleagues[8] reported successful defibrillation with threshold less than or equal to 14 J using an active abdominal can and a single subcutaneous array in a 2-year-old girl with a single chamber ICD using an epicardial bipolar rate-sensing lead.

Stephenson and colleagues[13] reported a larger, multicenter retrospective review of subcutaneous defibrillation (that is, not using transvenous high-voltage coils or epicardial patches) in children with mean age of 8.9 years and complex cardiac disease. Of 22 patients examined, 14 had a subcutaneous coil system while the remaining 8 had the coil placed on the epicardium; all patients had an epicardial or transvenous bipolar ventricular pace-sense lead and used an active can configuration. While a true DFT was not obtained in all patients, subcutaneous lead placement was associated with a higher DFT than the epicardial system (19 ± 7 vs 13 ± 4 J, P = .03). Though 7 of the 22 patients required system revisions, this study again demonstrated the feasibility of subcutaneous defibrillation in children.

### Experimental Models of Subcutaneous Defibrillation in Adults

There have also been studies examining a subcutaneous lead system in adults indicated for and receiving transvenous ICDs. Grace and colleagues[14] examined the DFT for subcutaneous ICD systems using various dual electrode configurations between the ICD can and subcutaneous electrode. In one study, 41 patients were enrolled in a multicenter, prospective study comparing DFT between a standard transvenous ICD system and a subcutaneous system. For the subcutaneous system, the active can be placed in the anterolateral axillary line at the sixth intercostal space and the subcutaneous electrode was placed 3 cm left of the sternum with the coil centered at the fifth intercostal space. The DFT for the subcutaneous system was 39 J. As expected, this was higher than the 12 J DFT of the transvenous system but still within a technically feasible range.

Optimal electrode configurations were further examined by Grace and colleagues[15] in a study of 10 patients undergoing standard transvenous ICD implantation. Four electrode configurations were tested: (1) 60 cc lateral can and 8 cm parasternal coil, (2) 60 cc lateral can with a 5 cm squared parasternal disk electrode, (3) 60 cc pectoral can with a 4 cm paraxiphoid coil, and (4) 60 cc pectoral can with a 8 cm inframammary coil electrode. In this study, though the optimal configuration appeared to require a lateral can position, all groups were thought to be in a technically feasible range of defibrillation with mean DFT for the four groups ranging between 27 to 39 J.

Similarly, Lieberman and colleagues[16] examined the efficacy of a nontransvenous defibrillation, this time using an anteroposterior shock pathway. Specifically, 33 patients undergoing standard transvenous ICD implantation had an anterior low pectorally-placed active can emulator and a 25 cm coil tunneled subcutaneously around the back of the left thorax between the 6th and 10th intercostal space. A standard electrophysiology catheter was placed for sensing and for ventricular fibrillation induction. Biphasic shocks with a 50%-50% tilt and total waveform time of 16 ms were delivered and defibrillation testing was performed using a stepwise protocol. Eighty one percent of patients had successful defibrillation using less than or equal to 35 J.

Likewise, Burke and colleagues[17] estimated the subcutaneous defibrillation energy requirement in 20 adults indicated for an ICD, this time using anterior-anterior vector. In their experimental model, a cutaneous electrode patch, acting as a surrogate for a subcutaneous electrode, was first placed at the inferior border and apex of the left heart. Next, a standard transvenous ICD was implanted and DFT testing was performed. The DFT using the standard transvenous system was 10.4 ± 6.5 J. The device was then removed (replaced at the end of study) and an emulator was placed in the device position. Defibrillation was retested for the investigational, nontransvenous configuration using an external defibrillator that delivered a shock between the pectoral subcutaneous emulator and the apical cutaneous electrode patch, 10 seconds after induction of ventricular fibrillation. Using the nontransvenous system, successful defibrillation at 50 J was achieved in 17 of 20 (85%) patients including 7 of 9 (78%) patients with successful defibrillation tested at 30 J. Only two patients required more than 70 J for successful defibrillation.

A follow-up study by Burke and colleagues,[18] again using cutaneous electrode patches as surrogates for subcutaneous electrodes, suggested that subcutaneous signals could distinguish ventricular fibrillation from sinus rhythm when using sensing and detection algorithms typical for ICDs. Gold and colleagues[19] also showed reliable arrhythmia detection in an experimental model using subcutaneous equivalent cutaneous electrode configurations that were compared with detection from single-chamber transvenous ICD systems. Based upon the recorded signals from 43 induced ventricular arrhythmias and 45 induced atrial arrhythmias with rate greater than or equal to 170 beats per minute, the subcutaneous system showed significantly improved specificity and not different, excellent sensitivity greater than 98% for the detection of ventricular arrhythmias. Unlike prior studies and case reports that demonstrated the feasibility of subcutaneous defibrillation, these experiments suggested that a subcutaneous ICD system could further be used to reliably detect ventricular arrhythmias. Studies such as these paved the way for investigations in humans using totally subcutaneous ICD systems.

### Totally Subcutaneous ICD Systems in Adults

Recently, early experience with a total-purpose, totally subcutaneous ICD system has been reported by Crozier and colleagues.[20] This device, manufactured by Cameron Health, Inc (San Clemente, CA) is an approximately 69 cc, 145 g defibrillator that is able to discharge 80 J and provide limited postshock pacing. The system consists of a subcutaneously placed pulse generator and a subcutaneous lead that is placed along the left side of the sternum (**Fig. 1**). Sensing occurs via one of three electrode configurations: from the distal subcutaneous lead to the can, from the proximal subcutaneous lead to the can, or from the distal to proximal subcutaneous lead. The device has a projected longevity of 5 years.

The initial clinical experience regarding this device was recently reported.[20] In a multicenter study, 55 patients with an indication for a standard ICD underwent implantation of a subcutaneous ICD without the use of fluoroscopy. The patients had a mean age of 56 years and mean ejection fraction of $34 \pm 13\%$ and the majority of individuals had ischemic heart disease (67%). Implant time and testing was $74 \pm 38$ minutes. Specifically, the procedure involved subcutaneous implantation of the pulse generator over the sixth rib in the anterior axillary line and tunneling of the subcutaneous lead in a parasternal position, 1 to 2 cm left of midline and midway between the xiphoid and sternomanubrial junction. The primary study objective was to describe device detection and conversion efficacy for induced ventricular fibrillation.

The subcutaneous ICD was able to successfully detect ventricular fibrillation in all 137 episodes of induced ventricular fibrillation among the 53 patients able to complete the protocol (100% sensitivity). Moreover, the device had 98% (52 of 53 patients) conversion efficacy, defined as two consecutive successful conversions of ventricular fibrillation using a 65 J shock per maximum four inductions. Thus, the majority of patients had a 15 J safety margin, as the device is able to deliver 80 J. Of note, the charge time to deliver a shock was $14 \pm 2.5$ seconds. In addition, over a brief follow-up period, there was one case of appropriate detection and treatment and two cases of inappropriate oversensing due to noise from a loose setscrew and from T-wave oversensing. The lead was also found to have moved in four patients, requiring repositioning in two individuals. Despite some initial encouraging results, the clinical experience with totally subcutaneous ICD systems remains preliminary and limited.

## LIMITATIONS WITH CURRENT ICD SYSTEMS

A primary drawback of epicardial ICD systems is that they require invasive procedures associated with higher periprocedural risk. The perioperative mortality associated with lead implantation via thoracotomy may be as high as 5%, acknowledging that heterogeneity exists between operators and patients (including for example need for concomitant cardiac surgery) within and between surgical series.[21,22] Epicardial systems may pose other unique challenges such as difficulty in removing fibrosed epicardial leads or patches, potential for triggering a restrictive pericardial process, possibility of complicating future cardiac surgery, or risk of hindering external cardioversion due to increased transthoracic impedance.[23]

Epicardial ICD systems have been largely supplanted by endocardial ICD systems using transvenous delivery of leads. Though the procedure is substantially safer, less expensive, and easier

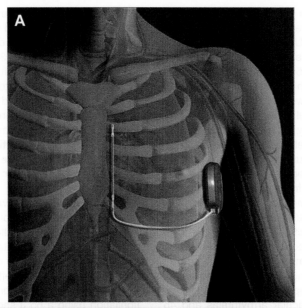

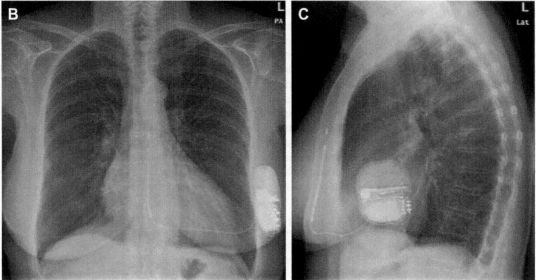

**Fig. 1.** (*A*) Schematic depiction. (*B*) Posterior to anterior chest radiograph. (*C*) Lateral chest radiograph of an individual implanted with a totally subcutaneous ICD system. The pulse generator is located approximately over the sixth rib in the anterior axillary line and is connected to a tunneled subcutaneous lead approximately 1 cm left of the sternum between the xiphoid and sternomanubrial junction. The subcutaneous electrode consists of a high-voltage, low-impedance, shocking coil electrode and low-voltage, high-impedance, sensing electrodes. (*Courtesy of* Cameron Health, Inc, San Clemente, CA, USA; with permission.)

to perform, procedural risks remain. For example, among a cohort of the ICD Registry of 111,293 initial ICD implantations reported between 2006 and June of 2007, Curtis and colleagues[24] reported that 1.5% of all patients experienced a major in-hospital procedural complication and 3.7% of all patients experienced any complication. In this study, complications stemming from transvenous lead delivery were prominent with reported complications specifically including hematoma (1.1%), lead dislodgement (1%), pneumothorax (0.5%), and cardiac arrest (0.3%) and a less than or equal to 0.1% rate of hemothorax, cardiac perforation, pericardial tamponade, stroke, conduction block, myocardial infarction, infection, phlebitis, transient ischemic attack, drug reaction, arteriovenous fistula, peripheral nerve injury, and cardiac valve injury.

Moreover, transvenous lead delivery can be technically challenging, potentially restricting dissemination of this technology to eligible patients. In the same study performed by Curtis and colleagues,[24] they reported that 70.9% of the 111,293 ICD implantations were performed by certified electrophysiologists. Interestingly, in comparison to electrophysiologists, the risk of complications in both unadjusted and adjusted analyses was higher when performed by nonelectrophysiologist cardiologists (who performed 21.9% of implants) or thoracic surgeons (who performed 1.7% of implants).

Beyond periprocedural risks of transvenous lead delivery, such leads pose long-term challenges. For example, late infection, vessel occlusion, lead dislodgment, and valvular dysfunction may be observed with endocardial leads.[25] Most notably, defibrillation lead failure is common, potentially leading to need for procedural revision, lead extraction with its attendant risks, accelerated battery depletion, failure to deliver appropriate therapy, or inappropriate shocks. For example, Kleemann and colleagues[26] examined 990 patients with first implantation of transvenous ICD between 1992 and May of 2005 from five manufacturers, excluding patients requiring device explant due to infection and patients with lead dislodgement. They estimated lead survival rates of 85% at 5 years and 60% at 8 years, and reported an annual incidence of lead failure up to 20% in 10-year-old leads. The majority of lead defects were due to insulation defects (56%). However, leads were implanted at a single center and approximately 95% of implantations were via the subclavian vein.

Eckstein and colleagues[27] reported a lower incidence of lead malfunction among a series of 1317 consecutive patients with transvenous ICDs implanted between 1993 and 2004 followed for a median 6.4 years. Specifically, they reported a cumulative incidence of lead failure requiring surgical revision of 2.5% at 5 years and 4.6% at 10 years. Though variable incidences of lead defects have been reported in smaller series, likely due to a combination of factors such as definitions of lead performance, ICD models examined, patient and physician characteristics, and tools used to detect lead failure, the rate of lead dysfunction remains clinically relevant.[28] Nonetheless, a vast clinical experience documenting the efficacy of transvenous lead technology along with continued technological advances have solidified its primary role in ICD therapy.

# POTENTIAL ADVANTAGES AND DISADVANTAGES OF SUBCUTANEOUS ICD SYSTEMS
## Advantages of Subcutaneous ICD Systems

Although clinical experience is required with subcutaneous ICD systems before meaningful comparisons can be derived with current transvenous ICD systems, they do offer multiple potential advantages and disadvantages. The primary potential strengths of subcutaneous ICD systems are that implantation and explantation may be easier and may be associated with fewer complications. In their pilot studies with a totally subcutaneous ICD system, Crozier and colleagues[20] reported implantation time including testing of $74 \pm 38$ minutes for the first three implants per operator, then $60 \pm 22$ minutes thereafter. Notably, fluoroscopy, intravascular access, and instrumentation in the heart are not required for implantation or explantation.

These features have significant implications in select populations for whom placing transvenous or epicardial leads is not possible or is especially unpalatable. This may include individuals in whom long-term device therapy is indicated and who are thus anticipated to have higher rates of lead-related complications or failure, leading to more potential device revisions or removals. This may include ICD-indicated pediatric patients with cardiac disease, younger patients with channelopathies (such as long or short QT, Brugada syndrome, or catecholaminergic polymorphic ventricular tachycardia), and younger patients with cardiomyopathies (such as hypertrophic cardiomyopathy, arrhythmogenic right ventricular cardiomyopathy, dilated cardiomyopathy, or acquired disease).[29] A subcutaneous ICD may also have a role in individuals at risk for ventricular arrhythmias though with potential for improvement, such as those individuals awaiting cardiac transplantation or high-risk individuals immediately postinfarction.[29]

Beyond potential indications in niche populations, subcutaneous ICD systems, by perhaps representing a simpler and safer method of implant, offers the potential for greatly expanding ICD therapy in the overall pool of potentially eligible patients. Though individual estimates of appropriate ICD use vary widely, with one analysis approximating the current prevalence of individuals in the United States eligible for, yet without, prophylactic ICD therapy to be 820,000,[29] all studies consistently demonstrate underutilization.[30,31] The reasons for low implantation are multifactorial and require further definition. However, challenges with transvenous implantation including its expense, requirement for access to technical expertise, and associated morbidity may all be contributory factors that may somewhat be ameliorated by use of subcutaneous ICD systems.

### Disadvantages of Subcutaneous ICDs

Notwithstanding, subcutaneous ICD systems have limited clinical experience and have several significant potential limitations. First, current subcutaneous ICD systems can provide temporary, but not long-term, pacing support. At present, such devices would not be appropriate for the significant pool of ICD-indicated patients requiring pacing for cardiac resynchronization therapy or bradycardia. Moreover, many of the patients requiring bradycardia support cannot be identified at implant owing to the development of drug-induced, progressive, or acquired disease.[32] In addition, current subcutaneous ICDs cannot deliver pacing support for ventricular tachyarrhythmias (eg, antitachycardic pacing [ATP]), a cornerstone of ventricular tachycardia management. Multiple studies have demonstrated high efficacy of ATP in terminating slow and fast ventricular tachyarrhythmias.[33,34] For example, Wathen and colleagues[34] demonstrated that for fast ventricular tachyarrhythmias with rates between 188 and 250 beats per minute, a strategy of initial empiric ATP therapy was effective in terminating 72% of fast ventricular episodes and was overall equally safe as a strategy of shock-only therapy.

In addition, intracardiac leads potentially offer advantages over subcutaneous leads with respect to (1) lower DFTs; (2) decreased charge times; and (3) improved sensing of intracardiac ventricular and atrial activity, thus enhancing tachyarrhythmia detection and discrimination using established algorithms. Data to establish the performance, reliability, and stability of sensing and defibrillation in subcutaneous ICDs will be critical before such comparisons can be made and before subcutaneous ICD technology can be adopted.

Whereas subcutaneous ICDs avoid intravascular access and potentially offer a safer method of implantation and explantation, operator skill is still critical and the potential for significant device-related complications remain. Subcutaneous systems do not mitigate pocket-related complications such as skin erosion; hematoma and seroma; infection; dehiscence; and device migration. In fact, if larger pulse generators were required to deliver more energy, the rate of such complications may in theory increase. In addition, leadless ICD is a misnomer for most current subcutaneous ICD systems, which employ subcutaneous leads. These leads are likewise subject to mechanical stress, albeit different from transvenous leads, and are vulnerable to failure, erosion, infection, and migration and may cause irritation to the patient. The optimal subcutaneous electrode configuration, size, shape, and material all require definition. Current data prospectively examining subcutaneous lead performance is also required, though an older study prospectively examining the performance of 398 patients with transvenous ICDs employing subcutaneous high voltage electrodes reported a 93.7%, 5-year cumulative survival of these leads.[35]

### SUMMARY

The advent of subcutaneous ICD systems represents a major paradigm shift for the detection and therapy of ventricular tachyarrhythmias. Despite critical advances in lead technology that have permitted widespread adoption of highly effective transvenous ICDs, problems remain including requirement for technical expertise; peri-procedural complications during implantation and explantation; and long-term lead failure. Although subcutaneous ICD systems may mitigate some of these risks, they provide new shortcomings, such as inability to provide pacing therapy for bradyarrhythmias, ventricular tachyarrhythmias, and cardiac resynchronization. Moreover, despite promising initial experimental studies and clinical reports, the safety, efficacy, cost, reliability, and long-term performance of subcutaneous ICDs require thorough investigation before adoption into clinical practice. Though promising, ongoing clinical evaluation and development are required before the role of subcutaneous ICDs as an adjunctive or primary therapy can be defined.

### REFERENCES

1. Mirowski M, Reid PR, Mower MM, et al. Termination of malignant ventricular arrhythmias with an implanted automatic defibrillator in human beings. N Engl J Med 1980;303:322–4.
2. Moss AJ, Hall WJ, Cannom DS, et al. Improved survival with an implanted defibrillator in patients with coronary disease at high risk for ventricular arrhythmia. Multicenter Automatic Defibrillator Implantation Trial Investigators. N Engl J Med 1996;335:1933–40.
3. Buxton AE, Lee KL, Fisher JD, et al. A randomized study of the prevention of sudden death in patients with coronary artery disease. Multicenter Unsustained Tachycardia Trial Investigators. N Engl J Med 1999;341:1882–90.

4. Moss AJ, Zareba W, Hall WJ, et al. Prophylactic implantation of a defibrillator in patients with myocardial infarction and reduced ejection fraction. N Engl J Med 2002;346:877–83.

5. Bardy GH, Lee KL, Mark DB, et al. Amiodarone or an implantable cardioverter-defibrillator for congestive heart failure. N Engl J Med 2005;352:225–37.

6. Schuder JC, Stoeckle H, Gold JH, et al. Experimental ventricular defibrillation with an automatic and completely implanted system. Trans Am Soc Artif Intern Organs 1970;16:207–12.

7. Gradaus R, Hammel D, Kotthoff S, et al. Nonthoracotomy implantable cardioverter defibrillator placement in children: use of subcutaneous array leads and abdominally placed implantable cardioverter defibrillators in children. J Cardiovasc Electrophysiol 2001;12:356–60.

8. Berul CI, Triedman JK, Forbess J, et al. Minimally invasive cardioverter defibrillator implantation for children: an animal model and pediatric case report. Pacing Clin Electrophysiol 2001;24:1789–94.

9. Thogersen AM, Helvind M, Jensen T, et al. Implantable cardioverter defibrillator in a 4-month-old infant with cardiac arrest associated with a vascular heart tumor. Pacing Clin Electrophysiol 2001;24:1699–700.

10. Madan N, Gayno JW, Tanel R, et al. Single-finger subcutaneous defibrillation lead and "active can": a novel minimally invasive defibrillation configuration for implantable cardioverter-defibrillator implantation in a young child. J Thorac Cardiovasc Surg 2003; 126:1657–9.

11. Greene AE, Moak JP, Di Russo G, et al. Transcutaneous implantation of an external cardioverter-defibrillator in a small infant with recurrent myocardial ischemia and cardiac arrest simulating sudden infant death syndrome. Pacing Clin Electrophysiol 2004;27:112–6.

12. Luedemann M, Hund K, Stertmann W, et al. Implantable cardioverter defibrillator in a child using a single subcutaneous array lead and an abdominal active can. Pacing Clin Electrophysiol 2004;27:117–9.

13. Stephenson EA, Batra AS, Knilans TK, et al. A multicenter experience with novel implantable cardioverter defibrillator configurations in the pediatric and congenital heart disease population. J Cardiovasc Electrophysiol 2006;17:41–6.

14. Grace AA, Smith WM, Hood M, et al. A prospective, randomized comparison in humans of defibrillation efficacy of a standard transvenous ICD system with a totally subcutaneous ICD system (the S-ICD system) [abstract]. Heart Rhythm 2005;2:1036.

15. Grace AA, Hood M, Smith WM, et al. Evaluation of four distinct subcutaneous implantable defibrillator (S-ICD) lead systems in humans [abstract]. Heart Rhythm 2006;3:S128–9.

16. Lieberman R, Havel WJ, Rashba E, et al. Acute defibrillation performance of a novel, non-transvenous shock pathway in adult ICD indicated patients. Heart Rhythm 2008;5:28–34.

17. Burke MC, Coman JA, Cates AW, et al. Defibrillation energy requirements using a left anterior chest cutaneous to subcutaneous shocking vector: implications for a total subcutaneous implantable defibrillator. Heart Rhythm 2005;2:1332–8.

18. Burke MC, Haefner PA, Gilliam R, et al. Feasibility of left chest cutaneous electrode configurations to distinguish ventricular fibrillation from sinus rhythm. Heart Rhythm 2006;3(Suppl 1):S156.

19. Gold MR, Theuns DA, Knight BP, et al. Arrhythmia detection by a totally subcutaneous S-ICD® system compared to transvenous single-chamber ICD systems with morphology discrimination [abstract]. Heart Rhythm 2009;6:S34–5.

20. Crozier I, Melton I, Park RE, et al. Clinical evaluation of the subcutaneous implantable defibrillator (S-ICD) system [abstract]. Heart Rhythm 2009.

21. Gartman DM, Bardy GH, Allen MD, et al. Short-term morbidity and mortality of implantation of automatic implantable cardioverter-defibrillator. J Thorac Cardiovasc Surg 1990;100:353–9.

22. Saksena. Defibrillation threshold and perioperative mortality associated with either endocardial and epicardial defibrillation lead systems. The PCD investigators and participating institutions. Pacing Clin Electrophysiol 1993;16:202–7.

23. Russo AM, Marchlinski FE. Engineering and construction of pacemaker and implantable cardioverter-defibrillator leads. In: Ellenbogen KA, Kay GN, Lau CP, et al, editors. Clinical cardiac pacing, defibrillation, and resynchronization therapy. 3rd edition. Philadelphia: Saunders Elsevier; 2007. p. 161–200.

24. Curtis JP, Luebbert JJ, Wang Y, et al. Association of physician certification and outcomes among patients receiving an implantable cardioverter-defibrillator. JAMA 2009;310:1661–70.

25. Gold MR, Peters RW, Johnson JW, et al. Complications associated with pectoral implantation of cardioverter defibrillators. Pacing Clin Electrophysiol 1997;28:208–11.

26. Kleemann T, Becker T, Doenges K, et al. Annual rate of transvenous defibrillation lead defects in implantable cardioverter-defibrillators over a period of >10 years. Circulation 2007;115:2474–80.

27. Eckstein J, Koller MT, Zabel M, et al. Necessity for surgical revision of defibrillator leads implanted long-term: causes and management. Circulation 2008;117:2727–33.

28. Maisel WH, Kramer DB. Implantable cardioverter-defibrillator lead performance. Circulation 2008; 117:2721–3.

29. Santini M, Cappato R, Andresen D, et al. Current state of knowledge and experts' perspective on the subcutaneous implantable cardioverter-defibrillator. J Interv Card Electrophysiol 2009;25:83–8.

30. Fonarow GC, Yancy CW, Albert NM, et al. Heart failure care in outpatient cardiology practice setting: findings from IMPROVE HF. Circ Heart Fail 2008;1:98–106.

31. Shah B, Hernandez AF, Liang L, et al. Hospital variation and characteristics of implantable cardioverter-defibrillator use in patients with heart failure: data from the GTWG-HF (Get With The Guidelines-Heart Failure) Registry. J Am Coll Cardiol 2009;53:416–22.

32. Saksena S. The leadless defibrillator or the return of the subcutaneous electrode: episode III in the ICD saga? J Interv Card Electrophysiol 2005;13:179–80.

33. Peinado R, Almendral J, Rius T, et al. Randomized, prospective comparison of four burst pacing algorithms for spontaneous ventricular tachycardia. Am J Cardiol 1998;82:1422–5.

34. Wathen MS, DeGroot PJ, Sweeney MO, et al. Prospective randomized trial of empirical antitachycardic pacing versus shocks for spontaneous rapid ventricular tachycardia in patients with implantable cardioverter defibrillators. Pacing Fast VT Reduces Shock Therapies (PainFREE Rx II) Trial Results. Circulation 2004;110:2592–6.

35. Pratt TR, Pulling CC, Stanton MS. Prospective post-market device studies versus returned product analysis as a predictor of system survival. Pacing Clin Electrophysiol 2000;23:1150–5.

# Index

*Note:* Page numbers of article titles are in **boldface** type.

Heart Failure Clin 7 (2011) 295–298
doi:10.1016/S1551-7136(11)00015-8
1551-7136/11/$ – see front matter © 2011 Elsevier Inc. All rights reserved.

# *Moving?*

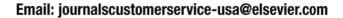

## *Make sure your subscription moves with you!*

To notify us of your new address, find your **Clinics Account Number** (located on your mailing label above your name), and contact customer service at:

**Email: journalscustomerservice-usa@elsevier.com**

**800-654-2452** (subscribers in the U.S. & Canada)
**314-447-8871** (subscribers outside of the U.S. & Canada)

**Fax number: 314-447-8029**

**Elsevier Health Sciences Division**
**Subscription Customer Service**
**3251 Riverport Lane**
**Maryland Heights, MO 63043**

*To ensure uninterrupted delivery of your subscription, please notify us at least 4 weeks in advance of move.

Printed and bound by CPI Group (UK) Ltd, Croydon, CR0 4YY

03/10/2024

01040355-0009